Hearing-Impaired Children and Youth with Developmental Disabilities

An Interdisciplinary Foundation for Service

Contributors

Editor/Author

Evelyn Cherow
> Director, Audiology Liaison Branch
> American Speech-Language-Hearing Association
> 10801 Rockville Pike, Rockville, Maryland 20852

Guest Editors/Authors

Noel D. Matkin, Ph.D.
> Professor of Audiology, Department of Speech and Hearing Sciences
> University of Arizona, Tucson, Arizona 85721

Raymond J. Trybus, Ph.D.
> Dean, Research Institute
> Gallaudet College, Kendall Green, Washington, D.C. 20002

Authors

Karoldene Barnes
> Special Education Resource Teacher/Consultant
> School Administrative District 64, East Corinth, Maine 04488

Holly A. Benson, M.Ed.
> Doctoral Candidate, Department of Special Education
> University of Kansas, Lawrence, Kansas 66045

Lynne Blennerhassett, Ed.D.
> Assistant Professor, School of Psychology
> Gallaudet College, Kendall Green, Washington, D.C. 20002

Pamela J. Cress, M.S.
Investigator, Sensory Assessment Projects
Bureau of Child Research, University of Kansas
Parsons Research Center, P.O. Box 738, Parsons, Kansas 67357

W. Scott Curtis, Ph.D.
Professor, Department of Speech Pathology and Audiology
University of Georgia, Aderhold Hall, Athens, Georgia 30602

Carl B. Feinstein, M.D.
Chief, Department of Outpatient Psychiatry
Children's Hospital National Medical Center
111 Michigan Avenue NW, Washington, D.C. 20010

Ronald S. Fischler, M.D.
Family Practice Office, Health Sciences Center
University of Arizona, 1450 North Cherry, Tucson, Arizona 85719

Brad W. Friedrich, Ph.D.
Chief of Audiology
The John F. Kennedy Institute, 707 North Broadway, Baltimore, Maryland 21205

Susan Harryman, R.P.T.
Director of Physical Therapy
The John F. Kennedy Institute, 707 North Broadway, Baltimore, Maryland 21205

Judith S. Johnson, Ph.D.
Assistant Professor of Education, Department of Education
Gallaudet College, Kendall Green, Washington, D.C. 20002

Michael A. Karchmer, Ph.D.
Director, Center for Assessment and Demographic Studies
Gallaudet College, Kendall Green, Washington, D.C. 20002

Robert R. Lauritsen
Director, Program for Deaf Students
St. Paul Technical Vocational Institute, 235 Marshall Avenue, St. Paul, Minnesota 55102

Mary Pat Moeller
Coordinator, Aural Rehabilitation Programs
Boys Town Institute for Communication Disorders in Children
555 North 30th Street, Omaha, Nebraska 68131

Kenneth L. Moses, Ph.D.
Psychologist
President, Resource Networks, Inc.
930 Maple Avenue, Evanston, Illinois 60202

Jerome D. Schein, Ph.D.
Professor of Deafness Rehabilitation
New York University, New York, New York 10003

Howard C. Shane, Ph.D.
> Director, Communication Enhancement Clinic
> Children's Hospital Medical Center, 300 Longwood Avenue, Boston, Massachusetts 02115

Charles R. Spellman, Ed.D.
> Senior Scientist, Bureau of Child Research
> University of Kansas, Parsons Research Center, P.O. Box 738, Parsons, Kansas 67357

David Tweedie, Ed.D.
> Dean, School of Communication
> Gallaudet College, Kendall Green, Washington, D.C. 20002

David R. Updegraff, Ph.D.
> Assistant to the Vice President, PreCollege Programs
> Gallaudet College, Kendall Green, Washington, D.C. 20002

Lana Warren, O.T.R.
> Director, Occupational Therapy Department
> The John F. Kennedy Institute, 707 North Broadway, Baltimore, Maryland 21205

Sandra Raymore Wright
> Director, Project PDQ
> American Speech-Language-Hearing Association
> 10801 Rockville Pike, Rockville, Maryland 20852

American Speech-Language-Hearing Association

Hearing-Impaired Children and Youth with Developmental Disabilities

An Interdisciplinary Foundation for Service

Editor
Evelyn Cherow

Guest Editors
Noel D. Matkin
Raymond J. Trybus

GALLAUDET COLLEGE PRESS
Washington, D.C.

This project was supported in part by the Administration on Developmental Disabilities, U.S. Department of Health and Human Services, under Grant No. 90DD0005/01. The views expressed in this book are solely those of the editors and authors and do not necessarily reflect official positions of the Administration on Developmental Disabilities or the American Speech-Language-Hearing Association.

Gallaudet College Press, Washington, DC 20002
© 1985 by Gallaudet College. All rights reserved
Published 1985
Printed in the United States of America

Library of Congress Cataloging in Publication Data

Main entry under title:
Hearing-impaired children and youth with developmental disabilities.

    At head of title: American Speech-Language-Hearing Association.
    "This project was supported in part by the Administration on Developmental Disabilities, U.S. Department of Health and Human Services, under Grant No. 90DD0005/01"—T.p. verso.
    Includes bibliographies and index.
    1. Hearing disorders in children. 2. Developmentally disabled children—Services for. 3. Children, Deaf—Services for. I. Cherow, Evelyn. II. Matkin, Noel D. III. Trybus, Raymond J. IV. American Speech-Language-Hearing Association. V. United States. Administration on Developmental Disabilities. [DNLM: 1. Child Development Disorders. 2. Community Health Services—United States. 3. Hearing Disorders—in adolescence. 4. Hearing Disorders—in infancy & childhood. 5. Social Service—United States. WV 271 H4353]
RF291.5.C45H319 1985   362.4'2   85-4356
ISBN 0-913580-97-X

Gallaudet College is an equal opportunity employer/educational institution. Programs and services offered by Gallaudet College receive substantial financial support from the U.S. Department of Education.

Contents

Foreword

I shall be telling this with a sigh
Somewhere ages and ages hence:
Two roads diverged in a wood, and I—
I took the one less traveled by,
And that has made all the difference.
      —Robert Frost, *The Road Not Taken*

The problems of providing humane and liberating service to hearing-impaired developmentally disabled people and to their families are at times overwhelming. Perhaps that is why we in the responsible professions have so often chosen the more traveled way and hence why services to hearing-impaired developmentally disabled people and their families have so often been limited in scope, poor in quality, or nonexistent.

But there is reason for hope. The last decade has brought us the legal and financial support of the Education for All Handicapped Children Act and the Developmental Disabilities Assistance and Bill of Rights Act at the federal level, and corresponding attention, sometimes, from the states and local communities. The two organizations responsible for the present volume, the American Speech-Language-Hearing Association and Gallaudet College, have been working together during that same decade to improve professional and scientific understanding of, and services to, hearing-impaired developmentally disabled people and their families. Planning conferences, training workshops, and dissemination programs have brought together professionals in the fields of deafness, mental retardation, psychology, medicine, education, mental health, and the human communication sciences. These experiences led to the understanding that, though more has been written on the subject recently than in years past, there is yet more we could do. This book is the result of that understanding and consequent sense of urgency.

Part of this book's message is that "we've come a long way, baby." Pioneering is always challenging and can often be fun—but with mixed emotions I must announce that we are past the pioneer era in this field. Pioneers have the advantage of being able to move into new territory safe in the knowledge that their efforts will be useful and will be remembered, despite their limitations. Who can challenge a pioneer without having been there? Pioneers need not read the maps of the territory; maps may not exist, for one, and are likely to be crude and perhaps misleading for another. But this territory has now been explored, and its boundaries charted. We must read the maps carefully lest our attempts at traveling the least traveled road lead us into familiar pitfalls. The authors and editors summarize much of what has been mapped out within this now well-explored territory and delineate for the reader where new investment is likely to prove fruitful.

We know now that consistently high quality service requires that professionals from many different fields make frequent expeditions into the domains of their fellow professionals. We must know each other's work from the inside, from firsthand experience, in order to move beyond the hollow "team" myths of the past two decades. The contemporary era is one of interactive interdisciplinary teams whose current successes and limitations are delineated in these pages. What is described here is happening now in the area of direct service, as professionals of diverse backgrounds interact daily, educate themselves, and provide the best service of which we are capable.

The next challenge will be to move this experience into the area of preservice, into the education programs in which up-and-coming professionals earn their entry-level credentials. Here the challenge is likely to be far more formidable. Do we mean that psychologists must actually learn something about education, about speech and language behavior, and about medicine? Do we mean that speech/language/hearing professionals must learn about family interaction and mental health? Do we mean that physicians-in-training have lessons to learn from teachers and curriculum writers? Yes, indeed! But our graduate curricula are already full; how can we add more? The means are not yet clear, but the need is unquestionable. There is hope that this challenge will be faced squarely, that we will be able to rise above our respective professional turfs and traditions. There is hope that our response to the challenge will truly be equal to the best of all our combined creative abilities.

Much has been done, and much remains to be accomplished. The challenge is humbling, as anyone can attest who has faced a family with a hearing-impaired developmentally disabled member and tried to inform, to support, to listen, to comfort, to help, and to liberate. In this new book on an old problem, the authors and editors have surely taken a road less traveled, and I hope it makes all the difference.

DAVID YODER
President, American Speech-
Language-Hearing Association,
1984

Preface

Over the past decade, there has been increasing concern for the issues surrounding service delivery to those individuals who have impaired hearing and additional disabilities. This book represents the fourth phase of a nine-year federal commitment to children and youth who have both hearing impairment and developmental disabilities. In 1975, the American Speech-Language-Hearing Association (ASHA) was awarded a grant from the Division of Developmental Disabilities, Rehabilitation Services Administration. The focus of the initial project phase was to delineate service and programmatic needs of hearing-impaired mentally retarded (HIMR*) people and then to recommend strategies for early intervention, deinstitutionalization, training, and policy development. The rationale for such action stemmed from concern that traditional legislative mandates on behalf of disabled citizens were categorically oriented. Advocacy and lobbying efforts tended to be specific to deafness, blindness, or cerebral palsy issues, for example. As a result, those people with multiple disabilities who could not be neatly categorized by a traditional diagnostic label were precluded from innovative programming mandates designed exclusively for those with a single disability.

A publication entitled *The Hearing-Impaired Mentally Retarded: Recommendations for Action* (Healey & Karp-Nortman, 1975) emerged from the initial ASHA project. In it the authors outlined in depth the perceived needs of individuals with hearing impairment and mental retardation. At the 1973 Airlie House Conference sponsored by the Office of Mental Retardation Coordination and the National Advisory Committee on Education of the Deaf, four broad recommendations were offered by the National Task Force on the Mentally Retarded Deaf.

- Recommendation 1: The following operational definition of mentally retarded deaf should be adopted by program planners at national, state, and

---

*This acronym is used by Healey and Karp-Nortman (1975, p. 9). The term refers to those individuals who have hearing impairment, sub-average general intellectual functioning, and deficits in adaptive behavior. The combination of these three factors requires services beyond those traditionally needed by people with either mental retardation or hearing impairment alone.

local levels of government: A mentally retarded deaf (MRD) person is an individual who has a combination of mental retardation and hearing impairment of sufficient degree that he or she cannot be appropriately served by traditional programming for the mentally retarded or deaf alone. The MRD person may have other handicapping conditions.

- Recommendation 2: The mentally retarded deaf should be designated as a priority target population by appropriate governmental agencies and professional organizations.
- Recommendation 3: Federal legislation should be enacted authorizing commitment of public resources specifically for MRD program development.
- Recommendation 4: Professionals, parents, and public officials should continue pressing American society and political institutions to guarantee equal rights for America's handicapped persons. (Healey & Karp-Nortman, 1975, p. 95)

These recommendations provided the bases from which detailed practical action plans were derived.

The second phase of activity following these recommendations was the 1976–79 Model Demonstration Project (MDP) funded by the Administration on Developmental Disabilities (ADD) and launched at the University of Arizona (Stewart, 1978). The main MDP goal was to develop innovative service delivery formats and materials for replication throughout the country. This project served to alert professionals working with a deaf clientele to the unique multidisciplinary and cross-agency program efforts required to adequately accommodate the mentally retarded deaf.

The third project phase consisted of a 1981 award of national significance from ADD to ASHA in partnership with Gallaudet College. This phase aimed at dissemination of materials using those models developed under the two previous projects. The materials and the literature in general were reviewed, and previous project staff and professionals in the field were interviewed. These activities revealed that past interpretations of legislative mandates, technological advances, and current economic factors had modified or altered the scope of application of the available materials. In addition, the federal definition of developmental disabilities had been revised to encompass more than those persons with mental retardation, cerebral palsy, epilepsy, or autism as the primary handicapping condition. For these reasons, an updated resource manual was compiled by project staff in 1981–82. That manual was a compendium of published articles and chapters in nine selected topic areas: demographics, assessment, communication, mental health issues, instructional management, programmatic options, personnel preparation, advocacy, and future trends.

The document was well received by those 1981 conference participants who attended either the national invitational seminar for University Affiliated Programs or one of four regional workshops conducted as part of grant activities. Repeated feedback praised the compendium as distinct in that knowledge from a variety of disciplines was merged into a single reference. Represented in the document were the fields of education of the hearing impaired, audiology, speech/language pathology, psychology, neurology,

special education, administration, pediatrics, and linguistics. Copies of a second printing of the manual were quickly depleted, and yet requests for it persisted. The message
seemed quite clear; professionals from diverse fields had a strong interest in current
theory and practice for optimal service delivery to the hearing-impaired developmentally
disabled population. Thus, phase four, the development of this multiauthored text on
the subject, was funded by a supplemental ADD award from October 1982 through
March 1984.

We have designed this book to present multiple perspectives on foundations of
service; those that are theoretical and practical, as well as those that, in some instances,
may be speculative in nature. Our intentions are first to define the issues and the
population; second, to put forth the philosophic foundations for subsequent recommendations; third, to emphasize and delineate the complex assessment and programmatic needs resulting from the combination of hearing impairment and developmental
disability; and last, to provide some unique solutions and to foster further thinking
about ways to enhance service delivery to a specific population, the hearing-impaired
developmentally disabled from birth to 21 years of age.

The reader will note that throughout the text inherent redundancy and occasional
divergent viewpoints have intentionally not been excluded. These were retained to
highlight differing views as possible "red flags" that require our attention in looking
toward revised models of service.

Part I opens with an overview of perceptions relative to the needs of individuals who
have hearing impairment plus one or more developmental disabilities, and a theoretical
perspective on optimal provision of services from the clinical and educational communities for addressing such needs. It is so structured to reiterate, rephrase, and reorganize
observations and recommendations from past projects and update these to reflect current
legislative, educational, mental health, and economic trends.

The current revised federal definition of developmental disabilities and interpretations of the mandate (Chapter 2) form the mortar that creates the foundations upon
which subsequent philosophical and practical constructs of this text are based.

In Chapter 3, Karchmer reports results from surveys of special education programs
for hearing-impaired children and offers an indepth description of children and adolescents who constitute the hearing-impaired developmentally disabled group. Current
findings are based on more explicit data than have been available heretofore. The
introduction, definition, and demographic overviews constitute Part I, the background
and rationale for this text.

Part II, "On Systems, Teams, and Families," offers, in one sense, a recapitulation of
the "no man is an island" theme. Trybus offers a systems approach to the provision of
services to hearing-impaired developmentally disabled individuals and their families
that incorporates interagency accountability. This perspective includes considerations of
cost-effectiveness and an examination of service-seeking vs. service-delivery models.
Geographic location, funding sources, availability of resources and personnel, and, in
particular, client awareness of agency resources are cited as factors impinging on program design and ultimately on effective delivery of services. Trybus proposes a rationale
for client "liberation" and self-sufficiency as desired end products of any program
implementation.

Despite years of advocacy for an intermeshing of professional expertise to expedite and facilitate programmatic efforts on behalf of hearing-impaired developmentally disabled people and others, the reality of "professional territorial imperatives" lives on. Chapter 5, "Effective Communication," is specifically positioned to emphasize our philosophic priority in this regard; that is, to reinforce programmatic models designed to minimize single discipline approaches to service and to maximize what we call the interactive interdisciplinary model. Matkin presents evidence in support of this conceptual framework as well as an outline of an effective service delivery model which is appropriate in either educational or clinical settings.

A holistic approach to working with the families of hearing-impaired developmentally disabled children is described by Moses as critical to effective intervention. Experience has shown that treatment modes which separate the client from the family breed enmity or apathy between the service provider and the primary caregivers. In Chapter 5, Moses urges a parent-professional interaction model that is based on a mutual understanding of the grieving issues which surround the rearing of a disabled child.

"Profiling Potential" (Part III) reflects our position that any individual has strengths upon which to capitalize and limitations which may be of the moment or permanent. Experienced professionals known to be steeped in the interactive teaming tradition were selected from a variety of disciplinary groups. These authors—Fischler, Friedrich, Cress, Spellman, Benson, Moeller, Harryman, Warren, and Blennerhassett—share knowledge and experience from their particular fields relative to the evaluation of and planning for hearing-impaired developmentally disabled children and youth. Their focus includes criteria for discipline-specific selection of appropriate instruments for use with hearing-impaired developmentally disabled youth (birth to 21 years of age); issues and techniques for assessment in each professional area; and interpretation of performance results relevant to personal, instructional, communication, and vocational planning for these clients and their families.

Part IV, "Bridging the Gap between Assessment and Programming," is designed to carve out topical areas that have an overt, and sometimes covert, impact on the growth of hearing-impaired developmentally disabled individuals in educational, clinical, personal, and, often, political arenas.

The psychiatric intervention chapter was inspired by my program planning experience with hearing-impaired developmentally disabled adolescents in a day school for the deaf. Teenagers with emerging recognition of their "differences" from hearing siblings and peers would instigate daily conflict. Counselors, social workers, and psychologists who were responsible for addressing the mental health needs of an entire school community—students, families, and professionals—found that "acting-out" adolescents required much of their time. Mounting frustrations for both the students and the professionals led to the addition of a new member of the team, the child psychiatrist. The psychiatric consultant served two purposes: first, to provide group therapy for an identified group of adolescents; and second, to provide consultation to the interdisciplinary team and supervisory staff on a regular basis. Feinstein, one of two psychiatrists who served in that capacity, offers his views and experiences regarding the role of the psychiatrist in programs serving hearing-impaired developmentally disabled individuals. Referral criteria for considering psychiatric intervention for such youth and/or their families are outlined, and a preventive model of service is described.

The need and rationale for specialized programming for students with combined hearing impairment and developmental disabilities cannot be overstated. Curtis and Tweedie clarify the parameters for choosing among available curricula and model programs. In addition, barriers that impede curriculum implementation are explored, with creative solutions offered to deal with traditional roadblocks. Similarly, Lauritsen and Updegraff review legislative mandates for incorporating career development and vocational training into programmatic formats for hearing-impaired developmentally disabled people. A philosophy underpinning such programming and examples of successful offerings are described.

Signed English, American Sign Language, and auditory/oral approaches have alternately been recommended as the preferred communication mode for hearing-impaired developmentally disabled individuals. Unfortunately, while the oral/manual/total-communication controversy raged, other avenues of communication, particularly in established programs geared for those with hearing impairment as the primary handicap, were often overlooked. Select unaided and aided augmentative communication systems have been utilized primarily with cognitively impaired persons and only in isolated communicative circumstances. Shane defines and reviews the application of augmentative communication devices as an alternate strategy worthy of consideration. He further outlines a decision-making process for assessing optimal receptive and expressive communication modes. Psychosocial ramifications of such alternative ways of communicating are explored through case illustrations.

Wright and Barnes address the manifold aspects of formal program evaluation and quality assurance. They describe several well-tested evaluation models for monitoring program effectiveness and individual client progress. Processes are suggested that ensure accountability in bridging gaps between diagnostic procedures and programmatic implementation and mesh evaluation formats with Individualized Education Program (IEP) mandates, cost-effectiveness concerns, and caseload accountability criteria.

In "Stress Management and Professional Burnout," Johnson then explores the phenomenon of stress as it influences professional burnout in those who serve hearing-impaired developmentally disabled individuals. The mental health needs of professionals in the workplace are an important factor affecting program delivery and deserve more attention than they typically get. Suggestions for dealing with professional stress and enhancing the interactive interdisciplinary team concept are offered as an integral part of the total picture of service delivery to hearing-impaired developmentally disabled individuals.

These two areas of concern, quality assurance and stress management, are juxtaposed deliberately to stress the inextricable relationship between effective service delivery and staff morale. Effective administrators are often those who gauge program success by attending to evaluation of client progress as well as to the needs of the professional staff serving those clients.

Service delivery to any disabled population cannot be broached without also addressing how to establish programming priorities through formal means. Schein presents a unique historical perspective on this subject of advocacy. The classic advocacy interpretation connotes efforts on behalf of the disabled. Although federal mandates influencing these efforts and judicial precedents are reviewed, Schein also presents the moral imperative underlying advocacy activities. In addition, he advises professionals on "sound advocacy practice" and cautions us from becoming so zealous as to ignore or overlook the attitudes, opinions, and self-advocacy role of those for whom we advocate.

"Networking: A Critical Strategy," the concluding chapter, urges readers to utilize available human and technological resources to meet the inevitable challenges ahead in providing optimal services for those individuals who experience both hearing impairment and developmental disabilities.

EVELYN CHEROW

References

Healey, W. C., & Karp-Nortman, D. S. (1975). *The hearing-impaired mentally retarded: Recommendations for action.* Rockville, MD: American Speech-Language-Hearing Association.

Stewart, L. (1978). *Severely handicapped deaf people: A perspective for program administrators and planners* [Monograph]. Tucson, AZ: University of Arizona, The Rehabilitation Center.

Acknowledgments

If this text has one prevalent theme, I would say it's that of fostering human growth through sharing—sharing skills, knowledge, and caring—and through commitment. The primary cast of characters involved in the evolution of this book, the guest editors and authors, is lengthy and, to no one's surprise, consists of those whose tendency toward commitment in an abundant fashion is well known. These individuals promote this theme daily by example; to them I extend my heartfelt gratitude.

At the ASHA National Office, Jim Gelatt, Jim Lingwall, Fred Spahr, and many in the Professional and Governmental Affairs Departments offered time, counsel, and expert review despite already over-burdened schedules.

Two Administration on Developmental Disabilities personnel, Thelma Lucas (Project Officer) and Jean Elder (Commissioner), encouraged and reinforced our efforts by providing funding and extensions so that "the job got done."

Jim Stentzel of Gallaudet College Press provided necessary and skillful editorial guidance. I appreciated the thorough and patient manner in which he worked with me to correct errors, omissions, and style inconsistencies. Right and left hands in manuscript preparation were provided by Anne "Penny" Watts (editorial assistant) and Bobbi Schroeder (typist). Their patience and fortitude were also limitless.

This book is dedicated first to my parents, Eli and Marianne Cherow, who were and are models for my own growth and involvement in human service professions; second, to my daughter, Jennifer, who reminds me daily of how capable, challenging, and deep human potential can be; and last, but never least, to my mentors and friends—Noel Matkin, Thomas Behrens, Bettie Waddy Smith, and Susan Weber—whose wisdom, humor, caring, futuristic outlooks, and availability for support have been ever-present throughout the years.

Evelyn Cherow

Part I
Introduction

Chapter 1

Through the Looking Glass

Evelyn Cherow

A series of philosophical principles constitutes the foundation of this text. Some reflect traditional beliefs and practices; others may seem, at first glance, to represent a radical shift in programmatic theory and management.

Public Law 94-142, the Education for All Handicapped Children Act of 1975,* has resulted in almost a decade of reviewing clinical and educational efforts on behalf of the disabled school-age population. Indelible and resounding effects have been felt in several quarters. For example, the nation's public schools have confronted the challenge of mainstreaming children and adolescents previously served in special schools, resource rooms, or institutions. Professionals working in settings influenced by the classic medical service delivery model have had to reconsider carefully the long-term ramifications of their assessment practices and findings for the individual consumer of their services. Families have been educated as to their legal rights for obtaining appropriate services, including assessment followed by educational and vocational programming, for their disabled children and adolescents. As a result, many parents have asserted themselves both informally and formally via due process procedures to ensure the availability and refinement of such programs. Educators and clinicians have looked to administrators for guidance, for inservice training, and for support in the workplace as they address their own needs for professional growth while designing and implementing programs for the population. In turn, administrators have had to justify and substantiate the use of personnel resources, child-find efforts, and budgetary allotments by way of novel evaluative and reporting mechanisms.

The synergistic effects of such legislative changes have been complex, slow to evolve, and often difficult to measure. Parallels can be drawn to the cognitive and behavioral synergies that result from the combined sensory deficits characteristic of the hearing-impaired developmentally disabled individual. For purposes of this text, distinct topic areas have been organized in such a way as to disentangle some of the important variables that influence individual and group change, and to present a philosophy for program development and service delivery.

---

*In December 1983, a new piece of legislation, Public Law 98-199, Secondary Education and Transitional Services for Handicapped Youth, was approved by Congress. This further amends PL 91-230, the Education for the Handicapped Act, of which PL 94-142 is a part.

The Background

The revised federal definition of developmental disabilities (1978) has brought about an expanded perception of which individuals constitute the hearing-impaired developmentally disabled. Mentally retarded persons with concomitant hearing loss initially were the target population, as this largely institutionalized group was, before enactment of PL 95-602 and PL 94-142, often overlooked, "misidentified," under-served, and classified only in terms of their primary handicap. As innovative diagnostic methodology has emerged, and secondary and tertiary disabilities have been attributed greater import in short- and long-range program planning, functional classifications have been added to the federal definition. These have replaced categorical labels and are considered to reflect more accurately an individual's potential to function as a member of our society (see Chapter 2).

Despite the usefulness of functional definitions, federal agencies continue to use traditional categorical terminology in describing the prevalence of disabled populations. In one recent report, the 1983 U.S. Department of Education's *Fifth Annual Report to Congress on the Implementation of Public Law 94-142,* categorical statistics and trend information relevant to our discussion are presented. First, the states' child-count efforts have revealed that the numbers of handicapped children (their terminology) continue to rise; an increase of one-half million was observed since 1976–77. Yet, 15 states reported fewer such children, particularly in the speech-impaired and mentally retarded categories. An overall increase was noted for those with learning disabilities, emotional disturbance, and multiple handicaps. The author's explanation that "the extent to which the changes reflect shifts in the characteristics of the population served as opposed to changes in the way states classify children is not known" emphasizes the ambiguity surrounding child-find activities and related categorization of students. The "learning disabled" label, seemingly more palatable to administrators, teachers, and families, may currently be the catch-all term applied to certain disability conditions (Polloway & Smith, 1983; Ysseldyke, Algozzine, & Epps, 1983). A 104.1 percent increase in learning disabled children 3–21 years old during 1977–82 and an additional 118,000 reported in 1982–83 substantiate concern in this matter. The National Association of State Directors of Special Education (NASDSE) attributed the substantial rise in the reported prevalence of learning disabled children to several factors.

- Improved procedures for identifying and assessing children with learning disabilities;
- Liberalized eligibility criteria;
- Cutbacks in other programs and lack of educational alternatives for children who experience problems in regular classes;
- Social acceptance/preference for the learning disabled classification relative to being classified as mentally retarded;
- Reclassification of minority children as learning disabled versus mentally retarded as a result of judicial decisions. (U.S. Department of Education, 1983, pp. I-6 to I-7)

The NASDSE also speculates that intensive efforts by many states to identify and serve previously underserved children account for increased counts of multihandicapped and emotionally disturbed children. In addition, many of those children now found in regular schools were previously served by private schools or programs administered by other than state education agencies, e.g., state supported schools for the retarded.

A second finding of the report to Congress shows personnel increases in special education have been made to accommodate the perceived rise in emotionally disturbed, learning disabled, and multihandicapped children found in the system. Third, despite the emphasis on mainstreaming, the overall percentage of handicapped children served in regular schools, whether in regular or self-contained classes, has remained relatively constant at slightly more than 92 percent since PL 94-142 was enacted.

The report to Congress is vague with respect to which individuals constitute the multihandicapped group. How many fit within the revised federal definition of developmental disabilities cannot be gauged due to the different nomenclature. Yet, these different methods of categorization may very well influence the quality of programs for such individuals.

For the first seven years after enactment, the federal government focused its attention on ensuring compliance with the procedural requirements of PL 94-142. Based on the data in the 1983 report to Congress, however, the Office of Special Education Programs, U.S. Department of Education, has now shifted its focus to improvement of the quality of special education programs. The five principal areas of technical assistance now will include (1) assessment of handicapped students, (2) development of services for adjudicated/incarcerated handicapped students, (3) supervision of other related agencies by the state education agency, (4) application of technological developments, and (5) preparation of personnel.

As formal counts of disabled children in the states have improved, long-needed scrutiny of the "homogeneity" of the hearing-impaired population has taken place almost simultaneously, both formally and informally. The fifth annual report clearly reflects that the population with normal hearing contains those who are gifted and retarded, learning disabled and motorically impaired, and visual and auditory learners. Acknowledgment and acceptance that the hearing-impaired population must also contain people with a wide and similar variety of characteristics are slowly emerging. This heterogeneity stems from multiple causes, all of which impose differing degrees of health, learning, communication, adaptive, and social disability that may interfere with the individual's ability to function in categorically oriented programs. Consequently, administrators of programs and agencies that traditionally serve the hearing-impaired population—as well as those responsible for programs for mentally retarded persons— have begun to search for models, methods, and materials more congruent with federally mandated individualized educational programming schemes. Of necessity, the goal has become the modification of program parameters to acknowledge and accommodate individual differences among people with hearing impairment and concomitant developmental disabilities.

Interactive Interdisciplinary Teaming

The revised definition of developmental disability (see federal definition, Chapter 2), together with national budgetary cutbacks, has created an incentive for states to strive toward interagency and cross-disciplinary forms of cooperation and consolidation to serve this heterogeneous population. The phrase employed here to describe coordinated services is "interactive interdisciplinary teaming." Though some may find the term to be inherently redundant, the desired perspective is that the reality of finely tuned interaction is optimal and yet to be achieved. Despite programmatic barriers, an interactive mechanism for service is the most appropriate approach to serving the hearing-impaired developmentally disabled population.

Teaming efforts provide a fertile milieu for adopting a holistic approach to profiling the individual client's strengths and *current* limitations. Assessment or diagnostic activities gain value in such a format by providing an opportunity for productive interdisciplinary dialogue and prioritization of service and program needs for a given individual. Stress can then be placed where it should be placed; that is, on designing a "custom" set of short- and long-range goals for a particular individual. Anything less than a custom fit is no fit at all for a variety of reasons which over time have become quite clear. In recent years, we have spent much energy on extricating both children and adults from educational and residential placements that were clearly inappropriate in view of the presenting disabling conditions. Well-intentioned policy makers in the past had set about creating categorical programmatic options that worked from the societal vantage point. Unfortunately, those program options often lacked the means for stimulating the individual's growth, and subsequently, furthering his or her place in society. From diagnostic activities resulting in categorical labels, permanent placements evolved, often out of view of the general public which knew and understood little of such problems.

Scientific progress and legislative and regulatory action of the past two decades have facilitated adoption of a broader view of the civil rights of persons with disabilities. Society has correspondingly sought ways to provide greater accessibility to the mainstream of life for such individuals. Advances in medicine and technology have combined to offer unprecedented life-sustaining and life-lengthening gains. The results of such strides are explained in a 1982 report of the Surgeon General's Workshop on Children with Handicaps and Their Families. Healy (1982) noted six distinct factors responsible for betterment of programs for the disabled.

1. Care became individualized. There was a shift in thinking from "All Down [sic] Syndrome children are alike," to "All Down Syndrome children require a continuum of evaluation services to document their individual strengths and deficits."

2. The settings for providing required services were critically examined and, in many instances, found to restrict the development of social, intellectual, and functional life skills. As a consequence, considerable numbers of children and adults moved from institutional settings and were placed in community-based residential homes and care facilities.

3. Parents and guardians became involved in decisions regarding their children's participation in educational programs and the provision of related services.

4. Patients and their parents or guardians were provided specific legal safeguards to ensure their participation in and knowledge of programs through

such legislation as PL 94-142, The Education for All Handicapped Children Act, and Section 504 of the Rehabilitation Act of 1973.

5. Statewide planning for coordination of services was mandated, and specific accountability was required of states to ensure the delivery of services. These changes were seen in PL 94-142 and in PL 95-602, The Developmental Disabilities Act, and in some aspects of the Health Block Grants.

6. Many programs were devised that implemented the interdisciplinary process, one that recognizes the need for a variety of professional expertise in the evaluation and care of disabled persons and that no one discipline has exclusive "rights" to a patient, irrespective of the problem or the "importance" of the discipline. (p. 42)

More recently, the Supreme Court's *Baby Doe* decision (1983) raised the consciousness of the public and of professional groups to the need to prioritize our professional responsibilities in the direction of life sustenance for those with multiple handicaps. In addition, liability decisions, such as *Evers v. Buxbaum* (1958), have set a precedent for viewing professional accountability and liability as belonging to all members of a "diagnostic and intervention team," not solely as the responsibility of a "case manager" or primary physician.

The teaming philosophy and rationale, then, can address the need to gather professional and societal forces in a proactive and advocative format. The pragmatics for bridging the gap between the initial and subsequent diagnostic processes and the use of diagnostic findings by educators, families, and other professionals have long been preached, yet implemented only sporadically. The mechanisms for achieving such interactive dialogue have been slow to develop and, in some cases, deemed financially prohibitive. But we have seen that single-discipline avenues of service delivery are ultimately more costly to society in both financial and human resources.

In 1976 the Bureau of Education for the Handicapped, Office of Education, funded a national demonstration and training consortium to improve services to severely handicapped hearing-impaired (SH/HI) individuals. The model design incorporated and capitalized on interdisciplinary cooperation and coordination (Campbell & Baldwin, 1982). A survey was undertaken in 1980 to investigate national goals of providers of training services to personnel serving the SH/HI child (Gage, Baldwin, & Campbell, 1980). This study sought to determine programmatic priorities chosen by professionals associated with the SH/HI consortium. Respondents not only included those professionals affiliated with the National Demonstration and Training Consortium for the Severely Handicapped Hearing Impaired, but also, for contrast, a sample of professionals associated with other preservice or inservice programs for SH/HI children. Consortium personnel chose as their top priority the need for an increased emphasis on improving means for identifying SH/HI children at an early age. The need to improve procedures for diagnosis and program planning were ranked second in order of importance. Nonconsortium professionals also gave first and second rank to these goals. Apropos of our discussion, those respondents who were *not* associated with the consortium indicated a need for increased interagency coordination in planning, management, and program evaluation at local, state, and federal levels as a critical priority. Conversely, consortium members felt that they were already part of a network that had a built-in exchange of ideas, methods, and materials.

Though it is often difficult to quantify, one could assume that interagency coordination would lead to increased cost-effectiveness, professional stimulation, and furtherance of the best interests of our clients—in this case, individuals with hearing impairment and accompanying disabilities. Of prime importance in such interagency exchange are the valuable increased resources upon which to draw for planning individualized assessment and intervention plans. The era of the classroom teacher who serves as a generalist utilizing a generic curriculum, or the isolated clinical practitioner, is fading. The advent of electronic mail and software program development and the concurrent relinquishing of "territorial turf" has effected a multifaceted training and service delivery model that is eclectic in its use of diverse personnel, technology, and resources. The payoffs in employing an interactive interdisciplinary model may be even more far-reaching than previously assumed.

The Human Factor and Program Management

Determination of long-term program effectiveness in the human services domain is nearly impossible to accomplish. Estimating whether our students or clients ultimately actualize their individual potentials and maximize their participation as citizens in our society is not possible. And yet, these goals underlie legislative efforts and continue to influence the shape of program development. One indicator of successful programming might be the longevity of employee tenure in our programs as it relates to personal job satisfaction. In recent years, the study of Japanese business management techniques by U.S. corporations has received much attention in the popular press. The reason for this increased U.S. attention has been linked primarily to economic motives. The Japanese economic recovery after World War II has not only been swift and expansive, but, as pointed out in *Business Week* (Staff, 1982), has also been of sufficient magnitude to threaten traditional U.S. markets. In looking at the critical variables influencing Japan's productivity and that country's ability to secure a strong foothold in the international marketplace, one particularly important aspect of Japanese corporate organizational structure has emerged: Companies there invest in the emotional well-being of employees and their families. Pascale and Athos (1981) drew a contrast between U.S. and Japanese cultural philosophies that account for the different management strategies.

> The Japanese see each individual as having economic, social, psychological, and spiritual needs, much as we do when we step back and think about it. But Japanese executives assume it is *their* task to attend to much more of the whole of the person, and not leave so much to other institutions (such as government, family, or religious ones). And they believe it is only when the individuals' needs are well met within the subculture of a corporation that they can largely be freed for productive work that is in larger part outstanding. U.S. executives, conditioned by a society which for good reason firmly separated church from state, and later the corporation from both, perhaps naturally assumed in the early years of this century that the mandate of the corporation was much more narrowly economic. Such a view, especially given the later technologies of mass production epitomized by the assembly line, led easily to an engineer's view of individuals as primarily interchangeable parts and units of production. (p. 132)

The authors further explain,

> The essence of Japanese success in these areas is rooted in assumptions that are rather fundamental to life. First, the Japanese accept ambiguity, uncertainty, and imperfection as much more of a given in organization life. Consequently, their staffing policies and skills at dealing with people in aggregates (as well as with one another) work from entirely different premises than do ours. . . . Second, the Japanese see themselves as far more *interdependent*. Thus, they are prepared to make far greater investments in people and in the skills necessary to be effective with others. (pp. 135–136)

While the theoretical applicability of these attitudes to human service agencies and educational institutions is just beginning to be explored in the U.S., the overall logic of applying such concepts can hardly be questioned by those who have chosen to work in the service professions. In fact, one might propose an application of the Japanese Quality Circles approach that would address the overall mental health needs of hearing-impaired developmentally disabled clients, their families, and the professionals who serve them (see Chapters 17 and 18).

Academic and clinical schedules as well as reimbursement criteria tend to dictate the nature and extent of client services. Time and formal mechanisms for dealing with the mental health needs of program staff as well as those of clients and their families or caregivers are typically in short supply on human service programs. And yet, the ramifications of neglect of psychosocial issues have been well documented (Darling & Darling, 1982; Gallagher, Beckman, & Cross, 1983; Meadow, 1981; Rose, 1983; Stedt & Palermo, 1983). A client's normal emotional development is often overlooked because of the narrow focus of professionals toward providing service in their specialty area—language development or mobility training, for example. Criticism has been leveled at special educators, pediatricians, and allied health professionals who have become so child- and task-oriented that they no longer have a sense of the gestalt. The needs of families initially immersed in "diagnostic crisis" and, later on, adjusting to modifying life goals and styles to accommodate a disabled child or adult cannot be neglected in planning intervention programs.

A new body of professional literature has emerged as a result of the increased interest in the structure and dynamics of family life in the U.S. over the past decade. Gallagher, Beckman, and Cross (1983) support the notion that professionals in special education have classically lacked preservice training in this area. Yet, experience has shown that to effect change for our students and clients requires cooperation and support from their families or caregivers. A family's ability and willingness to participate in a child's treatment may well be related to family members' perceptions of the additional stress imposed by the child's disabilities and their own coping strategies and support mechanisms. Gallagher et al. cite several studies that document common behavior patterns noted in families having children with disabilities. These patterns include increased divorce and suicide rates; child abuse; increased financial difficulties resulting from the need for special equipment, programs, and medical care; isolation and decreased social mobility; and depression, anger, guilt, and anxiety. Increased family stress correlates with the number of additional or unusual care-giving demands of, for example, older dependent children, those with autistic characteristics, children making slow progress, those with difficult temperaments, and those who are less socially responsive.

Sources of Stress

The effect of mainstreaming on perceived family stress (Turnbull & Blacker-Dixon, 1980), as cited in Gallagher et al. (1983), is also of relevance to our concerns in working with families of hearing-impaired developmentally disabled children. Turnbull and Blacker-Dixon indicated that parents, as a result of their child's mainstreamed placement, may experience increased family stress due to

- A daily reminder of the discrepancy between their child and the normal children around them;
- A shared "stigma" of handicap with their child, and a feeling of not being respected or accepted by other parents;
- A lack of common interests with other parents;
- A deep concern with the difficult social adjustment of their handicapped child;
- Worry that the normal school setting may lack the supportive services available in a special program for handicapped children. (p. 14)

Treatment modes for stress in the general population have been found to be equally applicable to families of handicapped children. Support networks have been very effective in alleviating the effects of crisis and change, and in creating needed access to information, resources, and intimacy. Professionals who may be the most accessible resource often are themselves sources of stress. Pieper (in Darling & Darling, 1982) wrote, "The pain, frustration and anxiety of professionals result in curtness to the point of rudeness, technical jargon to the point of insensibility, and other well-known behaviors that aid them in distancing themselves from us just when we need human contact the most" (p. vii). Typically, we as professionals are intent on achieving the goals outlined for the hearing-impaired developmentally disabled children we perceive to be our primary clients. As such, we often create an inability to see the forest for the trees within our programs. In adding to the demands placed on families, we alienate those whose influence on the child's growth provides the thread of continuity throughout that child's life. We can and do become the stressors in what we perceive as a battle against time and critical periods of learning. Gallagher et al. (1983) suggested that professionals should reflect on the role we ask parents to assume and, perhaps, rework our goals for parents to encompass providing sources of respite, sibling counseling groups, focus on fathers, and information and training for members of the extended family. Though the long-term benefits of such an approach are yet to be scientifically supported, it seems sensible and sensitive in a humanitarian framework.

At a 1983 National Institute of Handicapped Research conference (Karp, 1983) geared toward developing research priorities specific to parents' interaction with their disabled children, several directions were charted for exploration. These included (1) identification of positive behaviors and their effect on affective/emotional outcomes; (2) examination of changes in and interactions between child, family, and society over a

5-year period; (3) determination of the most effective and efficient early interventions; and (4) identification of strategies to develop links between agencies serving handicapped children for the purpose of coordinating efforts.

If, in fact, professionals can shift their perspective from a single-minded focus on client-oriented assessment, treatment, and instruction to a broader one in which overall family dynamics and support play a larger role, the outcome might well be worth the initial awkwardness and uncertainties.

Concern for burnout in the helping professions has also received increased attention in both the professional and lay literature. Again, the Japanese have established an effective precedent in industry by promoting an emotional climate conducive to quality service. From either a cost-effective or a humane perspective, those of us in the social service "business" cannot afford to overlook the comparable needs of professionals under stress.

One example of such concern is found in a recent study by Stedt and Palermo (1983) in which the Purdue Teacher Opinionaire was used in interviews of teachers of deaf and multihandicapped deaf children at a special school. Some researchers have found (e.g., Johnson, 1983; Meadow, 1981) that working with children with several disabilities is directly correlated with professionals' perceptions of job-related stress. To their surprise, Stedt and Palermo found the converse to be true; that is, responses of teachers of younger multihandicapped children reflected higher morale than those of teachers in both the regular program for the deaf and the program for older multihandicapped children. The authors surmised that strong administrative support of this group accounted for this finding. Such positive indicators as teacher rapport with the principal and with other teachers, a manageable teaching load, adequate facilities and services, and minimal community pressure received high ratings. Further, the fact that the school was recognized as an established institution with clearly defined entry criteria and curriculum for children with multiple handicaps might account for this unexpected result. The teachers perhaps were clearer about role expectations when hired and were supported by an administration committed to meeting the needs of this population. One could also speculate that professionals who serve younger children might have a more optimistic outlook on their ability to effect change and growth in their students. Exploration of these variables over the long term will have implications for professional preservice education as well as for the preparation and selection of special education and clinical administrators.

Program continuity for hearing-impaired developmentally disabled clients will best be ensured by preserving our personnel resources. Attitudinal shifts will be necessary in order to allot funds for activities that reduce staff stress. Large U.S. corporations such as Xerox and IBM have demonstrated an investment in staff by providing employee counseling and alcoholic and drug treatment programs. Why are human service programs so reluctant to follow suit? Are the years we have invested in training human service professionals so dispensable, and are our efforts so easily interchangeable? Professionals who have been involved in process-oriented seminars addressing these issues have later commented on the value and application of such knowledge and skills when brought to the client-therapist relationship (American Speech-Language-Hearing Association, 1983). Others who have received training in group consensus techniques for formal evaluation of programs or intervention strategies have also expressed an increased

individuals to enter the workforce and maximize their potential toward independent living. Cho indicates that 20 percent of households that include a disabled person were below the poverty line in 1972, compared to 12.3 percent for households with no disabled individuals. Families of mentally retarded people were poorest, with almost 90 percent below the poverty line. Cho notes that this group consists mostly of unmarried individuals.

How then can professionals serving the hearing-impaired developmentally disabled population modify these appalling statistics and build upon this legislative foundation?

Technological advances and research have not only provided professionals with the tools for making earlier diagnoses of individuals with multiple disabilities; these advances have also created vehicles for communication between those very professionals in need of rapid exchanges of ideas, materials, and moral support. The challenge now appears to be one of coordinating these skills and enhancing communication. Attitudinal change is a necessary prerequisite to attainment of such goals. As members of this society, we cannot afford either to cling to old habits or to procrastinate further when the main goal of fostering human independence and self-sufficiency is quite clear. Philosophical differences will and should persist in order to inspire growth and creativity. These differences must not, however, impede the dialogue essential to cooperative planning and programming for those people with hearing impairment and developmental disabilities.

Weintraub and McCaffrey (1976) outlined a compelling code of ethics for professionals working with exceptional children. They urged learning our own constitutional rights of free speech so well that ultimately we may advocate more effectively and in a cooperative spirit on behalf of our clients. To take this one step further, when we care for our clients and their families and for our professional staffs, then caring as a community and a society for the exceptional among us will be a natural outgrowth.

References

American Speech-Language-Hearing Association. (1983). *Social/emotional issues for clients and professionals* (Final Report). Rockville, MD: Author.

Baby Doe, 45 CFR 84; 48 *Federal Register* 30846 (1983).

Campbell, B., & Baldwin, V. (1982). Preface. In B. Campbell and V. Baldwin (Eds.), *Severely handicapped/hearing impaired students: Strengthening service delivery.* Baltimore: Paul H. Brookes.

Cho, D. W. (1982). *Labor market activities of disabled persons: An analysis of a national survey of disabled persons* (Rehabilitation Engineering Center Tech. Brief, Cerebral Palsy Research Foundation of Kansas). Wichita: Wichita State University.

Darling, R. B., & Darling, J. (1982). *Children who are different: Meeting the challenges of birth defects in society.* St. Louis: C. V. Mosby.

Evers v. Buxbaum, 253 F. 2d 356 (1958).

Gage, G., Baldwin, V., & Campbell, R. (1980). *Survey of national goals of providers of training services to personnel serving the SH/HI child.* Monmouth, OR: Teaching Research, Oregon College of Education.

Gallagher, J. J., Beckman, P., & Cross, A. (1983). Families of handicapped children: Sources of stress and its amelioration. *Exceptional Children, 50,* 10–19.

Healy, A. (1982). Children with disabilities: Implications for care. *Report of the Surgeon General's workshop on children with handicaps and their families.* Washington, DC: Public Health Service, U.S. Department of Health and Human Services.

Johnson, J. L. (1983). *Stress as perceived by teachers of hearing impaired children and youth.* Unpublished doctoral dissertation, Gallaudet College, Washington, DC.

Karp, N. (1983). *Parents' roles in the rehabilitation of their handicapped children: Research priorities.* Washington, DC: National Institute of Handicapped Research, U.S. Department of Education.

Meadow, K. (1981). Burnout in professionals working with deaf children. *American Annals of the Deaf, 126,* 13–22.

Pascale, R. T., & Athos, A. G. (1981). *The art of Japanese management: Applications for American executives.* New York: Warner Books.

Pieper, B. (1982). Foreword. In R. B. Darling & J. Darling, *Children who are different: Meeting the challenges of birth defects in society.* St. Louis: C. V. Mosby.

Polloway, E., & Smith, J. D. (1983). Changes in mild mental retardation: Population, programs, and perspectives. *Exceptional Children, 50,* 149–159.

Rose, D. S. (1983). The fundamental role of hearing in psychological development. *Hearing Instruments, 34,* 22–26.

Staff. (1982, November 1). Quality: The U.S. drives to catch up. *Business Week,* pp. 66–80.

Stedt, J. D., & Palermo, D. S. (1983). The morale of teachers of multihandicapped and nonhandicapped children in a residential school for the deaf. *American Annals of the Deaf, 128,* 383–387.

U. S. Department of Education. (1983). *Fifth annual report to Congress on the implementation of Public Law 94-142: The Education for All Handicapped Children Act.* Washington, DC: Author.

Weintraub, F., & McCaffrey, M. A. (1976). Professional advocacy. In F. Weintraub, A. Abelson, J. Ballard, & M. LaVor (Eds.), *Public policy and the education of exceptional children.* Reston, VA: Council for Exceptional Children.

Ysseldyke, J., Algozzine, B., & Epps, S. (1983). A logical and empirical analysis of current practice in classifying students as handicapped. *Exceptional Children, 50,* 160–166.

Chapter 2

The Federal Definition

Editor's Note: On November 6, 1978, the Amendments to the Developmental Disabilities Assistance and Bill of Rights Act (Public Law 95-602) was adopted by Congress. Encompassed in this act is the change in the definition of developmental disabilities from one that is categorically based to one that emphasizes an individual's functional limitations and accompanying need for services. In 1981 the government published findings that analyzed the impact of the definition change from three perspectives: the numbers of individuals served, the funds expended, and the quality of the services provided before and after passage of the 1978 law. That publication, *Special Report on the Impact of the Change in the Definition of Developmental Disabilities,* * was mandated by Public Law 95-602, Sec. 502(b)(2). The information that follows is adapted from that report. The legislative history, rationale for change, and the immediate outcomes are well documented therein. In addition, that discussion is integral to an understanding of the theoretical premises and practical strategies offered throughout this book. The statistical data and trends noted are valuable in planning optimal service delivery systems for hearing-impaired developmentally disabled people.

EVELYN CHEROW

[Executive Summary omitted here]

Part I: Introduction

Purpose of the Report

The purpose of this report is to inform the Congress of the impact of the functional definition of developmental disabilities incorporated into the Developmental Disabilities Assistance and Bill of Rights Act in 1978. The 1978 Amendments, contained in Public Law 95-602, specified that the Secretary submit a special report to the Congress on the impact of the newly enacted functional definition:

Sec. 502(b)(2) The Secretary of Health, Education and Welfare shall submit to Congress not later than January 15, 1981, a special report concerning the impact of the amendment of the definition of "developmentally disabled" made by paragraph (1). This report shall include—

---

*U.S. Department of Health and Human Services, Office of Human Development Services, Administration on Developmental Disabilities, Washington, D.C., May 1981.

(A) an analysis of the impact of the amendment on each of the categories of persons with developmental disabilities receiving services under the Developmental Disabilities Assistance and Bill of Rights Act before the date of enactment of this Act, and for the fiscal year ending on September 30, 1979 and for the succeeding fiscal year, including—

(i) the number of persons with developmental disabilities in each category served before and after such date of enactment; and

(ii) the amounts expended under such Act for each such category of persons with developmental disabilities before and after such date of enactment; and

(B) an assessment, evaluation and comparison of services provided to persons with developmental disabilities provided before the date of enactment of this act and for the fiscal year ending September 30, 1979 and for the succeeding fiscal year.

Overview of the Developmental Disabilities Program

The purpose of the Developmental Disabilities Program is to improve and coordinate the provision of services to persons with developmental disabilities, those severe and chronic disabilities which result in substantial functional limitations in the major activities of daily living.

The basic goal of the program is to provide for significant improvement in the quality, scope, and extent of the services for persons with developmental disabilities by means of

- Comprehensive planning for current and future service needs, including needs and resource assessment, analysis of resources against needs, and prioritizing objectives and unmet needs;
- Coordination and appropriate integrated utilization of services and resources at all levels of government and the private sector for more effective utilization of existing resources for developmentally disabled persons; and
- Demonstration of new programs designed to fill existing gaps in specialized services.

The developmentally disabled persons to be served comprise about 9 percent of the 29 million physically and mentally disabled in the country. Their disabilities are chronic and severe, with many having multiple handicaps due to other impairments and disorders such as blindness, deafness, absence of language, orthopedic defects, and emotional disturbance. About 150,000 reside in state public institutions for the mentally retarded. About 2.5 million, over age three, are noninstitutionalized and reside either with their families or in supervised alternative community-based living arrangements.

The aim of the program is to move the developmentally disabled individual from total dependency to his or her maximum level of independent functioning. This can be accomplished through the provision of a combination of specialized or generic services which are individually planned and delivered under the separate jurisdiction of a variety of service agencies all relying primarily or exclusively on states.

To accomplish these purposes, the Developmental Disabilities Program has four major program components.

- **Basic State Grant Program,** which provides grants to states for planning, coordination, and systems advocacy;

- **Protection and Advocacy System,** which provides grants to states to protect and advocate for the rights of developmentally disabled individuals;
- **University Affiliated Facilities Program,** which provides grants for administrative and operational costs related to the training and research programs conducted by the facilities; and
- **Special Projects,** which provide grants to public and nonprofit organizations to demonstrate improved methods of service delivery and protection and advocacy services.

More specific information on each of these program components will be presented in Part II of this report.

The Current and Previous Definitions of Developmental Disabilities

The current definition of developmental disabilities, as contained in Public Law 95-602, the "Developmental Disabilities Assistance and Bill of Rights Act," Section 102(7), is:

(7) The term 'developmental disability' means a severe, chronic disability of a person which—

(A) is attributable to a mental or physical impairment or combination of mental and physical impairments;

(B) is manifested before the person attains the age twenty-two;

(C) is likely to continue indefinitely;

(D) results in substantial functional limitations in three or more of the following areas of major life activity: (i) self-care, (ii) receptive and expressive language, (iii) learning, (iv) mobility, (v) self-direction, (vi) capacity for independent living, and (vii) economic sufficiency; and

(E) reflects the person's need for a combination and sequence of special interdisciplinary, or generic care, treatment, or other services which are of lifelong or extended duration and are individually planned and coordinated.

The definition of developmental disability contained in Public Law 95-602, sometimes referred to as the new definition of developmental disability, is based solely on an individual's functional limitations and need for services, rather than the diagnosis or nature of his or her disabling condition.

The previous definition of developmental disability contained in Section 102(a)(7) of Public Law 94-103, the one used by the Developmental Disabilities program until November 1978, generally applied to persons with one of the four handicapping conditions listed:

The term "developmental disability" means a disability of a person which—

(A)(i) is attributable to mental retardation, cerebral palsy, epilepsy, or autism;

(ii) is attributable to any other condition of a person found to be closely related to mental retardation because such condition results in similar impairment of general intellectual functioning or adaptive behavior to that of mentally retarded persons or requires treatment and services similar to those required for such persons; or

(iii) is attributable to dyslexia resulting from a disability described in clause (i) or (ii) of this subparagraph;

(B) originates before such person attains age eighteen;

(C) has continued or can be expected to continue indefinitely; and

(D) constitutes a substantial handicap to such person's ability to function normally in society.

In addition, the conference report on the 1978 Amendments carried a provision that the functional definition was intended to cover everyone covered under the PL 94-103 categorical definition. The conferees stressed that individuals currently receiving services should continue to receive those services irrespective of the revised definition. Data are not available to assess the impact of this "hold harmless" provision on the Developmental Disabilities Program.

This report contains the analysis of the impact of the change in the definition of developmental disabilities, in terms of both the numbers of individuals served and the federal expenditures before and after enactment of Public Law 95-602 and the assessment of services provided to individuals with developmental disabilities. The baseline for the data to be analyzed is fiscal year 1978, the last year that the categorical definition from Public Law 94-103 was in effect. The succeeding fiscal years, fiscal years 1979 and 1980, saw the introduction of a functional definition of developmental disabilities into the service network for individuals with developmental disabilities.

The basic assumption of the report is that the fiscal year 1978 funds were expended based on the categorical definition of developmental disabilities and that the fiscal year 1979 and fiscal year 1980 funds were expended based on the functional definition of developmental disabilities.

The mandate for this special study grew out of concern that the use of a functional definition of developmental disabilities could result in a diminution of services to individuals with the conditions specifically mentioned in Public Law 94-103. Part II of this report discusses the specific impact of the change in the definition.

Reasons for the Change in the Definition of Developmental Disabilities

The philosophy underlying the Developmental Disabilities Program is unique in its broad ecumenical approach to advocacy and planning for a target population with various disabilities and needs. Since the inception of the Developmental Disabilities Services and Facilities Construction Act of 1970, the Developmental Disabilities Program has attempted to bring together a variety of agencies traditionally serving disabled persons to develop a coordinated and comprehensive service delivery system for its target population.

Because of the unique broad-based approach to the program, it is not surprising that ambiguity has existed about the program's target population. The question of which groups of disabled persons fall under the term "developmentally disabled" and which groups do not qualify has been raised by various agencies, programs, and consumers. . . .

The bases for the changes reflected in PL 95-602 are, as determined by the National Task Force on the Definition of Developmental Disabilities who [sic] conducted the independent study, mandated in PL 94-103

- The need to focus scarce resources on that segment of the disabled population most in need of services;
- Developmentally disabled persons will require a combination and sequence of special interdisciplinary or generic care, treatment, or other services which are of lifelong or extended duration and are individually planned and coordinated;
- The target population of developmentally disabled individuals is substantially and chronically disabled;
- Service agencies' traditional approaches are not oriented toward meeting the unique needs of this population so that the following combination is required.
  Comprehensive planning;
  Improved leverage on existing monies;
  Increased access to existing services;
  Interdisciplinary services in a variety of service delivery modes;
  Advocacy to ensure the above; and
  Coordination of services at the delivery point to ensure that needs are met.
- Concern that individuals with conditions or disabilities other than the four listed in PL 94-103 might share the limitations and service needs of the four named conditions and because of the definition be denied services.

The purpose of the functional definition was to emphasize the complexity, pervasiveness, and substantiality of the disabling conditions to be addressed by the Developmental Disabilities Program by focusing on the individual's functional limitations and the resulting need for comprehensive services. Thus, the definition of developmental disabilities changed from one which was categorically based to one which is functionally based.

Summary of Key Findings on the Developmentally Disabled Population

Included as an appendix to this report [Appendix B] are the findings contained in the document entitled "Estimates of the Size and Characteristics of the Non-institutionalized Developmentally Disabled Population in the United States Based Primarily on an Analysis of the 1976 Survey of Income and Education" which was prepared by Morgan Management Systems, Inc., and Gollay and Associates.

These findings were derived from an analysis of the Survey of Income and Education (SIE) conducted in 1976 by the U.S. Bureau of the Census on the noninstitutionalized population over age three. Each of the criteria in the definition of developmental disabilities was operationalized for use with the data gathered. Since the SIE was not conducted with the definition of developmental disabilities in mind, the operationalization of the criteria was not easy or precise. However, as can be seen from the summarized findings, the methodology used produced results generally consistent with other estimates; provided considerable additional insight into the characteristics of the developmentally disabled population; and compared both nondevelopmentally disabled persons and nondisabled persons.

Resource Documents

The resource documents utilized by Departmental staff to develop this report are described in Appendix C [of this chapter]. . . .

Organization of the Report

The main body of the report, Part II, summarizes data on the effect of the definitional change and presents information on the impact of the change in each of the four components of the Developmental Disabilities Program. The final section of the report discusses the conclusions and findings of the analysis of the data.

Part II: Components of the Developmental Disabilities Program

The mandate for this special study requires an analysis of the impact of change in the definition of developmental disabilities, in terms of the number of individuals served, the federal expenditures, and an assessment of the services provided before and after enactment of PL 95-602 in 1978. Since the concern is that individuals with any of the previously listed categories of conditions continue to receive services, the data are displayed with the four categories specified: mental retardation, cerebral palsy, epilepsy, and autism. The category "other" is used for those conditions which are now included as a result of the change to a functional definition, such as spina bifida, tuberous sclerosis, osteogenesis imperfecta, multiple sclerosis, or Tourette's syndrome.

The following sections present the appropriations for the Developmental Disabilities Program for each of the three years by program component, summary findings on the impact of the change in the definition in terms of the developmentally disabled population planned for or served, the expenditures, and the assessment of quality and then a discussion of the impact within each program component.

Appropriation Levels for Program Components

Because the changes in funding levels which occurred between FY 1978 and FY 1980 had some impact on each of the program components, it is necessary to examine these appropriation levels when assessing the impact in the change of the definition. Table 1 [page 22] gives some perspective on the size of the total Developmental Disabilities Program and each of its components for the three fiscal years being analyzed. There was no increase in the appropriated funds from FY 1978 to FY 1979. In FY 1980 the amount appropriated for the program represented an increase of $3,311,000 or 5.6 percent increase over the FY 1979 level.

The Basic State Grants account for the major part of the program resources. In FY 1978 the $30 million represented just over 50 percent of program resources. In FY 1979 the amount for Basic State Grants was increased to just over $35 million without an increase of the total amount appropriated for the DD Program. The $35 million represented almost 60 percent of program resources. In FY 1980 the Basic State Grants received just over $43 million and represented 69 percent of the program resources. Special project funds were used to augment the Basic State Grant Program.

In fiscal year 1978, the Protection and Advocacy Program was modestly funded at $3,000,000 with a minimum allotment state receiving only $20,000 to implement a

Table 1. Developmental Disabilities Program Expenditures

Program Component	Fiscal '78 Amount	%	Fiscal '79 Amount	%	Fiscal '80 Amount	%
Basic State Grants	$30,058,000	50.8	$35,331,000	59.8	$43,180,000	69.2
Protection & Advocacy	3,000,000	5.1	3,801,000	6.4	7,500,000	12.0
Special Projects	19,567,000	33.0	12,573,000	21.3	4,756,000	7.6
University Affiliated Facilities	6,500,000	11.1	7,420,000	12.5	7,000,000	11.2
TOTAL	$59,125,000	100.0	$59,125,000	100.0	$62,436,000	100.0

statewide system of Protection and Advocacy. The $3 million represented only 5.1 percent of the total program budget. In fiscal year 1979 the allotment was increased to $3.8 million due to the fact that Public Law 95-602 required that each minimum allotment state receive no less than $50,000 for its system of Protection and Advocacy. In fiscal year 1980, the total allotment for Protection and Advocacy was $7.5 million and represented 12 percent of the total program budget.

In fiscal years 1979 and 1980, Special Project funds were used to increase the funds available for the Basic State Grant Program. Consequently, these funds represented only 21.3 percent and 7.6 percent of the total program funds for those two fiscal years compared with 33 percent of the total program allotment for fiscal year 1978.

Funding for the University Affiliated Facilities Program (UAF) in fiscal year 1978 was $6.5 million, or 11 percent of the program resources. The University Affiliated Facilities received $7.4 million in fiscal year 1979, which represented 12 percent of the program resources. The amount appropriated in fiscal year 1980 was $7.0 million, or 11.2 percent of the program budget and a decrease of $400,000, or 5 percent, from the fiscal year 1979 level of funding.

It must be remembered, however, that the Developmental Disabilities Program appropriation of $62 million is only 1.5 percent of the total $4.4 billion expended annually by federal programs which provide services to developmentally disabled individuals.

Summary of Information on the Developmental Disabilities Program

The observations that can be made from the summary data on the total program are presented below for each of the major areas of concern identified in the congressional mandate for this study: individuals planned for or served, expenditures, and assessment of services provided. The relevant charts follow the summary observations.

1. Individuals Planned for or Served—Summary Observations
   - Individuals planned for under the Basic State Grant Program are receiving services under the other three components (Protection and Advocacy, University Affiliated Facilities, and Special Projects).

- Increases or decreases in the total number served are more reflective of changes in funding levels than a change in the definition.

PASADENA CITY COLLEGE
SHATFORD LIBRARY

Patrons must have a valid PCC Picture ID or PCC Shatford library card to check out materials or use them inside the library. Education code 19911 cites willful detention of library property as a misdemeanor. Patrons must return materials promptly. Items checked out must be returned on or prior to:

Date Due:

OCT 1 8 1994

'93   (over)

'ice delivery, the number and per- component can be attributed to the noted, however, that the number of remained basically the same during

)thers" served in the Protection and the change in the definition as well ction and advocacy offices are man-)led. Although the funds from the

d

	Fiscal '79		Fiscal '80	
	Number	%	Number	%
	3,291,862	64.3	2,140,988	54.8
	623,909	12.2	558,688	14.3
	1,007,646	19.7	679,802	17.4
	75,431	1.5	62,510	1.6
	120,011	2.3	464,925	11.9
	5,118,859	100.0	3,906,913	100.0
	16,265	60.2	14,073	51.6
	1,756	6.5	2,236	8.2
	1,513	5.6	2,209	8.1
	865	3.2	927	3.4
	6,619	24.5	7,828	28.7
	27,018	100.0	27,273	100.0
	12,924	55.0	13,475	55.0
	1,880	8.0	2,009	8.2
	1,316	5.6	1,470	6.0
	752	3.2	833	3.4
	6,627	28.2	6,713	27.4
	23,499	100.0	24,500	100.0

am cover individuals planned for while the ils served.

Developmental Disabilities Program are used only on services to developmentally disabled individuals, the reporting systems may not distinguish the source of funding.

- Although the percentage of mentally retarded individuals served may have decreased in each of the components, the percentage component is still roughly equivalent to the 55 percent of the total developmental disabilities population represented by the mentally retarded.

2. Amounts Expended—Summary Observations
   - The amounts expended for each condition increased from FY 1978 to FY 1980 although the percentage of the total may have decreased.
   - Mental retardation remains the condition on which over half of the expenditures in each component in FY 1978 and FY 1980 were made.
   - There was a 6 percent decrease in expenditures for mental retardation in the four program components between FY 1978 and FY 1980.
   - The reduction in the mental retardation expenditures can be related to the focus on severity of the condition in the functional definition. Generally, the mildly mentally retarded are no longer included in the developmentally disabled population unless there are multiple handicaps which in combination substantially limit the individual's ability to function.
   - Expenditures in the category cerebral palsy increased approximately 44 percent between FY 1978 and FY 1980. There seems to be no clear explanation for this change at this time.
   - There was a 16 percent decrease in expenditures for the epilepsy category between FY 1978 and FY 1980. The epilepsy groups had been concerned when the functional definition was enacted that those individuals with epilepsy whose seizures could be controlled with drugs so that their limitations were minimal would no longer be defined as developmentally disabled.
   - Expenditures for autism increased approximately 17 percent between FY 1978 and FY 1980. The study did not reveal causal factors for this change.
   - The category "other" increased by 400 percent. The expenditures in this category quadrupled between FY 1978 and FY 1980. This is attributable to the change in the definition.

3. Quality Assessment—Summary Observations
   A primary concern of the Developmental Disabilities Program has been that developmentally disabled individuals receive needed services in humane environments, services which enable individuals with developmental disabilities to achieve their maximum potential. There are several current efforts that relate to the assurance of quality services.
   - **Individualized Habilitation Plans.** Each developmentally disabled individual who receives services through the Developmental Disabilities

Table 3. Expenditures by Program and Category

Program Component	Fiscal '78		Fiscal '79		Fiscal '80	
	Amount	%	Amount	%	Amount	%
Basic State Grants						
Mental Retardation	$21,290,812	70.8	$23,877,602	67.6	$26,363,863	61.1
Cerebral Palsy	2,673,606	8.9	4,389,011	12.4	5,283,336	12.2
Epilepsy	4,646,130	15.5	4,385,125	12.4	5,109,232	11.8
Autism	957,024	3.2	1,217,963	3.4	1,339,173	3.1
Other	490,428	1.6	1,461,299	4.2	5,084,396	11.8
TOTAL	$30,058,000	100.0	$35,331,000	100.0	$43,180,000	100.0
Protection and Advocacy						
Mental Retardation	$2,119,102	65.8	$2,269,407	60.2	$3,825,595	51.6
Cerebral Palsy	270,524	8.4	245,036	6.5	607,943	8.2
Epilepsy	305,949	9.5	211,108	5.6	600,530	8.1
Autism	103,057	3.2	120,633	3.2	252,074	3.4
Other	421,887	13.1	923,595	24.5	2,127,802	28.7
TOTAL	$3,200,519[a]	100.0	$3,769,779	100.0	$7,413,944	100.0
Special Projects						
Mental Retardation	$11,984,586	70.4	$8,164,079	65.3	$2,685,141	56.5
Cerebral Palsy	1,395,915	8.2	1,189,821	9.5	587,761	12.3
Epilepsy	2,795,349	16.4	1,610,778	12.9	696,678	14.6
Autism	398,790	2.4	299,433	2.4	121,763	2.6
Other	444,793	2.6	1,238,808	9.9	664,657	14.0
TOTAL	$17,019,433[a]	100.0	$12,502,919	100.0	$4,756,000	100.0
University Affiliated Facilities						
Mental Retardation	$3,575,000	55.0	$4,081,000	55.0	$3,850,000	55.0
Cerebral Palsy	546,000	8.4	593,600	8.0	574,000	8.2
Epilepsy	416,000	6.4	415,520	5.6	420,000	6.0
Autism	208,000	3.2	237,440	3.2	238,000	3.4
Other	1,755,000	27.0	2,092,440	28.2	1,918,000	27.4
TOTAL	$6,500,000	100.0	$7,420,000	100.0	$7,000,000	100.0

[a]Funds reprogrammed with congressional approval.

Program must have a plan developed which states long-term goals and objectives and the services to be provided to achieve those goals;

- **Protection and Advocacy System.** A function of the system is to assure that needed services are delivered, that the services delivered meet minimum standards for quality, and that the services produce the desired changes;

- **Professional and Paraprofessional Assessment.** An instrument has been developed to assess the skills and qualifications of the various groups of professionals and paraprofessionals serving individuals with developmental disabilities;

- **Comprehensive Evaluation System.** This is to be a state-operated, client-centered evaluation system designed to evaluate services provided to developmentally disabled individuals on the basis of the degree of developmental progress attained by clients of these services;

- **National Standards for Developmental Disabilities Services.** These standards have been available and in use for some years, and some programs also use the national compliance-assessment service offered by the developers of the standards, the Accreditation Council for Services for Mentally Retarded and Other Developmentally Disabled Persons.

Each of these activities either takes place or will take place at the state or provider levels, where the main responsibility for assuring the delivery of quality services rests. Although the intensity of quality related activities has increased in the years following enactment of PL 95-602, few of these activities can be related directly to the change in the definition of developmental disabilities.

Basic State Grant Program

The comprehensive state plans for services to individuals with developmental disabilities for fiscal years 1978, 1979, and 1980 were reviewed for the data necessary to provide information on the Basic State Grant Program. The information gathered was returned to the states for verification and provided the main portion of the data included in the report entitled "The Impact of the Amendment of the Definition of 'Developmentally Disabled' on the Developmental Disabilities Program in FY 1979 and FY 1980."

The states reported their estimated developmental disabilities population by category of disability in fiscal year 1978, and most of the states continued to report their estimated population by the category of disability in fiscal year 1979. Only 10 states, or 19 percent of the programs, reported their fiscal year 1980 estimated population by disability in their State Plans.

Individuals Planned For. Table 4 shows the estimated developmental disabilities population by disability for each of the three fiscal years, based on data compiled from the plans developed by the State Planning Councils.

Ten states estimated in their fiscal year 1980 State Plans their developmental disabilities population, identifying these four causes of disability: mental retardation, cerebral palsy, epilepsy, and autism. Seven states did utilize a fifth category of the cause of disability, the composition of which varied from state to state. Five of the states have some combination of multiple handicapping conditions in this category, while two states considered the population of learning disabled as a separate category.

It appears from an analysis of these data that states are focusing on the substantially handicapped to a greater extent in estimating the developmental disabilities population in fiscal year 1980 than when they estimated the developmental disabilities population in fiscal year 1978. Additionally, the elimination of the mildly mentally retarded and

Table 4. Estimated Disability Populations

Disability Group	Fiscal '78 Number	%	Fiscal '79 Number	%	Fiscal '80[a] Number	%
Mental Retardation	3,518,742	65.5	3,291,862	64.3	2,140,988	54.8
Cerebral Palsy	505,269	9.4	623,909	12.2	558,688	14.3
Epilepsy	1,064,479	21.8	1,007,646	19.7	679,802	17.4
Autism	79,866	1.5	75,431	1.5	62,510	1.6
Other	97,490	1.8	120,011	2.3	464,925	11.9
TOTAL	5,265,846	100.0	5,118,859	100.0	3,906,913	100.0

[a]The numbers are extrapolated from the percentages provided by the 10 states that provided categorical information in their fiscal year 1980 state plans.

the ability to control seizures in persons with epilepsy accounted for a substantial reduction in the number of individuals considered developmentally disabled. . . .

Table 5 reveals that individuals with conditions described in Public Law 94-103 composed 88.2 percent of the developmental disabilities population in fiscal year 1980; 11.8 percent were newly eligible.

Table 5. Disability Populations with Definition Changes

Disability Group	Fiscal '78 %	Fiscal '79 %	Fiscal '80 %
Mental Retardation, Cerebral Palsy, Epilepsy, & Autism	98.4	95.8	88.2
All Others	1.6	4.2	11.8
TOTAL	100.0	100.0	100.0

Expenditures. The fact that the Basic State Grant monies are distributed according to population and size and the analysis of need in the Hill Burton formula is reflected in the distribution of the monies through the three fiscal years covered by this report. There was not a dramatic change in the percentage received by the various states from the Basic State Grant Program with the exception of the shift caused by the increase to minimum allotment states in fiscal year 1979.

Table 6 [page 28] contains the distribution of all Basic State Grant funds by disability group for FY '78, FY '79, and FY '80.

Although there has been a decrease in the percentage of funds expended related to mental retardation, the amount of funds increased each year. In addition, the percentage

Table 6. Basic State Grant Funding

Disability Group	Fiscal '78		Fiscal '79		Fiscal '80	
	Amount	%	Amount	%	Amount	%
Mental Retardation	$21,290,812	70.8	$23,877,602	67.6	$26,363,863	61.1
Cerebral Palsy	2,673,606	8.9	4,389,011	12.4	5,283,336	12.2
Epilepsy	4,646,130	15.5	4,385,125	12.4	5,109,232	11.8
Autism	957,024	3.2	1,217,963	3.4	1,339,173	3.1
Other	490,428	1.6	1,461,299	4.2	5,084,396	11.8
TOTAL	$30,058,000	100.0	$35,331,000	100.0	$43,180,000	100.0

expended related to mental retardation continues to be greater than the percentage of the total developmental disabilities population represented by mental retardation.

Generally, a similar trend is noted in the other categories of conditions. The exception is epilepsy, for which consistently less funds have been expended as a percentage of total program funds expended for the developmental disabilities population. In addition, there was a slight decrease in the amount of funds expended for epilepsy in FY 1979. A factor which could explain this is that seizure disorders or epilepsy often accompany other conditions, such as mental retardation, and the primary diagnosis is a condition other than epilepsy. There is some question whether the population counts by category are discrete. Nonetheless, efforts are currently underway to analyze further this information related to epilepsy and to determine future courses of action.

The annual increase in funds expended for "other" categories of conditions indicates that states are expanding the target population beyond the previously named four conditions. It could be expected that the "other" category would continue to grow as experience with the use of the functional definition grows.

Table 7 contains a comparison of the percentage of expenditures for each category of disability for the fiscal years under analysis. The data indicate changes have occurred in the amounts of funds expended for each category, changes that can be attributed generally to the change in the definition.

Table 7. Expenditure Changes by Disability Group

Disability Group	Percent Expended Fiscal '78	Percent Change Fiscal '78-'79	Percent Change Fiscal '79-'80
Mental Retardation	70.8	-3.2	- 9.7
Cerebral Palsy	8.9	+3.5	+ 3.3
Epilepsy	15.5	-3.1	- 3.7
Autism	3.2	+ .2	+ .1
Other	1.6	+2.6	+10.2

Assessment of Quality. Public Law 95-602 requires that "an assessment, evaluation and comparison of services provided to persons with developmental disabilities" be included in the mandated report.

It may be concluded that the quality of services provided with Basic State Grant funds to individuals with developmental disabilities remained constant or improved from the period of October 1, 1978, to September 30, 1980. There is nothing in the analysis of the project and program information indicating that the quality of service deteriorated during this period of time. The efforts of the State Planning Councils and their administering agencies in the area of standards and quality assurance have significantly increased between fiscal year 1978 and fiscal year 1980.

Protection and Advocacy System

The legal and individual client advocacy and protection of the rights of developmentally disabled individuals is the function of the Protection and Advocacy System. The Protection and Advocacy System is outside of the service system and is supported with a grant in aid which is separate from the Developmental Disabilities Basic Grant Program allotment. Designated agencies receiving allotments for protection and advocacy of the rights of the developmentally disabled must be independent of any state agency which provides services to the developmental disabilities population.

The state Protection and Advocacy offices are characterized by a diversity of organizational structures. Among the key factors serving to differentiate offices are the nature of implementation, i.e., public, private, established by Executive Order, established by statute; nature of facilities (single site, multiple sites); philosophy of organization (emphasis on legal model or on advocacy model); staffing patterns (numbers and types of professionals and paraprofessionals employed); and resources (state and agency funding).

Services provided by Protection and Advocacy offices include outreach, hotlines, information and referral, counseling and legal services, advocacy activities (individual, systems, and legislative) and training.

Individuals Served. The Protection and Advocacy System has been less oriented to the categorical concept than the Basic State Grant and the Special Projects. The definition contained in Public Law 95-602 appears to have influenced service to a broad target population by the Protection and Advocacy System.

The effect of the change has been an increase in the number of individuals, with conditions other than the four specified in the previous definition, receiving protection and advocacy services. However, the total number of individuals who are mentally retarded receiving protection and advocacy services did not significantly decrease in either fiscal year 1979 or fiscal year 1980.

Table 8 [page 30] contains the number and percent of individuals served by Protection and Advocacy offices in fiscal year 1978, fiscal year 1979, and fiscal year 1980 by cause of disability.

The increase of individuals with other handicaps who were served by Protection and Advocacy offices could originate from factors other than the change in the federal definition of developmental disabilities. Sixteen states received state monies for the operation of the Protection and Advocacy Program. Eligibility criteria for handicapped

Table 8. Populations Served by Protection and Advocacy Offices

Disability Group	Fiscal '78		Fiscal '79		Fiscal '80	
	Number	%	Number	%	Number	%
Mental Retardation	9,542	65.8	16,265	60.2	14,073	51.6
Cerebral Palsy	1,218	8.4	1,756	6.5	2,236	8.2
Epilepsy	1,377	9.5	1,513	5.6	2,209	8.1
Autism	464	3.2	865	3.2	927	3.4
Other	1,900	13.1	6,619	24.5	7,828	28.7
TOTAL	14,501	100.0	27,018	100.0	27,273	100.0

persons were changed in some states with the provision of state monies for protection and advocacy. The state contribution to protection and advocacy increased $1.2 million in fiscal year 1979 from fiscal year 1978. Some states required their Protection and Advocacy offices to serve all handicapped.

The number of individuals served by Protection and Advocacy offices in fiscal year 1980 was 27,273. Of this number, 51.6 percent of the individuals served were mentally retarded. There were 2,236 individuals with cerebral palsy served in fiscal year 1980, which represented 8.2 percent of the total clientele. Individuals with epilepsy represented 8.1 percent of the clientele, and 3.4 percent of those served were autistic individuals. The individuals in the category of "other" served in fiscal year 1980 increased significantly.

Table 9 shows the changes in individuals served who were mentally retarded, cerebral palsied, epileptic, and autistic and all other individuals served by Protection and Advocacy agencies for fiscal year 1978, fiscal year 1979, and fiscal year 1980.

One could conclude from these data that the impact of the change in the definition of developmental disabilities in Public Law 95-602 was to shift the clientele of the Protection and Advocacy system approximately 15 percent from individuals with mental retardation, cerebral palsy, epilepsy, or autism to individuals with other types of handicapping conditions. However, it is not known what part state requirements in those states which received state funds played in the shift of Protection and Advocacy

Table 9. Changes in Populations Served by Protection and Advocacy Offices

Disability Group	Fiscal '78 %	Fiscal '79 %	Fiscal '80 %
Mental Retardation, Cerebral Palsy, Epilepsy, & Autism	86.9	75.5	71.3
All Others	13.1	24.5	28.7
TOTAL	100.0	100.0	100.0

clientele over fiscal year 1979 and fiscal year 1980. It can be concluded for the purposes of this report that the definition in Public Law 95-602 was the major factor in the shift of clientele.

Expenditures. The data compiled on expenditures for the Protection and Advocacy system reflect the percentage a particular category of disability is of the total developmental disabilities population served by the Protection and Advocacy system in a given fiscal year. The reporting system does not capture expenditures by category of condition. Table 10 distributes the expenditures by the categorical percentage of the total developmental disabilities population served by the Protection and Advocacy system in each of the three fiscal years.

Table 10. Expenditures of Protection and Advocacy Offices

Disability Group	Fiscal '78		Fiscal '79		Fiscal '80	
	Amount	%	Amount	%	Amount	%
Mental Retardation	$2,119,102	65.8	$2,269,407	60.2	$3,825,595	51.6
Cerebral Palsy	270,524	8.4	245,036	6.5	607,943	8.2
Epilepsy	302,949	9.5	211,108	5.6	600,530	8.1
Autism	103,057	3.2	120,633	3.2	252,074	3.4
Other	421,887	13.1	923,595	24.5	2,127,802	28.7
TOTAL	$3,220,519	100.0	$3,769,779	100.0	$7,413,944	100.0

In terms of expenditures, however, it should be remembered that the resources for protection and advocacy continued to grow from a $5.3 million program in fiscal year 1978 to a $12.6 million program in fiscal year 1981. Protection and Advocacy offices have consistently attracted 40 percent of their resources from alternative funding sources other than the grants received from Section 113 of Public Law 95-602.

The clientele of the Protection and Advocacy agencies is increasingly becoming those multihandicapped individuals who have no specific service resource in the generic service system.

Assessment of Quality. A primary function of the Protection and Advocacy system is to assure the provision of quality services to individuals with developmental disabilities. The data do not indicate that the change in the definition of developmental disabilities had any measurable effect on the Protection and Advocacy offices as they carried out this responsibility.

Special Projects

Special Projects grants are made to public or nonprofit organizations for demonstration projects establishing programs which hold promise of expanding or otherwise improving

- Services to persons with developmental disabilities, especially those who are disadvantaged or multihandicapped;

- Program linkages with other agency programs which impact on developmentally disabled individuals; and
- State capacities to enlarge personnel resources and enhance the knowledge and skills of all persons, professionals and paraprofessionals, working with developmentally disabled persons in specialized or generic services.

Individuals Served. The apparent effect of applying the functional definition of developmental disabilities on the number of individuals involved in Special Projects is a decrease in the percent of individuals with mental retardation by almost 25 percent, an increase in the other three previously named categories of conditions, and an increase of 11.1 percent in the number of individuals with "other" handicapping conditions.

Table 11 contains a comparison of the percentage of individuals involved in Special Projects by disability for each of the three fiscal years. The percentage change is against the FY 1978 base year.

Table 11. Changes in Populations Served by Special Projects

Disability Group	Percent of Disability Group Fiscal '78	Percent of Change Fiscal '79	Percent of Change Fiscal '80
Mental Retardation	79.0	-5.8	-24.9
Cerebral Palsy	3.3	+ .9	+10.4
Epilepsy	12.0	+3.7	+ 3.1
Autism	1.5	+ .4	+ .3
Other	4.2	+ .8	+11.1

Expenditures. Table 12 contains the expenditures for Special Projects by category of condition.

Table 12. Expenditures for Special Projects

Disability Group	Fiscal '78 Amount	%	Fiscal '79 Amount	%	Fiscal '80 Amount	%
Mental Retardation	$11,984,584	70.4	$8,164,079	65.3	$2,685,141	56.5
Cerebral Palsy	1,395,915	8.2	1,189,821	9.5	587,761	12.3
Epilepsy	2,795,349	16.4	1,610,778	12.9	696,678	14.6
Autism	398,790	2.4	299,433	2.4	121,763	2.6
Other	444,793	2.6	1,238,808	9.9	664,657	14.0
TOTAL	$17,019,433[a]	100.0	$12,502,919	100.0	$4,756,000	100.0

[a]Does not include over $2 million spent for employment and vocational development.

[End of Part II plus Part III and Appendix A omitted here]

Appendix B
Summary of Key Findings on the Developmentally Disabled Population in the United States

The key findings of the analysis are:

- There were a total of approximately 2.5 million non-institutionalized developmentally disabled individuals over age three in the United States in 1976 who comprised about 1.2 percent of the total population:

DD Population	2,487,000	1.23%
Non DD Disabled Population	26,578,000	13.13%
Total Disabled Population	29,065,000	14.36%
Non Disabled Population	173,368,000	85.65%
Total Non-Institutionalized Population	202,433,000	100.01%

- The developmentally disabled population comprises 8.5 percent of the over 29,000,000 disabled people in the United States.

- Of the total developmental disabilities population, about 35 percent is mentally retarded, 10 percent is seriously emotionally disturbed, 17 percent is sensory impaired, and the remaining 38 percent is physically impaired.

DD MR Population	870,000	35.00%
DD seriously emotionally disturbed population	259,000	10.42%
DD sensory impaired	427,000	17.17%
DD physically impaired	931,000	37.41%
Total DD Population	2,487,000	100.00%

- Over half the developmental disabilities population is under age eighteen, compared with the total population of which only about 30 percent is under age eighteen.

- A higher proportion of Blacks and Native Americans are reported to be developmentally disabled than are other ethnic/racial groups. More Blacks are reported to be mentally retarded or developmentally disabled physically impaired and more Native Americans are reported to be mentally retarded or developmentally disabled sensory impaired.

- About 25 percent of the developmentally disabled individuals come from families that are below the poverty level, compared to only about 19 percent for the non-developmentally disabled population and 11 percent for the non-disabled population. This was true quite consistently for sub-groups within the developmental disabilities population.

- Over three quarters of the total developmental disabilities population over age 18 has had no previous work experience, compared with less than one quarter of the remainder of the population.

- The annual income in 1975 of the developmental disabilities population is about one quarter the average of the non-disabled population, and about one third of the income of non-developmentally disabled persons. While non-disabled persons receive only about 1 percent of their total income from public assistance, and non-developmentally disabled persons receive about 14 percent, developmentally disabled individuals receive about 67 percent from public assistance. Conversely, developmentally disabled individuals receive less than 20 percent of their income from earnings compared to 65 percent for other disabled persons and 92 percent for non-disabled persons. Social security benefits are received by the largest number of developmentally disabled individuals compared to other sources of public assistance.

- The proportion of a state's population that is developmentally disabled varies from a low of .6 percent in Alaska to a high of 2.04 percent in West Virginia. The states that reported .90 percent or less of their total population to be developmentally disabled were

Alaska	Oregon
Colorado	Utah
Nevada	Wyoming
North Dakota	

- The states that reported having 1.5 percent or more of their total population to be developmentally disabled were

Alabama	Mississippi
Arkansas	Tennessee
Georgia	West Virginia
Louisiana	

Appendix C
Primary Resource Documents

1. *The Impact of the Amendment of the Definition of "Developmentally Disabled" on the DD Program in FY '79 and FY '80* (December 1980): This report was the major resource used for the data contained in this report on the clients, services, and expenditures of the Developmental Disabilities Program components. The report was written and produced by the Institute for Comprehensive Planning under a contract with the Accreditation Council for Services for Mentally Retarded and Other Developmentally Disabled Persons (AC/MRDD).

2. *A Study of the Potential Impact of the Definition Recommended by the National Task Force on the Definition of Developmental Disabilities* (September 1978–January 1981): A contract was awarded in September 1978 to Morgan Management Systems, Inc., to study the *potential* impact of a functional definition of developmental disabilities. After the passage of the functional definition in November 1978, however, the study focused instead on the ability of the program components to use the definition and on tools which might aid in utilizing the functional definition. The study products, listed below, were completed by Gollay and Associates, Inc.

   - Estimates of the Size and Characteristics of the Non-Institutionalized Developmentally Disabled Population in the United States Based Primarily on an Analysis of the 1976 Survey of Income and Education;
   - Operational Definition of Developmental Disabilities;
   - Description of Major New Categories of Disabilities; and
   - Summary Final Report.

3. *Secretary's Report to Congress on the Definition of Developmental Disabilities* (1978): This Report was mandated in Public Law 94-103, Section 301, to be submitted annually to the Congress. The Act required an annual report on the conditions which the Secretary had determined should be included and not included under the statutory definition of developmental disabilities. This Report recommended retention of the definition stated in Public Law 94-103.

4. *Final Report of the Special Study on the Definition of Developmental Disabilities* (November 1977): This was the report of the National Task Force on the Definition of Developmental Disabilities described earlier. In addition to the Final Report, several of the background papers prepared for the Task Force by the contractor's staff were used as resource documents.

[Appendix D omitted here]

Chapter 3

A Demographic Perspective

Michael A. Karchmer

In this chapter, developmental disabilities among hearing-impaired children and youth will be discussed from a population perspective by broadly examining the group of hard-of-hearing and deaf students across the United States who were receiving special education and support services as of the spring of 1982. The chapter describes the extent to which these students have disabilities in addition to hearing impairment and characterizes the groups of hearing-impaired students with specific conditions.

Two main themes underlie the analyses here. The first pertains to the magnitude of the phenomenon. As will be shown later, a sizeable minority—more than 30 percent—of all hearing-impaired students in special education is reported to have at least one additional condition that has educational impact. The fact that hearing impairment in children is often accompanied by other disabilities emphasizes the importance of understanding this group and, in fact, offers the strongest rationale for a book such as this. A complementary theme relates to diversity. The extent and the nature of particular handicapping conditions vary enormously. There is no such thing as a "typical" hearing-impaired student with additional handicaps. Service providers face a challenge in dealing with the diversity of characteristics found among hearing-impaired students with developmental disabilities.

The focus of this chapter is to examine some of the major concomitants of additional handicaps among hearing-impaired students. Specifically, what kind of additional disabilities are reported, and what is their relative frequency of occurrence within the population of interest? The chapter includes a consideration of characteristics of students with specific handicapping conditions. Etiologies of hearing loss also are examined in relation to the extent of additional handicapping conditions. Finally, the extent to which specific handicaps occur together is analyzed.

Source of Data

The information presented in this chapter comes from a continuing national study of hearing-impaired students in the U.S., the Annual Survey of Hearing-Impaired Children and Youth. This study has been conducted on a national basis since 1968 by the Gallaudet Research Institute's Office of Demographic Studies (now the Center for Assessment and Demographic Studies). The information collected constitutes the largest known data base on individual hearing-impaired children and youth. Each year, all educational programs known to be providing preschool, primary, or secondary school services to hearing-impaired students are asked to participate. All types of educational programs are contacted, ranging from special schools for the deaf to public schools offering both regular and special education service options.

The Annual Survey gathers from each program, on an individual child basis, educationally relevant information about characteristics of the students and the instructional and support services they receive. Specific items on the survey pertain to such background characteristics of the student as age, sex, and ethnic status. Other items, including audiological findings, etiology, and age at onset of hearing loss, attempt to describe the type and extent of the unaided hearing loss. Another section of the survey, the one of particular importance to this chapter, solicits information on educationally significant handicaps which the hearing-impaired student may have in addition to hearing loss. Finally, data are also gathered on special- and regular-education instructional and support services which the student is receiving.

The Annual Survey data used here were collected in the spring, 1982, as part of the 1981–82 school year project, the most recently available national information. The 1981–82 Annual Survey contains information on 54,774 hearing-impaired students in more than 6,000 schools across the U.S. Within the survey, information on additional handicapping conditions or lack thereof was provided for 51,962 students or 94.9 percent of the total. This is the group analyzed here.

Although the Annual Survey is the largest educational data base on individual hearing-impaired children and youth, it is by no means a complete head count of students with hearing impairments. The 1981–82 handicapped child figures provided to the U.S. Department of Education by the states in compliance with Public Laws 89-313 and 94-142 state that there are more than 76,000 "hard-of-hearing and deaf" students and another 2,600 children in the "deaf-blind" category who are receiving services under these laws (U.S. Department of Education, 1983). This suggests that the coverage of the Annual Survey is in the 70 percent range. However, assuming that the federal figures accurately represent the total is not entirely warranted. In many cases, it would appear that states report estimates rather than actual head counts for specific handicap categories. Whatever the exact relationship between the Annual Survey and the federal figures, where the actual numbers of children are of interest, the totals in this report should be increased by at least one-third.

In considering the generalizability of the information reported here, it is important to emphasize again the nature of the data base. The Annual Survey is an educational data base in that it deals primarily with students from 3 to 21 years old who are identified as receiving educational and support services in relation to their hearing impairment and other possible disabilities. It represents the broad group of hard-of-hearing and deaf students who are receiving special education and related support services in preschool, primary, and secondary educational programs across the country. Because of its special education orientation, the survey does not cover all segments of the hearing-impaired school-age population equally. This unevenness of coverage qualifies the data reported in this chapter to the degree that they relate to additional handicaps. On one hand, students who are educated in regular classes with minimal or no support services are not likely to be well represented in the data. Generally, these are students with mild hearing losses, and the fact that they receive no special services implies that they are unlikely to have additional handicaps. On the other hand, there are hearing-impaired children and youth who have multiple disabilities so severe that the primary services they receive are other than educational. Specifically, individuals with hearing impairments who attend residential facilities for the multihandicapped or programs for deaf-blind children are proportionately underrepresented in the Annual Survey.

Handicapping Conditions

The disabilities discussed in this chapter are listed in Table 1 according to the way they are categorized in the Annual Survey. The table also gives definitions of the additional handicapping conditions. (In this chapter, the terms *disability* and *handicapping condition* are used synonymously.) Conditions are noted on the Annual Survey form only if they are judged to be educationally significant. As the instructions on the survey form state, an educationally significant handicapping condition is one "which places additional demands or requirements upon instructional arrangements, causes modification of teaching methods, or alters or restricts the student's activities or learning in ways additive to those occasioned by the hearing loss alone."

Table 1. Additional Handicapping Conditions: Categories and Definitions

Condition	Definition or Explanation
Group 1: Physical Conditions	
Legal blindness	condition in which corrected vision in the better eye is less than 20/2000, and/or a specialist designates legal blindness
Uncorrected visual problem	uncorrected or uncorrectable visual problem, including blindness in one eye, muscular imbalance or paralysis, and retinitis pigmentosa
Brain damage or injury	condition verified by abnormal EEG or physican's neurological findings
Epilepsy (convulsive disorder)	condition in which the student is subject to uncontrollable seizure behavior
Orthopedic	condition which restricts use of extremities as a result of permanent injury, paralysis, or polio
Cerebral palsy	checked if this condition has been medically diagnosed
Heart disorder	malfunction of the heart which restricts physical functioning and requires monitoring by a physican
Other health impaired	any other physical condition which restricts functional ability, such as asthma, diabetes, kidney defects
Group 2: Cognitive/Intellectual Conditions	
Mental retardation	condition that is documented by scores within defective limits from individually administered scale(s) of intelligence (a measured IQ at least two standard deviations below the mean); degree of hearing impairment and communication level should determine whether verbal or performance scale scores would be appropriate
Emotional/behavioral problem	condition in which inappropriate behaviors interfere with normal academic progress (behaviors include passive/withdrawn; aggressive/abusive; rapid mood

	changes/sudden outbursts; bizarre, unexplainable actions; and chronic, unfounded physical complaints and symtoms)
Specific learning disability	condition in which normal general intelligence is present, but specific learning deficits restrict accomplishments; these restrictions may be attributable to difficulty in visual/auditory perception, perceptual/motor functioning, as well as to a lack of control of attention, impulse, or motor function
Other	this category would include any other observed condition which would restrict functioning, such as nutritional deficits, educational deprivation, neglect

Note. Unpublished material from the Annual Survey of Hearing-Impaired Children and Youth, 1981-82. Copyright 1983 by Gallaudet College Center for Assessment and Demographic Studies. Used by permission.

The handicapping conditions are classified under two headings for purposes of some of the analyses in this chapter: Those conditions which fall into Group 1 (according to Table 1) will be termed *physical* conditions, and those in Group 2 will be termed *cognitive/intellectual* conditions. In general, physical conditions are reported only if they are documented by medical diagnosis; the other conditions are noted on the Annual Survey only if they are diagnosed by appropriate assessment personnel.

In the analysis and discussion of the data which follow this section, a few qualifications and limitations should be noted. First, there is no indication on the data file as to the severity of a disability that a student may have, only whether or not it is present to the degree that it interferes with the educational process. Second, it is not possible to distinguish among the relative impacts that various handicaps may have on an individual. Hence, the data do not permit us to say which disability is primary and which is secondary.

Basic Findings

Figure 1 (page 40) summarizes information from the 1981–82 Annual Survey on 51,962 hearing-impaired students across the United States on whom handicapping information was reported. As shown by the figure, 30.6 percent of the students were reported to have at least one additional educationally significant handicap beyond hearing loss; 9.6 percent of the entire group had two or more additional handicapping conditions. It is clear from these data that efforts at understanding and providing services that meet the needs of the nation's hearing-impaired young people must take into consideration the high likelihood that these children will have additional handicapping conditions. The percentage of students reported to the Annual Survey as having one or more additional handicapping conditions has stayed relatively stable over the past 15 years at somewhat more than 30 percent of the total (Gentile & McCarthy, 1973). Further, a 1979 study of the Canadian hearing-impaired school-age population placed the percentage with additional handicaps at approximately 30 percent of the total (Karchmer, Petersen, Allen, & Osborn, 1981).

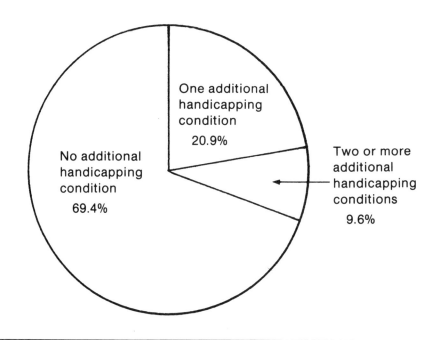

Figure 1. Additional handicapping condition(s) among hearing-impaired students. This represents information on 51,962 students. Information on additional handicapping conditions was not available for 2,812 or 5.1 percent of the 54,774 total. Unpublished data from the Annual Survey of Hearing-Impaired Children and Youth, 1981-82. Copyright 1983 by Gallaudet College Center for Assessment and Demographic Studies. Used by permission.

Table 2 lists specific handicapping conditions and percentages of the students who were reported to have each condition. The number of conditions, of course, totals more than the number of additionally handicapped students, because nearly 10 percent of the students had more than one additional handicap. As shown in Table 2, cognitive/intellectual disabilities were far more common than physical disabilities. Mental retardation (8.4 percent of the total sample), specific learning disabilities (7.5 percent), and emotional/behavioral problems (6.1 percent) were the three most common conditions. Of the physical conditions, students with uncorrected visual problems or vision deficits severe enough to have the individuals classified as legally blind accounted for 6.2 percent of the total. Epilepsy, orthopedic problems, and brain damage were less common conditions, each being reported in 1 to 3 percent of the cases.

It is helpful, for purposes of analysis, to define four categories of hearing-impaired students, according to whether the individuals were reported to have (1) no additional handicapping conditions, (2) one or more physical handicaps in addition to hearing impairment, (3) one or more cognitive/intellectual handicaps in addition to hearing impairment, or (4) both physical and cognitive/intellectual handicapping conditions in addition to hearing impairment. Table 3 shows the Annual Survey sample thus divided. These data again make the point that disabilities in the cognitive/intellectual category were the most common.

Table 2. Additional Handicapping Condition(s) of Hearing-Impaired Children and Youth

Condition	Number of Students	Percentage of 51,962[a]
Physical Conditions		
Legal blindness	960	1.8
Uncorrected visual problem	2,264	4.4
Brain damage or injury	1,149	2.2
Epilepsy (convulsive disorder)	640	1.2
Orthopedic	1,343	2.6
Cerebral palsy	1,570	3.0
Heart disorder	1,150	2.2
Other health impairment	2,047	3.9
Cognitive/Intellectual Conditions		
Mental retardation	4,353	8.4
Emotional/behavioral problem	3,157	6.1
Specific learning disability	3,874	7.5
Other	1,052	2.0

Note. Unpublished data from the Annual Survey of Hearing-Impaired Children and Youth, 1981-82. Copyright 1983 by Gallaudet College Center for Assessment and Demographic Studies. Used by permission.

[a]Information on handicapping condition was not provided for 2,812 students or 5.1 percent of the 54,774 students.

Table 3. Extent of Additional Handicapping Condition(s) among Hearing-Impaired Students by Category of Disability

Category	Number	Percentage of 51,962[a]
No additional handicap	36,083	69.4
One or more physical handicaps	5,045	9.7
One or more cognitive/intellectual handicaps	7,610	14.6
Both physical and cognitive/intellectual handicaps	3,224	6.2
TOTAL	51,962	99.9

Note. Unpublished data from the Annual Survey of Hearing-Impaired Children and Youth, 1981-82. Copyright 1983 by Gallaudet College Center for Assessment and Demographic Studies. Used by permission.

[a]Information on handicapping condition was not reported for 2,812 students or 5.1 percent of the 54,774 students.

Age (Year of Birth) in Relation to Disability

Viewed from the national perspective of the Annual Survey of Hearing-Impaired Children and Youth, year of birth (age) has a marked influence on the extent of additional handicapping conditions reported. There is a clear overall trend that higher percentages of older students have an additional handicap. This information is given in Figure 2, which shows the numbers of hearing-impaired students reported according to year of birth. The number of students in each age group who were reported to have additional handicaps is depicted by the shaded portions of the figure, the percentage of the total is noted above the shaded portion. In general, about 3,000 hearing-impaired students were reported to the Annual Survey for a typical birth year. Fewer are reported for the younger age groups, reflecting to some degree the reality that in their early years

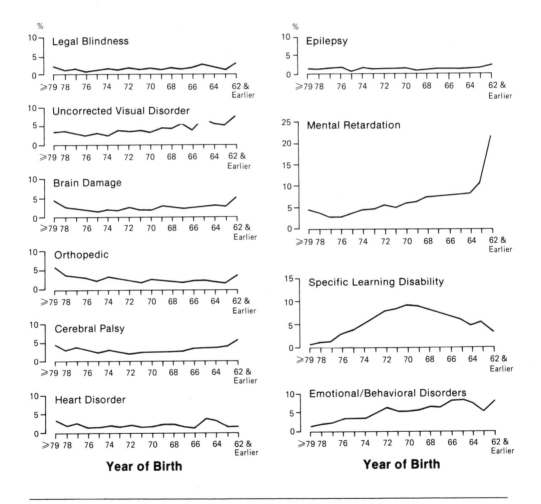

Figure 2. Additional handicapping condition(s) of hearing-impaired students by age (as of December 31, 1981). Unpublished data from the Annual Survey of Hearing-Impaired Children and Youth, 1981-82. Copyright 1983 by Gallaudet College Center for Assessment and Demographic Studies. Used by permission.

not all hearing-impaired children are identified or receiving educational or support services. Similarly, the sizes of the older age groups decline as students graduate from or leave secondary school programs. Of course, the most noteworthy feature of Figure 2 is the large size of the 1964 and 1965 birth-year groups compared with other birth years. As has been discussed elsewhere (e.g., Trybus, Karchmer, Kerstetter, & Hicks, 1980), the increase was due to maternal rubella contracted during the epidemic of 1964–65. During that period, approximately double the number of children were born with hearing impairments as would be expected during a comparable nonepidemic period. As Trybus et al. (1980) have described, maternal rubella-caused deafness is an etiology associated with the increased likelihood of specific additional conditions, among which are heart disorders, visual problems such as cataracts, and emotional and behavioral problems. Hence, the numbers of additionally handicapped students in the 1964–65 birth groups also increased dramatically.

In discussing the findings of the extent of additional handicapping conditions by age group, one must bear in mind the cross-sectional nature of the data. The 1981–82 Annual Survey provided a snapshot of the hearing-impaired special education population at a single point in time. This makes it difficult to separate what may be age-related effects from what may be cohort effects, that is, those influenced by events that may have happened during a specific period of time. The findings for 1964 and 1965, for example, were clearly dictated by the large percentage of students in the group with maternal rubella-caused hearing loss.

Another factor in interpreting the age data is that some conditions may not be identified or diagnosed until the child is older and they begin to impair educational function. Conditions that are present may not be disabling until the child is asked to function in a particular context. For example, children with specific perceptual/motor or other specific learning dysfunctions may not be considered handicapped in that domain until they are required to read.

Figure 3 (page 45) shows the percentages of students who were reported to have specific handicapping conditions by year of birth. With the exception only of specific learning disability and emotional/behavioral problems, increased rates for the specific handicapping conditions were noted for the youngest age groups. Hearing-impaired children with additional disabilities may be diagnosed or perhaps require services earlier than children without additional conditions. Similarly, all specific handicapping conditions with the exception of heart disorders and learning disabilities showed increases at the oldest age groups (19 years or older). This no doubt reflects the fact that multi-handicapped individuals are liable to continue to require significant special education and support services after the time most hearing-impaired youth have left or graduated from special education programs at the secondary level.

Beyond the age effects noted for the oldest and youngest groups, there are three

Two figures in Chapter 3 were inadvertently transposed:

Figure 3 on p. 45 should be Figure 2 as described on pp. 42-43
Figure 2 on p. 42 should be Figure 3 as described on pp. 43-44

conditions (e.g., heart disorders and visual abnormalities) associated with maternal rubella-caused hearing loss.

A second pattern obtains for mental retardation and emotional/behavioral problems. For these two categories there can be noted a steady increase of the percentage with additional handicaps by age group. For mental retardation, the pattern may be observed beyond age four (birth year 1977). For emotional/behavioral problems, the pattern may be observed beginning in the youngest age groups. However, it is not clear from these data whether the relatively high percentages of emotional/behavioral problems in 1964 and 1965 were related to age or to cohort effects, since it has been observed that students with maternal rubella etiologies are more likely to be reported to have such disabilities (Trybus et al., 1980).

Finally, the percentage of children reported to have specific learning disabilities (including perceptual/motor disorders) showed a distinct age-related pattern: There was a systematic increase in the percentage of students diagnosed as having these disorders through ages 10 and 11 and then an equally systematic decline after age 11. This pattern appears to be an age-based phenomenon, since a similar pattern was found on the Annual Survey for 1971–72 (Gentile & McCarthy, 1973, p. 26). Again, the reasons for the changes in rates of learning disabilities by age are open to speculation. While it is straightforward enough to attribute the age rate increases to diagnoses or identification on the basis of changing educational demands, it is harder to speculate as to the cause of the decline by age. Whether the cause for the declining rates for the older groups is remediation of the problem, students' "outgrowing" the condition, or changing diagnoses is beyond the power of these data to explain.

Student Characteristics

In this section, three student characteristics are described in relation to handicapping condition. Distributions of *sex, degree of hearing loss,* and *ethnic background* are compared for the groups of students with and without specific additional handicapping conditions.

Table 4 shows the percentage distribution by sex for the groups of students with and without additional handicaps. The overall results are clear. Hearing-impaired students

Table 4. Distribution of Additional Handicapping Condition(s) by Sex

Sex	No Additional Handicapping Condition		One or More Additional Handicapping Conditions	
	Number	%	Number	%
Male	18,474	51.7	9,191	58.3
Female	17,237	48.3	6,569	41.7
TOTAL[a]	35,711	100.0	15,760	100.0

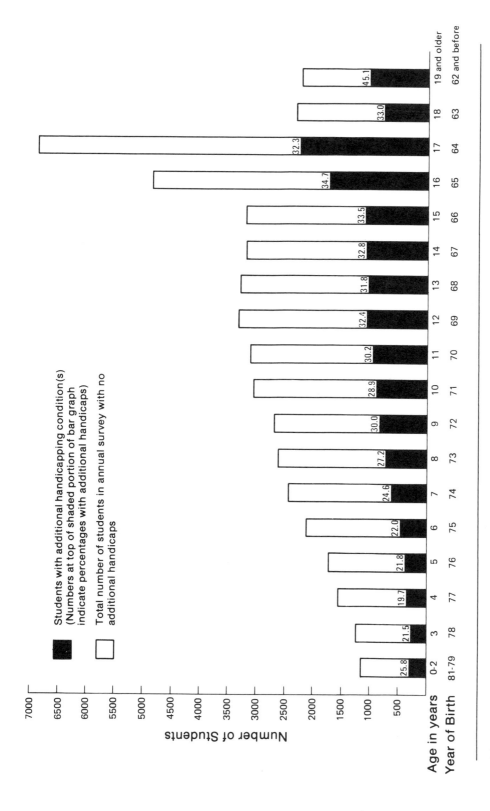

Figure 3. Percentage of hearing-impaired students with specific additional handicapping condition(s). Unpublished data from the Annual Survey of Hearing-Impaired Children and Youth, 1981-82. Copyright 1983 by Gallaudet College Center for Assessment and Demographic Studies. Used by permission.

with at least one additional disability were more likely to be male than students without additional disabilities. A slight plurality of the group without additional handicaps was male, 51.7 percent, whereas 58.3 percent of the additionally handicapped group were male. The exact percentage of males varied considerably (Table 5). The overall finding of male predominance is consistent for each handicapping condition except heart disorders. As noted above, heart disorders are associated largely with an etiology of maternal rubella; this etiology has affected a higher percentage of females than have most other causes of hearing loss (Trybus et al., 1980).

Table 6. Degree of Hearing Loss and Additional Handicapping Condition(s)

Degree of Hearing Loss (Hearing Threshold)	No Additional Handicapping Condition		One or more Additional Handicapping Conditions	
	Number	%	Number	%
Less-than-severe (70 dB, ISO, or below)	11,364	31.8	5,959	38.0
Severe (71-90 dB, ISO)	7,764	21.7	3,226	20.6
Profound (91 dB, ISO, or above)	16,607	46.5	6,503	41.5
TOTAL[a]	35,735	100.0	15,688	100.1

Note. Unpublished data from the Annual Survey of Hearing-Impaired Children and Youth, 1981-82. Copyright 1983 by Gallaudet College Center for Assessment and Demographic Studies. Used by permission.

[a]Information on degree of hearing loss is missing for 539 or 1.0 percent of the 51,962 students about whom information was reported regarding additional handicapping condition(s) or lack thereof.

Group differences also were found between hearing-impaired students with and those without additional handicaps on the basis of degree of hearing loss. As shown in Table 6, the general finding was that individuals with additional handicaps are more likely than the others to have less-than-severe hearing losses (38.0 percent vs. 31.8 percent, respectively). Conversely, those with additional handicaps are less likely than the others to have profound losses (41.5 percent vs. 46.5 percent, respectively). Actually, the pattern is somewhat more complicated when the distributions are broken down for specific handicapping conditions. Table 7 displays this information. The groups with physical conditions were similar to the group without additional handicaps. The distributions that differed were those for the groups of students diagnosed as learning disabled or mentally retarded. For these groups, 47.4 percent and 43.3 percent of the students, respectively, had less-than-severe hearing losses (unaided pure tone hearing thresholds of <70 dB, ANSI, in the better ear across the speech range).

A Demographic Perspective   47

Table 5. Percentage Distribution of Selected Additional Handicapping Conditions by Sex

Sex	Physical Conditions					Cognitive/Intellectual Conditions		
	Legal blindness	Brain damage	Orthopedic	Cerebral palsy	Heart disorder	Mental retardation	Emotional/ behavioral problem	Learning disability
Male	54.2	60.0	53.4	55.9	48.0	55.	69.2	63.7
Female	45.8	40.0	46.6	44.1	52.0	44.4	30.8	36.3
	100.0	100.0	100.0	100.0	100.0	100.0	100.0	100.0

Table 7. Percentage Distribution of Selected Additional Handicapping Conditions by Hearing Loss

Degree of Hearing Loss (Hearing Threshold)	Physical Conditions					Cognitive/Intellectual Conditions		
	Legal blindness	Brain damage	Orthopedic	Cerebral palsy	Heart disorder	Mental Retardation	Emotional/ behavioral problem	Learning disability
Less-than-severe (70 dB, ISO, or below)	28.6	35.6	34.0	28.5	27.1	43.3	28.7	47.4
Severe (71-90 dB, ISO)	23.2	20.9	20.8	25.9	24.5	18.9	22.4	18.0
Profound (91 dB, ISO or above)	48.2	43.5	45.2	45.6	48.4	37.9	48.9	34.6
	100.0	100.0	100.0	100.0	100.0	100.1	100.0	100.0

Note. Both tables based on unpublished data from the Annual Survey of Hearing-Impaired Children and Youth, 1981-82. Copyright 1983 by Gallaudet College Center for Assessment and Demographic Studies. Used by permission.

Ethnic background is also related to additional handicapping condition, as summarized in Tables 8 and 9. A breakdown for each ethnic group shows that, in comparison with other students, Black students are more likely to have one or more additional disabilities (Table 8). Table 9 shows the ethnic distribution for each handicapping condition. The mental retardation category is particularly noteworthy; nearly 30 percent of the students reported to be mentally retarded were Black, a percentage much higher than the overall percentage of Black students in the population.

Table 8. Ethnic Background and Additional Handicapping Condition(s)

Ethnic Status[a]	Total	%	No Additional Handicapping Condition		One or More Additional Handicapping Conditions	
			Number	%	Number	%
White	35,177	100.0	24,870	70.7	10,307	29.3
Black	8,839	100.0	5,481	62.0	3,358	38.0
Hispanic	5,014	100.0	3,486	69.5	1,528	30.5
Other	1,433	100.0	1,032	72.0	401	28.0
Multi-ethnic	352	100.0	234	66.5	118	33.5
All ethnic groups	50,815	100.0	35,103	69.1	15,712	30.9

Note. Unpublished data from the Annual Survey of Hearing-Impaired Children and Youth, 1981-82. Copyright 1983 by Gallaudet College Center for Assessment and Demographic Studies. Used by permission.

[a]Information on ethnic background is missing for 1,147 or 2.2 percent of the 51,962 students about whom information was reported regarding additional handicapping condition(s) or lack thereof.

Educational Services

The nature of instruction received by hearing-impaired students varied markedly according to whether students were reported to have additional handicapping conditions. Table 10 (page 50) gives an overview from the 1981–82 Annual Survey of the types of academic instruction being received by hearing-impaired students. Slightly more than half, 52.4 percent, received classroom instruction in special education settings only. The sites of these services varied considerably, ranging from residential or day schools for the deaf to special education classes in local public schools. Another 38.9 percent were reported to be receiving a mixture of special education services and regular education in settings with hearing students. A much smaller group (6.4 percent of the total) were reported to be receiving regular academic instruction services only. (A majority of these students did, however, receive such support services as notetaking, tutoring, interpreting, and speech/hearing therapy in relation to their hearing impairment. See Karchmer, 1983.)

Table 9. Percentage Distribution of Selected Additional Handicapping Conditions by Ethnic Background

Ethnic Background	Total Sample	Physical Conditions					Cognitive/Intellectual Conditions		
		Legal blindness	Brain damage	Orthopedic	Cerebral palsy	Heart disorder	Mental retardation	Emotional/ behavioral problem	Learning disability
White	69.2	65.5	70.1	69.5	73.2	65.3	59.2	68.3	67.3
Black	17.4	23.7	19.5	19.3	17.5	20.9	29.8	19.4	17.9
Hispanic	9.9	8.7	8.7	8.3	6.6	10.9	8.3	8.9	11.4
Other	2.8	1.3	1.2	2.2	2.2	1.4	2.2	2.3	2.7
Multi-ethnic	0.7	0.8	0.5	0.7	0.4	1.5	0.5	1.1	0.6
	100.0	100.0	100.0	100.0	99.9	100.0	100.0	100.0	99.9

Note. Unpublished data from the Annual Survey of Hearing-Impaired Children and Youth, 1981-82. Copyright 1983 by Gallaudet College Center for Assessment and Demographic Studies. Used by permission.

Table 10. Type of Classroom Instruction Received by Hearing-Impaired Students

Type of Instruction	Number of Students	Percentage of Total
Special education only	22,518	52.4
Both regular and special education	16,713	38.9
Regular education only	2,761	6.4
Neither regular nor special education	954	2.2
TOTAL	42,946[a]	99.9

Note. Unpublished data from the Annual Survey of Hearing-Impaired Children and Youth, 1981-82. Copyright 1983 by Gallaudet College Center for Assessment and Demographic Studies. Used by permission.

[a]Complete information on type of instructional setting was not reported for 11,828 students or 21.6 percent of the 54,774 students.

The type of special education settings in which hearing-impaired students receive services is summarized in Table 11. It is of great interest to observe that more than 14 percent of the hearing-impaired students in special education (i.e., the sum of categories 2 and 5 in the table) were receiving at least part of their academic instruction in situations designed for multihandicapped hearing-impaired students.

Table 11. Special Education Settings for Hearing-Impaired Students

Setting Designed for or with:	Number of Students[a]	Percentage of Total
Hearing-impaired students (not multihandicapped)	27,444	73.9
Multihandicapped hearing-impaired students	3,317	8.9
Students with various handicaps (not all of whom are hearing-impaired)	3,158	8.5
Home instruction	305	0.8
Part-Time in each of the categories 1 and 2	2,082	5.6
All other combinations of the above categories	838	2.3

Note. Unpublished data from the Annual Survey of Hearing-Impaired Children and Youth, 1981-82. Copyright 1983 by Gallaudet College Center for Assessment and Demographic Studies. Used by permission.

[a]A specific setting was not reported for 2,583 or 6.5 percent of the 39,727 students who were reported to be receiving special education services.

Tables 12A and 12B show, by type of instructional placement, the percentage distributions according to general category of disability. In general, the data demonstrate clearly that having a disability in addition to hearing loss decreases the likelihood that a student will be receiving any academic instruction outside of a special education setting. Few students with both physical and cognitive/intellectual disabilities were integrated into regular classroom instructional settings with hearing students.

Table 12A. Percentage Distribution of Instructional Placement for Hearing-Impaired Students in Four Handicapping Categories

Type of Classroom Instruction	Additional Handicapping Category			
	No additional handicapping conditions	Physical conditions	Cognitive/ intellectual conditions	Both physical and cognitive/ intellectual conditions
Special education only	49.2	59.5	53.4	69.8
Both special education and regular education	40.6	34.0	41.3	27.1
Regular education only	8.0	4.2	3.4	0.7
Neither	2.2	2.3	1.9	2.4
	100.0	100.0	100.0	100.0

Note. Unpublished data from the Annual Survey of Hearing-Impaired Children and Youth, 1981-82. Copyright 1983 by Gallaudet College Center for Assessment and Demographic Studies. Used by permission.

Table 12B. Percentage Distribution of Handicapping Category for Hearing-Impaired Students in Four Instructional Placements

Handicapping Category	Instructional Placement			
	Special education only	Both regular and special education	Regular education only	Neither
No additional handicapping conditions	65.5	71.7	85.3	70.7
Physical conditions only	11.1	8.5	6.3	10.1
Cognitive/intellectual conditions only	15.2	15.7	7.8	12.6
Both physical and cognitive/intellectual conditions	8.1	4.2	0.6	6.6
	100.0	100.1	100.0	100.0

Note. Unpublished data from the Annual Survey of Hearing-Impaired Children and Youth, 1981-82. Copyright 1983 by Gallaudet College Center for Assessment and Demographic Studies. Used by permission.

Etiology

Perhaps the strongest influence on whether a hearing-impaired child has an additional disability is the nature of the etiology. Table 13 lists the probable causes of hearing loss and the percentage of cases in which each is reported. Unfortunately, the data from the Annual Survey on probable cause of hearing loss need to be interpreted with some caution. For 38.5 percent of the students, the cause of hearing loss could not be determined or was not available in the student's records. For another 3.8 percent of the cases, no information on etiology was reported. Another problem was that several of the listed probable causes are factors that have diverse origins. Heredity, trauma after birth, and complications of pregnancy are examples.

It should be mentioned that the hearing-impaired special education population consists primarily of individuals who have lost their hearing at birth or early in life.

Table 13. Probable Causes of Hearing Loss of Hearing-Impaired Students

Probable Cause	Number[a]	Percentage of Total
Onset at birth		
Maternal rubella	9,135	17.3
Trauma at birth	1,286	2.4
Heredity	6,148	11.7
Prematurity	2,125	4.0
Rh incompatibility	862	1.6
Other complications of pregnancy	1,737	3.3
Onset after birth		
Meningitis	3,942	7.5
High fever	1,667	3.2
Mumps	142	0.3
Infection	1,460	2.8
Measles	455	0.9
Otitis media	1,392	2.6
Trauma	430	0.8
Other	4,207	8.0
Cause cannot be determined or data not available	20,302	38.5

Note. Unpublished data from the Annual Survey of Hearing-Impaired Children and Youth, 1981-82. Copyright 1983 by Gallaudet College Center for Assessment and Demographic Studies. Used by permission.

[a]Information on etiology was missing for 2,065 students or 3.8 percent of the 54,774 students. More than one cause was given for 4.1 percent of the 52,709 students for whom information was reported.

More than 60 percent of the students for whom this information was reported to the Annual Survey were said to have an onset of hearing loss at birth; more than 90 percent were reported to have lost their hearing before the age of three, that is, prelingually.

Despite the caution needed in examining the data on cause, several tentative observations can be made. Table 14 (page 54) shows for each reported cause the percentage distributions by type of additional handicapping condition. As a group, students with hereditary causes of hearing loss were less likely to have additional disabilities than students whose hearing losses arose from other etiologies. Whereas 30.6 percent of the entire sample had at least one additional handicapping condition, this was true for less than 19 percent of the students with deafness due to hereditary causes. Causes with onsets at birth (with the exception of hereditary causes) tended to be associated with higher rates of physical handicapping conditions than causes with onsets after birth.

Co-occurrence of Disabilities

As described previously, more than 30 percent of the hearing-impaired students reported to the Annual Survey were reported to have additional disabilities. Nearly one-third of this group (9.6 percent of the total sample) were reported to have at least two disabilities in addition to deafness. Multiple additional handicaps, when present, are not likely to be random combinations of conditions. Table 15 (page 55) shows for each specific handicapping condition the percentage of cases in which the condition was reported alone or in combination with other disabling conditions. The first conclusion to be drawn from this table is that there is a great deal of variation in the extent to which specific disabilities are found alone. In general, specific learning disabilities and emotional/behavioral problems were the only conditions more likely than not to be reported alone. A student reported to have any of the other specific conditions also usually had another handicapping condition. Legal blindness, brain damage, epilepsy, and orthopedic disorders were particularly extreme examples. Hearing-impaired students with these conditions also were reported to have other disabilities more than two-thirds of the time.

Only one additional handicapping condition, learning disability, was relatively independent of the other conditions. That is to say, the distribution of additional handicapping conditions was similar to the overall distribution (Table 2, page 41). Even so, students diagnosed as learning disabled were more likely to have emotional/behavioral problems. Those with brain damage and epilepsy also tended to have increased occurrence of learning disability.

In general, the most often reported concomitant of a specific condition was mental retardation. This was true for each of the specific additional handicapping conditions other than learning disability. In fact, for several of the additional handicapping conditions (legal blindness, brain damage, epilepsy, and orthopedic disorders), the number of students with mental retardation reported outnumbered those with the condition alone.

Table 14. Percentage Distribution of Additional Handicapping Condition(s) by Probable Cause of Hearing Loss

Handicapping Category[a]	Onset at Birth						Onset after Birth								
	Maternal rubella	Trauma at birth	Heredity	Prematurity	Rh incompatibility	Other complications of pregnancy	Meningitis	High fever	Mumps	Infection	Measles	Otitis media	Trauma	Other	Cause cannot be determined or data not available
No additional handicapping condition	60.9	50.0	81.4	55.2	63.7	54.7	74.1	75.2	70.2	69.5	75.5	59.1	60.7	59.9	73.8
One or more physical conditions	15.4	18.9	6.1	18.5	17.3	16.7	8.3	6.6	8.2	5.0	8.0	4.7	7.7	14.7	6.6
One or more cognitive/intellectual conditions	13.4	17.1	10.0	15.6	10.0	16.3	12.9	14.2	16.4	21.2	13.0	31.3	19.2	14.8	15.4
Both physical and cognitive/intellectual conditions	10.3	14.0	2.6	10.7	9.0	12.3	4.8	4.0	5.2	4.3	3.4	4.8	12.4	10.6	4.1
	100.0	100.0	100.1	100.0	100.0	100.0	100.1	100.0	100.0	100.0	99.9	99.9	100.0	100.0	99.9
Percent of students with no information provided regarding probable cause of or lack of additional handicap(s):	(3.4)	(3.0)	(3.4)	(3.8)	(2.2)	(5.2)	(5.0)	(5.1)	(5.6)	(4.8)	(4.0)	(3.0)	(6.5)	(4.6)	(4.5)

Note. Unpublished data from the Annual Survey of Hearing-Impaired Children and Youth, 1981-82. Copyright 1983 by Gallaudet College Center for Assessment and Demographic Studies. Used by permission.

[a]See Table 3 for applicable number for each category.

Table 15. Percentage of Hearing-Impaired Students for Whom Specific Additional Handicapping Condition(s) Were Reported Alone or in Combination with Another Condition

Condition(s) Reported	Physical Conditions							Cognitive/Intellectual Conditions		
	Legal blindness	Uncorrected visual problem	Brain damage	Epilepsy	Orthopedic	Cerebral palsy	Heart disorder	Mental retardation	Emotional/ behavioral problem	Specific learning disability
Alone	26.7	44.4	20.5	23.6	31.3	41.7	33.0	44.2	50.2	66.5
In combination with:										
Legal blindness	----	8.0	14.2	11.3	9.0	4.5	12.6	11.8	4.6	1.1
Uncorrected visual problem (but not legally blind)	1.9	----	18.0	15.6	15.3	12.6	23.3	11.8	8.2	5.2
Brain damage or injury	17.0	9.1	----	22.0	13.8	10.1	7.9	11.1	8.5	4.6
Epilepsy	7.5	4.4	12.3	----	8.2	7.6	3.1	6.3	3.2	2.6
Orthopedic	12.6	9.1	16.1	17.2	----	12.6	10.3	10.2	3.5	4.0
Cerebral palsy	7.4	8.7	13.8	18.6	14.7	----	5.9	10.6	3.6	3.7
Heart disorder	15.1	11.8	7.9	5.6	8.9	4.3	----	7.0	3.8	2.0
Other health impaired	8.2	10.1	12.5	12.5	13.9	6.1	15.5	8.6	5.8	5.2
Mental retardation	53.3	22.7	42.0	43.1	33.2	29.4	26.3	----	20.0	6.8
Emotional/behavioral problem	15.1	11.4	23.3	15.8	8.1	7.3	10.3	14.4	----	13.6
Specific learning disability	4.5	8.9	15.6	16.0	11.5	9.1	6.6	6.1	16.7	----
Other	2.5	1.8	3.2	3.1	2.4	2.0	3.1	1.8	2.8	3.2
Total number of students with additional handicapping condition(s)	960	2,264	1,149	640	1,343	1,570	1,150	4,353	3,157	3,874

Note. Columns will total more than 100 percent because the number of conditions exceeds the number of students. Unpublished data from the Annual Survey of Hearing-Impaired Children and Youth, 1981-82. Copyright 1983 by Gallaudet College Center for Assessment and Demographic Studies. Used by permission.

Summary

As of spring 1982, nearly one-third of all hearing-impaired students in special education had additional disabilities that significantly affected the educational process. The specific conditions varied widely, ranging from physical or health disabilities to impairments of learning, cognitive, or intellectual function. Almost 10 percent of the group had at least two additional handicaps in combination. Cognitive and intellectual disabilities were more frequently reported than physical conditions. The percentage of students with additional handicaps increased with age, though different patterns were found for specific conditions. Blacks were more likely than nonblacks to have additional handicaps; this was particularly the case for mental retardation. Degree of hearing loss and sex also showed distinct relationships to additional handicapping condition. Multi-handicapped hearing-impaired students were less likely than students without additional handicaps to be integrated with hearing students for their academic instruction. Finally, the etiology of hearing loss was shown to be related strongly to the presence of reported additional handicaps.*

References

Gentile, A., & McCarthy, B. (1973). *Additional handicapping conditions among hearing-impaired students, United States: 1971–1972* (Series D, Number 14). Washington, DC: Gallaudet College, Office of Demographic Studies.

Karchmer, M. A. (1983). Hearing-impaired students and their education: Population perspectives. In W. Northcott (Ed.), *Introduction to oral interpreting: Principles and practices.* Baltimore: University Park Press.

Karchmer, M. A., Petersen, L. M., Allen, T. E., & Osborn, T. I. (1981). *Highlights of the Canadian survey of hearing impaired children and youth, spring, 1979* (Series R, Number 8). Washington, DC: Gallaudet College, Office of Demographic Studies.

Trybus, R. J., Karchmer, M. A., Kerstetter, P. P., & Hicks, W. (1980). The demographics of deafness resulting from maternal rubella. *American Annals of the Deaf, 125,* 977–984.

U.S. Department of Education. (1983). *Fifth annual report to Congress on the implementation of Public Law 94-142: The Education for All Handicapped Children Act.* Washington, DC: Author.

---

*The author gratefully acknowledges the assistance of staff members at the Center for Assessment and Demographic Studies: Susan Jablonski carried out many of the computer analyses; Sue Hotto prepared the manuscript for publication; Gail Ries, Dorothea Bateman, and Henry Young helped prepare the tables and figures.

Part II

On Systems, Teams, and Families

Chapter 4

Beyond Service Delivery: Enabling Systems

Raymond J. Trybus

This chapter will pay attention to several general or *systems* issues in providing services for hearing-impaired developmentally disabled individuals.

- Points of entry into the service system;
- Interdisciplinarity as a way of life; and
- A critique of service systems in general as a useful counterpoint to more common professional themes.

Points of Entry into the Service System

It is in the nature of clinical work for a particular professional worker to pay primary attention to the needs of, and the services to be provided to, a particular client. While the quality and effectiveness of services ultimately depend upon these many client-provider contacts, such contacts occur as points or moments in an overall system embedded in society at large. Within this system, disabled individuals or their families recognize the existence of an anomalous situation; seek clarification in understanding the nature of the problem; and seek assistance in obtaining treatment, support, and remediation. Experience has made it increasingly clear that the potential benefits of client-practitioner contacts can be realized effectively only by coordinating these service-seeking and service delivery systems in an interactive mode.

Much has been written about service delivery systems in the human services fields; much less attention has been paid to the opposite side of the coin, namely, the service-seeking systems. Therefore, this chapter will address service delivery issues largely from the point of the client's service-seeking system rather than from the point of view of the professional service delivery system. Many of our professional pronouncements and writings use the term *client-centered,* reflecting a completely appropriate direction of professional attention to the needs and desires of the client rather than of the practitioner. However, the very notion of the service *delivery* system focuses professional attention on the professionals and their issues, rather than on the intended clients or service recipients and their needs, preferences, and behaviors.

The nature of service provision for hearing-impaired developmentally disabled people is, if anything, more complex than many other human service delivery systems, because of the interactive effects of the individual's disabilities and the limited knowledge and technology available for addressing those situations. As a result, service provision to these individuals must take account of both interagency issues and interdisciplinary issues within a particular agency.

An exceptionally instructive approach to assessment of this situation in a given locality may also be extremely simple in concept. The author was invited to participate in a statewide conference for providers of service to another special population group. In that setting, he had the advantage of having both professional knowledge of the typical needs of the client group and of the services usually provided to that group, as well as the added benefit of complete naivete about the specifics of the agency structure and service delivery system in that state. In the course of the day's discussions, the local participants continually referred to a series of personal names and agency acronyms which were well known to them but were completely unfamiliar to the author as an out-of-state visitor. An impromptu role play then developed, in which I was the legal guardian of a 19-year-old deaf boy with a variety of obvious but poorly understood secondary disabilities. The discussion group participants agreed that the hypothetical client would be eligible for continued special education services (until age 22), vocational rehabilitation services, developmental disability services, welfare and income supplement assistance, food stamps, housing assistance, and the like.

We then began to imagine the possible entry points of the client's guardians to the public service system. Such guardians, lacking extensive experience with public social service agencies, might approach a private medical or audiological practitioner, a hospital or speech and hearing clinic, the state welfare agency, city hall, the governor's office, the offices of state legislators or federal congressional representatives, or yet other sources. They were probably less likely to contact the educational system, assuming that education had nothing to offer for a person 18 or older. Similarly, they were not likely to contact the developmental disabilities or vocational rehabilitation service, since the very existence of these services is not well known to the general public. A counseling or mental health service for deaf people might also be a possible entry point, depending on the availability of their listings in the telephone book.

The idea of telephone contact then led to a discussion of how the various agencies that might be called upon are listed in public sources, notably the telephone book. Under what headings might the hypothetical legal guardians look in the telephone book, and what would they find under those headings? Since the client is deaf, one might look under the heading "deaf." Similarly, a few moments of thought might lead one to such headings as "handicapped," "disabled," "jobs" or "employment services" (because the guardians' perspective is that the boy primarily needs a job), or maybe "speech and hearing." An examination of the local telephone books, both the white and yellow pages, including the recently developed index to the yellow pages, proved extremely disappointing when these headings were sought.

No listings existed under "deaf," "handicapped," "disabled," or "jobs." The "speech and hearing" listing, carried as "speech and hearing therapy," contained only a cross-reference to "audiologist." Under this heading, only three agencies and two individual practitioners were listed, with no description of services except for hearing aid dispensing and hearing tests. "Employment services" seemed a potentially more fruitful title, with several subheadings and 10 pages of listings, but not a single listing made any mention of disability or handicap. Only two listings were governmental or public service in nature: the U.S. military recruiting office and the state employment service, neither of which made any mention of disability, handicap, or any other suggestion that they might be of help to the client in question. There can be little doubt that the service-seeking efforts of potential clients are significantly hampered and delayed by this lack of availability of the most elementary sort of information.

The discussion then turned to possible responses to such a client/guardian pair, assuming that they somehow were able to locate and approach the offices of the various service agencies mentioned earlier. What services would each agency describe itself as being able to offer to this client? What referrals to or information about other service agencies would the agency in question have and convey to this client and the guardian? As we worked through these issues, it became increasingly clear to all present that this was a significant aspect of access to the service system which had hardly been examined. What emerged clearly from the hour's exercise with the agency representatives described above was that, despite the professionals' view that the state had a well-planned and well-integrated service delivery system, this system might not be at all apparent or easily accessible to the service-seeking consumer, client representative, or guardian.

This should be a major concern for any agency providing services to hearing-impaired developmentally disabled individuals. While we certainly must think in terms of service delivery systems and, through contact with other professionals and service agencies, develop an appropriate and well-integrated service delivery system, the mere existence of such a system is by no means adequate to meet the needs of clients. Those developing programs and planning services must pay equal, and perhaps greater, attention to the service-seeking system, attempting to understand and delineate its possible variations, quirks, and inconsistencies. The goal is to maximize the possibility that the service-seeking activities of potential clients will, quickly and expeditiously, mesh with the service delivery system that has been developed in a given locality.

This consideration of the service-seeking system will necessarily lead to significant attention to the marketing aspects of human services. This in turn means attention to a wide variety of essentially mundane matters. While the term *marketing* may have an unfamiliar ring in the nonprofit context, the concept is rapidly gaining acceptance and recognition of its value in other nonprofit settings (Keller, 1983). This will probably include such procedures as

- Making information about services for hearing-impaired developmentally disabled persons available in printed and therefore distributable form (such as pamphlets and brochures).

- Identifying a wide variety of professional individuals and service agencies as potential recipients of such printed information, not because they are necessarily part of the service *delivery* network, but because they are likely components of the service-*seeking* network.

- Giving careful attention to the service agencies' listings in the telephone book, with special attention to the precise way in which listings appear in the white pages, in the yellow pages, and in the cross references in the yellow pages index. Agencies will almost certainly find that their current listings are quite inadequate from a service-seeking point of view and will probably decide to devote increased funds to telephone book listings and cross listings. This will be money exceedingly well spent.

- Using the contact networks of agency staff and board members to obtain occasional but regular coverage in local print and broadcast media. This informs the general public about both the existence of individuals with combined hearing impairment and developmental disabilities as well as the availability of professional services for such individuals.

- Developing active liaisons with local schools, churches, service clubs (Rotary, Lions, etc.) as vehicles for further dissemination of information both on people with impaired hearing and developmental disabilities and on services. Such liaison may involve membership and/or formal presentations by agency staff and board members.

- Encouraging and supporting staff to participate in local professional organizations, particularly those which include a broad range of service providers in the community (local medical and psychological societies, local social work and mental health associations, etc.). In this way, the existence of services and the identities of the service providers become known to the local professional community, which includes potential referral sources.

Because population characteristics vary from place to place, and because different groups of individuals would go about service seeking in different ways, this process can be usefully begun by conducting an interview poll of perhaps 50 to 75 local residents. The interviewer would present the hypothetical client problem and ask where the residents would turn for information. The results of this simple survey can then be used to guide the nature and extent of information dissemination, telephone book listings, and the like. The key issue throughout this process is that of keeping an eye on the needs of the client population; that is, focusing not only on the substantive kinds of information or services required, but also on the ways in which clients are likely to seek services. In our society, the provision of professional service is a respected and valued function. Therefore, one must expect to have to earn the right to serve. This can be done, in part, by continually seeking expressions of preference, need, and desire from our intended clients and their families, and trying as much as circumstances will permit to be responsive to those indications of need or desire.

Interdisciplinarity as a Way of Life

One of the major challenges facing humanity, including human service professionals, is that of simply knowing about, and then making use of, knowledge that already exists. Though many questions remain and there is much intellectual and investigative work to be done, a great amount of knowledge already exists in every human service field. One of the major tasks facing professionals, especially those of us who work in interdisciplinary situations, is that of simply learning something about the kinds of information already available in disciplines represented on the staff, or which might be so represented in an ideally staffed service agency.

Each of us receives basic professional training in some discipline. Each field or discipline takes care to see that its newest members are thoroughly immersed in the facts and myths, the approaches and problems that make the field distinctive. There is never enough time in the graduate curriculum to include all that the faculty wishes were there, much less to devote more than passing attention to what other, even closely related, fields have to offer. Each of us thus begins professional practice blessed with a vast and varied ignorance of most of what lies beyond the purview of our particular field.

At the same time, adequate provision for hearing-impaired developmentally disabled people depends upon detailed assessment and program design conducted from a wide variety of viewpoints: anatomy; functional residual auditory capacity; communication, speech, and language skill development in a variety of modes; educational and academic progress; psychological status; mobility; and so on. In one way or another, each member of the interactive interdisciplinary team must become acquainted with at least the basics of the other team members' work, including the concepts and vocabulary, the perspective and approach, typical issues or problems, and the essential areas of current knowledge and new development in each field.

This is one overall purpose for the design of this book—to identify the major points of view that might be brought to bear on the complexity of a particular hearing-impaired developmentally disabled client. In addition, an interdisciplinary team needs to develop this awareness in its members, periodically refreshing and expanding such consciousness and paying special attention to the enlightenment of newly appointed members of the team. Why is this so critical? There are many reasons.

First, as Matkin discusses (Chapter 5), the primary value of the interactive interdisciplinary team lies in the multifaceted, composite approach to assessment and individualized program design. Constructing an overall view of a particular person's situation and recommending an integrated program design are the primary tasks of such teams. Actual provision of the recommended services, however, is generally a matter for individual client-practitioner contact. It may be the psychologist, or the activity therapist, or the special educator, who actually sits in the consulting room with the client and/or the client's family. Each such professional must be in a position to provide basic information and advice to the client/ parent at an appropriate time, i.e., when it is asked for or when the individual service plan calls for a next step.

Does the psychologist know what special education approach is used in school X by comparison with school Y? Can the activity therapist help with the problem of locating a more functional chair for a mobility-limited individual? One can almost guarantee that most such questions about services and resources will require knowledge about fields other than one's own. For this reason, each member of the interactive interdisciplinary team must attempt to build bridges with the "service-seeking system" so that, no matter at what point the service seeker enters the service delivery system, there is a high likelihood that the needed information can be made available.

Particularly important are such programs as the rehabilitation research and training centers and the rehabilitation engineering centers at various universities supported by the National Institute of Handicapped Research. These programs, especially the engineering centers (listed in Chapter 20), are established to work in very pragmatic ways to improve the everyday comfort and effectiveness of each disabled individual. These facilities are one example of a significant resource that can provide useful support to hearing-impaired developmentally disabled individuals but are not likely to be well known to those working with such clients.

A major responsibility of professional workers and managers in programs for hearing-impaired developmentally disabled individuals is to develop comprehensive information about the existence and availability of the widest possible set of such resources, whether located in the immediate vicinity or not. While resources for the provision of direct services generally need to be in the immediate geographical area to be of benefit to particular clients, information sources can be and often are located throughout the U.S. A wise program administrator will invest in the necessary telephone service to allow frequent and in-depth contact with major information sources that may be located at some distance from the service agency. Over the course of time, the program director will develop relationships with key individuals in various and widely geographically dispersed service agencies. Given simple demographics, one can reasonably expect to find a wide range of knowledge and skills with respect to elementary education of able-bodied children even in relatively small municipalities. However, with such a small and widely dispersed population as the hearing-impaired developmentally disabled, it is unrealistic to expect that all the necessary information and services will be available in anything smaller than a major region of the country; in any particular situation, the needed information or service may exist only in other regions of the country.

Once the program head has developed a network of contacts and acquaintances, professional time and energy will be well spent on behalf of clients by keeping abreast of the work of those individuals and conferring with them from time to time, in person, by telephone, by teleconference, or perhaps by means of one of the newer computer conferencing networks such as SpecialNet. In this way, the program administrator and other senior professionals will be exercising the most valuable sort of leadership: improving direct client service at the same time that they are improving the knowledge, skills, and abilities of the program staff. This sort of investment in program staff can almost be guaranteed to pay off handsomely, both by improving the morale and effectiveness of the professional staff and by facilitating the provision of the best available professional service and pragmatic information to clients and their families.

Interdisciplinarity, then, means far more than simply working in physical proximity to individuals whose background involves training in disciplines other than one's own. (See Chapter 5 for further description of the interactive interdisciplinary team concept.) The meaning of the interactive interdisciplinary team is that all members of the team, under the direction of the program head and other senior professionals, (1) actively learn from each other about their respective bodies of knowledge and information of potential value to clients and then (2) establish continuing networks of contact and communication, not only within the local service agency, but throughout the region and the nation. All service professionals, if they are worth their salt, are keenly aware of the limits of their knowledge and skill; they are easily debilitated by feeling isolated from fellow professionals and the additional knowledge and insights they may have to offer. Being required to provide services to individuals with very complex disabilities and sets of needs can be an impossible task if the service professional does not have adequate support networks of the sort described here. Some attention has been paid in the professional literature to the issue of interpersonal, emotional, and social support networks among service professionals (Crowell, 1982). This is certainly necessary and desirable. However, there is an equally pressing need for interactive communication networks with other professional individuals in one's own and other disciplines. This can aid in broadening one's sights and increasing one's skills and abilities, drawing upon the best available knowledge in order to provide the best possible service.

A Sobering Critique

One of our particular limitations as service professionals is that, since our work is so clearly aimed at improving the lot of individuals with multiple problems and their families, we too easily identify our professional exertions with unmitigated virtue, certainly in intention if not entirely in effect. A very sobering critique of the drawbacks of professionalism is provided by Illich in his various writings, but perhaps most clearly in *Toward a History of Needs*.* The following remarks draw heavily upon Illich's work, even where specific reference or quotation is not indicated.

Illich's first chapter, entitled "Useful Unemployment and Its Professional Enemies," provides a scathing critique of the ways in which various professional groups have defined the population, or some sector of it, as having a particular need which has hitherto been unidentified, then setting forth its own more or less exclusive prerogative to provide services designed to meet that new need. The underlying concept in this chapter as well as in more of Illich's work is the distinction between what he terms "use values" and "commodity values." A *use value* arises in the situation in which an individual develops a wish, preference, or need, such as the need to fix a broken bicycle, which is satisfied by a self-initiated and more or less self-directed activity. In the case of the broken bicycle, the individual may tinker with the bicycle in hands-on fashion, trying to understand how it operates and, in the process, learning how to do the necessary repair. He or she then satisfies the felt need through actually repairing the bicycle. A *commodity value*, by contrast, arises typically in a situation in which one is informed by an expert that one has a particular need, a need that one has not previously felt or been aware of. Thus, for example, the individual may be told that his or her automobile needs a tune-up, though it seems to be running well and shows no sign of malfunctioning. In addition to having the need defined by an expert, the need can be satisfied only by purchasing a commodity, in this situation, the services of a trained mechanic. Only the mechanic, one becomes convinced, is capable of understanding the complexities of the machine, the consequent need for the tune-up, and the appropriate procedures to perform this function. Illich's overall critique is that the direction of

---

Toward a History of Needs by Ivan Illich, 1978, New York: Pantheon. Copyright 1978 by Pantheon Books. Excerpts reprinted by permission of Pantheon Books, a Division of Random House.

Western industrial society has largely been a progression from the suppression and denial of use values to the creation and debilitating multiplication of commodity values. He said, for example:

> So persuasive is the power of the institutions we have created that they shape not only our preferences but actually our sense of possibilities. We have forgotten how to speak about modern transportation that does not rely on automobiles and airplanes. Our conception of modern health care emphasizes our ability to prolong the lives of the desperately ill. We have become unable to think of better education except in terms of more complex schools and of teachers trained for ever longer periods. Huge institutions producing costly services dominate the horizons of our inventiveness. . . . We conceive of improving the general well-being as increasing the supply of doctors and hospitals, which package health along with protracted suffering. We have come to identify our need for further learning with the demand for ever longer confinement to classrooms. In other words, we have packaged education with custodial care, certification for jobs, and the right to vote, and wrapped them all together with indoctrination in the Christian, liberal, or communist virtues. (pp. 55–56)

In an example, Illich said:

> The point is well illustrated by a woman who told me about the birth of her third child. Having borne two children, she felt both competent and experienced. She was in the hospital and felt the child coming. She called the nurse, who, instead of helping, rushed for a sterile towel to press the baby's head back into the womb and ordered the mother to stop pushing because "Dr. Levy has not yet arrived." (p. 14)

In very powerful language, Illich proposed that the mid-twentieth century should be called the "age of disabling professions." His objection is that though professionals may be people of excellent intention who have devoted substantial personal time and effort to acquiring the necessary knowledge to diagnose and serve their fellow humanity, they nevertheless "incapacitate people's autonomy through forcing them . . . to become consumers of care." He said further:

> Let us first face the fact that the bodies of specialists that now dominate the creation, adjudication, and satisfaction of needs are a new kind of cartel. . . . The new specialists, who are usually servicers of human needs that their specialty has defined, tend to wear the mask of love and provide some form of care. (p. 23)

Illich's point is that the overall trend of professionalism is not only towards defining new needs which can be met by their services, but also a tendency to coerce, whether through law, regulation, or monopoly, those who are defined as needing their services to obtain it only from them. Over time, professional-consumer relationships of this sort reinforce the individual and social understanding that the matters which form the professional's subject competence are too specialized or complex for the average individual to understand or handle competently. As a result, the professional becomes defined as the only legitimate provider of care, and the consumer is once again relegated to the status of attempting to satisfy a newly defined need through the purchase of a commodity, the services of the professional individual. The professional group therefore becomes more elite and powerful, while the society at large comes more and more to believe in its own inadequacy to deal with a variety of human situations. Illich came very close to describing the situation we have been addressing in this book when he said:

> Finally, the client is trained to need a team approach to receive what his guardians consider "satisfactory treatment." . . . Time scarcity may soon turn into the major obstacle to the consumption of prescribed, and often publicly financed, services. . . . Already in kindergarten, the child is subjected to management by a team made up of such specialists as the allergist, speech pathologist, pediatrician, child psychologist, social worker, physical education instructor, and teacher. . . . Why are there no rebellions against the coalescence of late industrial society into one huge disabling service delivery system? The chief explanation must be sought in the illusion-generating power that these same systems possess. Besides doing technical things to body and mind, professionally attended institutions function also as powerful rituals which generate credence in the things their managers promise. Besides teaching Johnny to read, schools also teach him that learning from teachers is "better" and that without compulsory schools, fewer books would be read by the poor. (pp. 33, 35–36)

As devastating as Illich's critiques can be, perhaps they are especially well timed in light of our current economic limitations, particularly in the publicly funded human services sphere. Until now, our professional prescriptions have in essence called for greater and greater quantities of a greater and greater variety of professional services and therapies. These services and therapies, not coincidentally, are provided by the very same professionals who insist that the services are needed for a full and humane life. Perhaps our greatest contributions as professionals will occur when we convince developmentally disabled individuals and their families that they are not incompetent to deal with their problems; that they can and legitimately should use their own creativity to address the problems of disability in their midst; and that they are more, rather than less, human and humane if they are able to provide adequately for hearing-impaired developmentally disabled individuals without frequent or extensive sanction from the professional service-providing community.

Perhaps we can begin to develop evaluation models in which we measure our effectiveness by the extent to which our initial interventions help our clients and their families to operate with a minimum of future professional assistance. Perhaps our most valuable service can be to liberate hearing-impaired developmentally disabled individuals and their families from the illusion that they are faced with an unmanageable problem which can only be handled adequately by scarce and high-priced professional workers. We should regard as the greatest technological advances in human services those things that require the least amount of professional involvement, that can most effectively be applied by individuals in their daily lives with an absolute minimum of introduction and professional supervision.

Perhaps another contribution we can make is to assist our clients to be nearly as critical as Illich of the professional services which are thrust upon them. To the extent that a professional service engenders the need for further professional service, it may be a disabling activity. To the extent that a service liberates the client from the need for further professional attention, it may be a healthful and enabling service. Could this approach, suggested by Illich on the basis of a radical social critique, become our model of operation for the present and future, when the ability of both individuals and the public sector to support ever-increasing quantities of professional service has declined dramatically?

At the same time, we know that parents do experience shock and grief at the suspicion and discovery of disability in their child. We also know that parents are not always ready or able to take satisfying, effective, autonomous action during those critical early months (see Chapter 6 for further discussion of this point). Perhaps our message to parents can shift from "You must learn to accept the child's disability" to "When you do learn to accept the reality of your child's disability, you will become capable of autonomous action and will be freed from the necessity to deal with me any further." This will constitute a great test for ourselves and any other professional group, for the obvious reason that our own economic well-being depends upon "repeat customers." Perhaps it is time to remind ourselves of that old proverb which says that, given a fish, one is fed for a day; if taught how to fish, one is fed for a lifetime.

A fact that we often overlook but which is frequently true in technological advance is that, as understanding and technology improve, the use of the more sophisticated technology requires less knowledge and prior ability on the part of the user.

Recent advances in microcomputers underscore this point dramatically. The deliberate and increasingly successful approach of microcomputer designers has been to increase the sophistication of both hardware and software in such a way that the device becomes more and more "user-friendly." In practice this means that the user needs less and less prior knowledge and skill in order to make use of a very powerful tool. The challenge to us in the human service professions is to take a similar approach to making our services user-friendly. We need to find ways to *enable* our clients on the basis of less and less contact with us; that is, to enable them to take charge of their lives and take primary responsibility for the disabled children in their families. This may very well be one of the reasons for the success of self-help groups and parent groups—the focus is not on a dependency relationship with a professional person, but on pragmatic actions and objects that can liberate the disabled person, family members, and those in society at large with whom the disabled person interacts.

Again, there may be a lesson for us from some of the computer software developers. The initial tendency was not to reveal the actual programs in the software package and to make the computer floppy disks noncopiable, so as to protect the developer's special knowledge and allow it to be sold again and again at relatively high prices. More recently the tendency has been the opposite—to reveal openly the underlying programs, so that the individual user can modify them as needed. Instead of reducing the developer's financial recompense, this has, in most cases, actually enhanced it. Users are eager to acquire a package which has done most of their work for them but which still allows customizations; they are less willing to buy a package on an all-or-nothing basis.

We professional service providers have been in something of the same position. We have been afraid to let others in on our special knowledge, asserting that "a little knowledge is a dangerous thing" and that no other person could perform our tasks or functions as well without our extensive professional training and therefore without our personal presence. The lesson of the software developers, however, is that an open approach can generate increased markets for our services, thus increasing both our humane professional influence and our personal economic situation. Surely we are creative enough to find ways, without endangering our economic survival, of developing more humane, peer-to-peer, liberating relationships with our clients as well as with our professional colleagues.

The Three Major Issues

In summary, then, at least three major issues need our attention as we attempt to formulate and improve a system-wide approach to service provision for hearing-impaired developmentally disabled individuals and their families. First, we must devote our attention to the service-seeking system as much as, or perhaps more than, to the service delivery system. In other words, the major focus needs to be on the needs, desires, and preferences of our clients rather than on the needs and desires of ourselves and our professional colleagues. Second, we can be of exceptionally useful service if we expand interdisciplinarity from a fact of our staffing patterns to a deliberate professional strategy. Third, and most generally, we need to be keenly aware of the criticisms made by Illich and seek new ways of providing professional service which can have the effect of being liberating rather than enslaving, creating independence on the part of our clients and their families rather than continued dependence upon our professional interventions. Paradoxically, this may become possible as well as necessary in the current economic climate, which has made it very apparent that the expansion of professional services both in sophistication and in quantity cannot continue unchecked and unchallenged.

References

Crowell, J. (1982). Understanding clinical staff's views of administration. In M. Austin & W. Hershey (Eds.), *Handbook on mental health administration*. San Francisco: Jossey-Bass.

Illich, I. (1978). *Toward a history of needs*. New York: Pantheon.

Keller, G. (1983). *Academic strategy: The management revolution in American higher education*. Baltimore: Johns Hopkins University Press.

Bibliography

Austin, M. J., & Hershey, W. E. (Eds.). (1982). *Handbook on mental health administration*. San Francisco: Jossey-Bass.

Backer, T., & Gordon, N. (1982). Consulting to mental health agency boards of directors—Progress report on a pilot project. *Consultation, 1*(2), 57–58.

Bevilacqua, J. (1982). The changing federal-state human service system: Perspectives from a state commissioner of mental health and mental retardation. *Consultation, 1*(3), 18–22.

Cummings, T. G. (Ed.). (1980). *Systems theory for organizational development.* New York: John Wiley.

Cyert, R. M. (1975). *The management of non-profit organizations, with emphasis on universities.* Lexington, MA: Lexington Books.

Ferguson, M. (1980). *The Aquarian conspiracy: Personal and social transformation in the 1980's.* Los Angeles: J. P. Tarcher.

Fraser, R. T. (1982). Serving the developmentally disabled. In M. J. Austin & W. E. Hershey (Eds.), *Handbook on mental health administration.* San Francisco: Jossey-Bass.

Gordon, N., & Backer, T. (1983). Consulting with mental health agency boards of directors. *Consultation, 2*(2), 33–40.

Murphy, E. F. (1983). Development of rehabilitation engineering. *RESNA a.r.t. works* (newsletter of the Rehabilitation Engineering Society of North America), *2*(2), 4–7.

Naisbitt, J. (1982). *Megatrends: Ten new directions transforming our lives.* New York: Warner Books.

Nash, K. B. (1982). Managing interdisciplinary teams. In M. J. Austin & W. E. Hershey (Eds.), *Handbook on mental health administration.* San Francisco: Jossey-Bass.

Chapter 5

Effective Communication: Interactive Interdisciplinary Teamwork

Noel D. Matkin

One belief prevalent among many members of the professional community is that hearing-impaired children represent a homogenous group with similar needs. Unfortunately, adherence to this false assumption can prevent children with significant hearing loss and additional handicaps from reaching their full potential. The use of a term such as "the deaf child," which is frequently encountered in the literature, implies that youngsters with hearing loss are more alike than different. As a consequence, routine assessments and traditional educational programming are commonly encountered, regardless of a particular child's profile of strengths and limitations. Surprise is then expressed later when the child does not achieve as anticipated while using traditional approaches. In other words, we unintentionally continue, in my judgment, to support a failure-based model. That is, our best resources are mobilized only when a child demonstrates failure, most often in the areas of language learning, academic achievement, and social interaction.

In 1953 Myklebust said, "A close cooperative effort is essential in order to meet the needs of hearing-impaired children, especially those with other handicaps." He further stated that only through a team endeavor will knowledge of individual differences and educational needs among children with hearing impairment continue to grow.

In the intervening 32 years—with the advent of neonatal intensive care units, the development of new antibiotics and vaccines, and improved pediatric care—an increasing number of hearing-impaired children have survived high-risk pregnancies, traumatic births, or serious childhood illnesses. As a result, many such youngsters have multiple problems. Current literature suggests that the presence of one or more additional handicapping conditions may be encountered in as many as one out of every three hearing-impaired children. Teamwork thus becomes even more critical.

In 1973 the Rand Corporation, under contract with the Department of Health, Education, and Welfare, published a study on the delivery of services to handicapped children, including those with hearing impairment (Brewer & Kakalik, 1973). This study concluded that uncoordinated, fragmented programs often tax the parents' ability to secure adequate services for their handicapped child. It was further stated that current service delivery systems tend to be specialty oriented, when they need to become child-oriented. Various professionals and agencies often provide only one or a limited range of services. As a consequence, each single service meets only one aspect of the child's total needs. In other words, the report urged specialists who deal with handicapped children to work together and to look at each child as a total human being.

With the passage of the Education for All Handicapped Children Act (Public Law 94-142), the issue of fragmented services and reactive rather than proactive evaluations was addressed. Recall that the Individualized Education Program (IEP) requires that each child be evaluated by a team, so that current developmental status is ascertained before program placement is determined. While the rules and regulations of PL 94-142 represent a major step forward, it still appears, in many instances, that evaluation teams are limited in both the developmental areas evaluated and the number of different professionals who are included on the primary team.

Effective Communication

Whether one refers to teamwork in a generic sense or is considering a specific group of individuals who routinely work together, the issue of effective communication among professionals is a primary consideration. In my judgment, there are five major deterrents that consistently impair effective communication among professionals during service delivery and, consequently, limit the effectiveness of teamwork.

First, there is a trend in this country for increased specialty training as reflected both by accreditation standards for training programs and by certification requirements for individual professionals. As a result, the student is often locked into an extensive curriculum exclusively within his or her own specialty area. Such students often graduate with advanced degrees but with little appreciation of the broad scope of the literature in child development or the competencies of individuals from allied professions.

Second, there is a lack of common terminology among various professionals who work with handicapped children. In other words, each professional discipline tends to develop its own lexicon. As a result, evaluation reports are often written to communicate effectively with a colleague, rather than to communicate with other specialists who may also be evaluating the child, with educators, or with parents.

Third, many professional training programs do not include either education or clinical experience in interactive teamwork. As a consequence, territorial defensiveness and paranoia develop with respect to being observed and evaluated by co-workers from other disciplines as we provide professional services. As noted by Holm and McCartin (1978), bringing together a group of child development specialists does not automatically create a functional team. Fortunately, there have been several publications which suggest issues that need to be addressed, as well as potential training models, with respect to education in interactive teamwork (Brill, 1976; Crisler, 1979; Golin & Ducanis, 1981; Gray, Coleman, & Gotts, 1981; Lyon & Lyon, 1980; Pfeiffer, 1980, 1981; Yoshida, 1980).

Fourth, among the various pediatric specialties there tends to be a professional pecking order which has developed over the years. Unfortunately, the physician, who may spend the least amount of time with the child and the parents, often has the most clout when it comes to making professional decisions relative to diagnosis and recommendations for follow-up services, including educational placement. In sharp contrast, the teacher and parents, who often spend the most time with the child, have minimal if any input as a team evaluates a particular child.

The fifth and final issue which often impairs the effectiveness of teamwork is the lack of time. Obviously, in a society where time is equated with money and where there is a major effort to contain costs for professional services, the expense of assembling a team for prestaffing and poststaffing activities, as well as for evaluations, must be a major consideration. For this reason, to be stressed later, very careful preselection of cases must be undertaken to assure that the full array of specialists represented on a particular developmental team is needed to evaluate effectively and plan for the child's future therapy and educational placement.

Despite these five deterrents, a number of benefits can accrue if effective multidisciplinary team services are available. Certainly, early identification and description of each child's strengths and current limitations are of paramount importance, especially when one considers the variety and combinations of handicapping conditions that may be encountered in the hearing-impaired pediatric population.

The obvious advantage of identifying at the outset the full array of handicapping conditions is that more appropriate initial planning and intervention can be undertaken. Further, and in response to the concerns expressed in the Rand report, there is an increased probability of more effective parental management when a team evaluation, rather than a number of unrelated specialty assessments, is undertaken. By having coordinated feedback, there is less probability that parents will feel fragmented and subsequently not follow through on a variety of recommendations for medical, educational, and related clinical services.

Another obvious benefit of a team evaluation is that a proactive, rather than a reactive, approach is taken to program modification. In other words, one benefit of teamwork is that such children are monitored over time by the group of specialists working together. Each team member thus has an opportunity to assess the validity of the initial recommendations as the child matures and develops. As soon as it becomes apparent that the child is not making adequate progress, it is then possible to reconvene the team and establish a new set of short- and long-range objectives.

Finally, one of the major advantages of participating as a member of a child development evaluation team, and one that is rarely mentioned, is the professional stimulation and growth that accrue over time. Typically, by listening to each specialist present his or her findings, by discussing the evaluation procedures employed, and by generating recommendations for future management, each member of the team develops a heightened sensitivity to the various aspects of child development and the potential impact that various deficits have upon total development. In short, effective teamwork is informative and stimulating and, further, represents the best in continuing professional education. As a consequence, the issue of burnout, which is currently discussed in numerous professional arenas, becomes much less of a problem among members of an interactive interdisciplinary team.

Variables That Influence Teamwork

My experiences, while serving on three different evaluation teams over the past 15 years, suggest that there are at least six major issues which merit consideration when formulating a child study team to serve hearing-impaired children and their families. Each of the six considerations, which directly influence the efficiency of interactive teamwork, will be noted and then discussed briefly.

The first consideration is adoption of a philosophy regarding the manner in which the team functions and the role of various team members. The second is recognition of the broad spectrum of children who fall in the general classification of hearing impaired. Adoption of an admissions procedure which assures that only children are selected who need such a concerted (and expensive) approach to evaluation is a third consideration. The fourth is the adoption of a structure to guide the sequence of the team's clinical activities. A fifth consideration is determination of the team's composition regarding members of the primary team versus consultants to the team. The sixth is adoption of a developmental model which will be used both to guide various aspects of the team evaluation and to determine referrals for additional specialty assessments.

I. Team Philosophy

With respect to adopting a philosophy to guide the team's function, a book by Brill (1976), *Teamwork: Working Together in the Human Services,* is quite informative. Briefly, Brill notes that there are essentially two philosophies that underlie and influence the manner in which the team will function.

One model is the leadership team where the same member of the team serves as the chair and directs the team's activities. Each team member essentially serves as a consultant to the team leader with final decisions regarding further evaluations and management delegated to the responsibility of one person—the team leader. In medical settings, this role is often assumed by the physician on the team. In contrast, a psychologist often fills the leadership role in the educational setting. While efficient in terms of time, such a team structure can reinforce the traditional professional pecking order and result in team members feeling that they have a relatively minor role to play. Further, the leadership team often uses a medical model which yields a diagnosis but little input relative to development of a comprehensive intervention plan.

The alternative is to develop a fraternal team. With this structure, the basic philosophy is that each member assumes equal responsibility for assessment and has equal input into the diagnostic process. Further, the generation and prioritizing of final recommendations are guided by group decisions. The fraternal team structure has proven most beneficial in building transdisciplinary teamwork. While more time consuming, the fraternal team structure tends to minimize territorial defensiveness and to facilitate interactive professional communication. In either case, it is essential that team members agree at the outset upon the philosophy that will guide the function of the team. Otherwise, each member may view his or her potential role somewhat differently, and conflict inevitably will develop.

II. The Spectrum of Impairment

Members of the team must recognize that a broad spectrum of hearing-impaired children will be referred to a team. This is particularly important when making critical decisions about tests, measures, and procedures to be used. The bulk of clinical investigations and research efforts in past years has focused on the so-called deaf child; that is, the child with a severe or profound bilateral sensorineural hearing loss. Yet, current surveys indicate that five or six youngsters with mild-to-moderate impairment exist for every child with a severe-to-profound loss (Berg & Fletcher, 1970). In other words, it must be anticipated that the preponderance of referrals will be hard of hearing, not deaf. As Davis (1977) has pointed out, it is the hard-of-hearing youngster who often represents our forgotten children in terms of diagnostic and educational services.

One further issue relative to hearing loss merits careful consideration. That is, the largest group of children will be those with a history of recurrent otitis media and a fluctuating conductive hearing loss which may be either unilateral or bilateral. At present, there is disagreement within the professional community as to the short- and long-range effects of such transient impairments. On one hand, it has been suggested that such hearing loss will have minimal impact on language learning in most children. In contrast, other investigators conclude that the impact may be pervasive in many cases, with long-term language and subsequent academic difficulties as the end result. The adverse effects of recurrent otitis media upon language and learning among children with additional handicapping conditions has not been adequately addressed. This is a topic which merits longitudinal study because the prevalence of middle ear dysfunction is relatively high among multihandicapped youngsters (Anderson, 1965).

III. Admissions Procedure

The time and effort, not to mention the cost, involved in each evaluation by a child study team are substantial. A rigorous admissions procedure, therefore, should be established to ascertain whether or not each child referred needs a comprehensive multidisciplinary evaluation. Obviously, no single tool will serve as an adequate admission screening strategy. As a minimum, a comprehensive parent questionnaire should be available which provides three types of information: (1) the parents' chief concerns; (2) the child's developmental history across the areas of motor, cognitive, communication, and social/emotional development; and (3) a medical history covering the pre-, para-, and postnatal periods. Some parents, especially those with limited educational backgrounds or those for whom English is a second language, may require assistance in completing the parent questionnaire. Further, with preschoolers, the completion of the Minnesota Child Development Inventory (Ireton & Thwing, 1974) has been fruitful for establishing a profile of strengths and limitations as perceived by the primary caregiver. If the child is older and enrolled in an educational program, either a teacher's report or completion of the Myklebust Pupil Rating Scale (Myklebust, 1981) can contribute additional key information. Input from an educator further serves as a cross-check on the reliability of the parents' perceptions as to the child's level of function and profile of strengths and current limitations.

Obviously, copies of all previous medical, audiological, speech/language, and psychoeducational reports should be obtained and carefully reviewed. Otherwise, the same tests and measures may inadvertently be administered in a relatively short period of time if the child is admitted for a team assessment. Not only should such duplication be avoided for financial reasons, but the test results may be of questionable validity due to the learning effect. Finally, making a home visit to collect observational data on both the child's behavior and interaction within the family is invaluable. If the family lives in the vicinity of the team's base of operation, it is best for a member of the team to complete the home visit. Otherwise, a community health nurse will often cooperate with the team if the family is from out of town. Use of the Home Observation for Measurement of the Environment (HOME) scale (Caldwell & Robert, 1970) in such instances will ensure that the nurse collects key observations in a systematic manner. The use of this scale, which is easy to interpret, serves to facilitate communication with the team while limiting the need for the visiting nurse to prepare a long, detailed written report.

IV. Team Coordination

The efficiency of a team's function is further enhanced if a routine schedule of activities is developed and maintained. As a minimum, it is essential that prestaffing be scheduled before initiating each evaluation. Otherwise, a good deal of duplication in testing may be encountered among the various team members. Another pitfall is that critical areas may not be assessed, since each member may assume that someone else on the team will complete such evaluation.

Without adoption and adherence to a few basic procedural guidelines, prestaffing can become very time consuming. To facilitate discussion during the prestaffing, a case summary should be developed and distributed to all team members prior to the meeting. The task of preparing and distributing this key document may be assigned to a caseworker or may be completed by various members of the team on a rotating basis. The case summary should be concise, yet contain the highlights from previous evaluations, all pertinent medical and developmental history, and a clear statement of the parents' and/or referring agency's concerns. A review of the case summary allows each team member to generate specific questions and concerns, as well as a basic assessment plan, *before* rather than during the prestaffing. With such preparation, an overall plan for evaluation, including the need for outside consultation, often can be agreed upon within 15 to 20 minutes.

It is ideal if the day and time for both the pre- and poststaffing meetings are mutually agreed upon and maintained over time. Otherwise, coordinating the work schedules of the different individuals on the team becomes a major hassle. Once a schedule of activities is set, each team member becomes personally responsible for attending the staffings or for identifying a colleague who can substitute on the team during schedule conflicts or vacations. Of equal importance is the development of a plan for conducting poststaffings. Such a meeting should be conducted before presenting the findings to the parents or representatives from the referring agency, to ensure that an integrated and comprehensive plan of action has been developed. Again, lack of preparation can result in long, verbal, and relatively nonproductive staffings. Ideally, each team will come to the poststaffing with a document which succinctly summarizes the child's strengths and current limitations.

There are two important points to be made here. First, all team members should initially focus upon the child's relative strengths—an issue that can easily be overlooked, especially when evaluating multihandicapped children. Second, use of the term "current limitations" rather than "weaknesses" is preferable since the former term implies that change may occur over time with appropriate intervention.

While each team member should come to the meeting with a plan of action in mind, recommendations for further assessment or for intervention should be tentative until the findings from all members of the team have been presented. For example, a child may appear substantially delayed in language development if only the results from such testing are considered. However, a comparison of the child's mental and language ages may reveal that a significant difference between the two areas of development does not exist. Certainly, such a finding will substantially alter the type of recommendation that is made relative to specific language intervention.

Prior to the termination of the poststaffing, each team member should finalize recommendations, and the list of strengths, current limitations, and recommendations should be given to the case manager. Such lists from the various specialists on the team are invaluable during feedback to the parents and later, when a master evaluation summary is prepared.

A strategy to communicate effectively the findings from the various team specialists in a printed format that facilitates use of the diagnostic information by clinicians, teachers, and program administrators must be selected. To explain, it is not uncommon for each specialist to prepare a report of three to five pages describing test procedures, findings, and recommendations. If the referring agency receives five to eight such specialty reports from the team without a unifying cover document, there is every reason to believe that the various reports will never be read in their entirety.

Two strategies have been found useful to overcome this potential breakdown in communication. First, plotting all objective scores from the various tests on a profile yields a visual display of the child's strengths and limitations. Either the profile can be organized with a bell-shape curve as the reference and the various scores converted to percentiles, or the child's chronological age can serve as a reference with all test results converted to developmental age scores. In my experience, using percentile scores has been found most productive for older children while developmental age scores are more easily interpreted with preschool youngsters. Second, the various specialty reports should be preceded by a cover document in which all findings and recommendataions are succinctly summarized in a page or so under the headings: strengths, current limi-tations, and recommendations. With this master summary and the attached profile, a coordinated overview of the child's present developmental status and needs is provided to anyone who receives the team's report. Each specialty report then serves to expand, to provide details, and to clarify the statements in the master summary.

V. Team Composition

The composition of the interdisciplinary team is the fifth consideration. Ideally, the developmental model which is discussed in the following section will influence the inclusion of certain specialists as primary team members. Obviously, the setting in which the team will be working may dictate the availability of various specialists to serve on the team. Nevertheless, my experience in working with a broad spectrum of hearing-impaired children suggests that the primary evaluation team ideally will include

- a pediatrician with a developmental orientation;
- either a social worker or pediatric nurse with skills in evaluating both the home environment and family dynamics;
- a psychologist experienced in the administration of performance measures to children with limited communication skills;
- an audiologist with clinical competencies in administering a pediatric battery of behavioral and, as appropriate, electrophysiologic measures of hearing;
- a speech/language pathologist familiar with the procedures and special precautions in test administration that are relevant to hearing-impaired children;
- an occupational therapist familiar with the manual skills needed to communicate effectively through the use of signs and fingerspelling;
- a physical therapist with a developmental orientation;
- a special educator (ideally the child's classroom teacher) who is competent both in the administration of achievement tests to school-age hearing-impaired children and in determining appropriate educational placement;
- the child's primary caregiver.

In addition to the primary team, there are key individuals who should be identified and be readily available as consultants to the team when deemed appropriate. The specialists most frequently needed for consultation include

- a pediatric ophthalmologist skilled in eye examinations with children having limited communication skills;
- a pediatric neurologist;
- a geneticist familiar with the various etiologies and syndromes related to sensorineural hearing losses;
- a child psychiatrist with diagnostic skills as well as experience in developing behavioral management programs for home and school implementation; and
- an otolaryngologist both to confirm that the hearing loss is not reversible and to treat any subsequent middle ear infection.

It is ideal, yet unrealistic, for the primary team members as well as the consultants to have basic manual communication skills so that children from total communication programs are managed efficiently during all evaluations. Recognizing that this is rarely the case, it has been helpful to utilize the child's teacher as an interpreter during the various evaluations. The obvious advantage of this strategy is that the child is more at ease with the teacher and is more familiar with the manual communication system being used. Both factors serve to improve the reliability and the validity of the findings from the various evaluations.

A spinoff from this approach is that including the teacher in the evaluation process provides an opportunity to compare "clinical behaviors" with those encountered by the teacher in the classroom. For example, it is not unusual to find that some hearing-impaired children function relatively well in a structured one-to-one learning environment. Yet these same children may fail to keep their attention to the task at hand when placed in a classroom where there are multiple activities and distractions. Finally, including the teacher as an active participant in the evaluation process makes the possibility much greater that recommendations made by the team will be implemented and evaluated in the educational setting. Without such implementation, one must question whether the theoretical advantages of a team evaluation offer any real benefits to the child, the family, or the school.

VI. A Developmental Model

The final issue, one that merits consideration during the organization of a team, is the adoption of a developmental model. A variety of developmental models, some quite elaborate, have been proposed for diagnostic use. In my experience, a simple model proposed by Myklebust (1954) has been found to be adequate and yet comprehensive. He suggests that four major development areas should be the points of focus during the case history, during clinical observations, and during formal testing. Those areas are motor development, cognitive development, language development, and social/emotional development. Obviously, each developmental area can be broken into as many component parts as deemed necessary for the child under study.

It should be kept in mind that knowledge of each child's visual and auditory functions should be established before formal assessment in the various areas outlined above is undertaken. Vision should be corrected and hearing should be aided if the goal of the evaluation is to establish optimal performance in the various developmental areas. One persistent problem which highlights this point is the use of verbal intelligence scales with children having undetected hearing loss. Obviously, the child's inability to follow verbal instructions and the language delay associated with the hearing loss interact to invalidate the score obtained on a verbal measure. The same problem may be encountered if pencil-and-paper tests are administered to a child with uncorrected vision.

Finally, an understanding of the child's physical status, and any related health problems, as well as environmental influences, is important before attempting to interpret test findings. Certainly, the interpretation of language scores will be modified if the child is ill and relatively nonresponsive during testing, or if the youngster comes from a non-English-speaking or bilingual home. Thus, completion of both the pediatrician's examination and a home visit should be given priority as the evaluation schedule is finalized. Further, hearing and vision testing should be scheduled early in the evaluation so that, if an impairment is identified, appropriate modifications can be made by other evaluators in the selection of further tests and procedures.

In short, one can visualize the preceding points by reviewing Figure 1. The child's current level of daily function is best understood if each of the components of the model is considered.

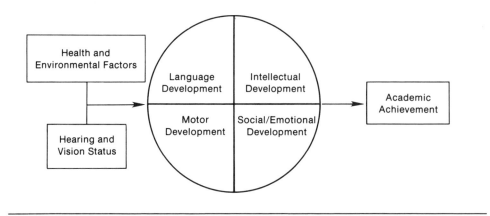

Figure 1. A developmental model for guiding interactive team evaluation.

Summary

In summary, the need for effective communication among various professions has been highlighted and identified as the basic consideration in teamwork. Implicit in the preceding discussion is the belief that as the population of hearing-impaired children becomes more varied and complex, the need for interactive interdisciplinary teamwork, whether in a clinical or school setting, becomes more imperative. To assume that any group of hearing-impaired children is a homogeneous sample with similar needs and limitations will lead to a substantial number of youngsters who fail to reach their optimal level of functioning across the various developmental areas.

Five deterrents to effective teamwork have been discussed, and six considerations for improving the function of any team, regardless of setting, have been reviewed. While there are numerous advantages in coordinating the services of various specialists, there are pitfalls that must be recognized and avoided. Otherwise, fragmented service delivery and conflicting recommendations from various specialists will continue to undermine the development of a comprehensive service delivery model for developmentally disabled hearing-impaired children and youth. Finally, and importantly, interactive interdisciplinary teamwork should not be viewed as a topic relevant only to evaluation clinics or medical centers. The key for improving ongoing services for all hearing-impaired children is the development of effective communication and teamwork among various specialists and educators in the school setting during such activities as IEP meetings, support service staffings, and annual progress reviews.

References

Anderson, R. (1965). Hearing impairment and mental retardation: A selected bibliography. *The Volta Review, 67*, 425–432.

Berg, F., & Fletcher, S. (1970). *The hard of hearing child.* New York: Grune and Stratton.

Brewer, G., & Kakalik, J. (1973). *Improving services to handicapped children* (R-1420, HEW). Santa Monica: Rand Corporation.

Brill, N. (1976). *Teamwork: Working together in the human services.* Philadelphia: Lippincott.

Caldwell, B. M., & Robert, H. B. (1970). *Home observation for measurement of the environment (HOME).* Little Rock: University of Arkansas Center for Child Development and Education.

Crisler, J. R. (1979). Utilization of a team approach in implementing Public Law 94-142. *Journal of Research and Development in Education, 12,* 101–108.

Davis, J. (1977). *Our forgotten children: Hard of hearing pupils in the schools.* Minneapolis: University of Minnesota Audio Visual Library Service.

Golin, A. K., & Ducanis, A. J. (1981). *The interdisciplinary team: A handbook for the education of exceptional children.* Rockville, MD: Aspen Systems.

Gray, N. M., Coleman, J. M., & Gotts, E. A. (1981). The interdisciplinary team: Challenges to effective functioning. *Teacher Education and Special Education, 4*(1), 45–49.

Holm, V. A., & McCartin, R. E. (1978). Interdisciplinary child development team: Team issues and training in interdisciplinariness. In K. E. Allen, V. A. Holm, & R. L. Schiefelbusch (Eds.), *Early intervention—A team approach.* Baltimore: University Park Press.

Ireton, H., & Thwing, E. (1974). *Minnesota child development inventory.* Minneapolis: Behavioral Science Systems.

Lyon, S., & Lyon, G. (1980). Team functioning and staff development: A role release approach to providing integrated educational services for severely handicapped students. *Journal of the Association for the Severely Handicapped, 5,* 250–263.

Myklebust, H. (1953). Toward a new understanding of the deaf child. *American Annals of the Deaf, 98,* 496–499.

Myklebust, H. (1954). *Auditory disorders in children.* New York: Grune and Stratton.

Myklebust, H. (1981). *The pupil rating scale revised.* New York: Grune and Stratton.

Pfeiffer, S. I. (1980). The school based interprofessional team: Recurring problems and some possible solutions. *Journal of School Psychology, 18,* 388–394.

Pfeiffer, S. I. (1981). The problems facing interdisciplinary teams: As perceived by team members. *Psychology in the Schools, 18,* 330–333.

Yoshida, R. K. (1980). Multidisciplinary decision making in special education: A review of the issues. *School Psychology Review, 9,* 221–227.

Chapter 6

Dynamic Intervention with Families

Kenneth L. Moses

My interests and concerns are related to the prevention of mental illness or, more specifically, to the enhancement of mental health. This area of emphasis is not restricted to working with parents of impaired children and the professionals who work with them, but with people in general crisis, trauma, grief, and loss. My main goal is one of enhancing mental health and growth in the face of crisis. You might say, "That's great, who cares; I've got troubles of my own," or "I have my own areas of specialty and I'm trying to get a job done; I don't need somebody else telling me I have more to do." After getting involved in the prevention of mental illness, it has become very clear to me that in the enhancement of health—mental, physical, or social—there is an overlap in all fields. Everything networks together. If you don't attend to all the parts, you're missing the boat in some fashion.

Early intervention is a case in point. This concept has revolutionized the fields of habilitation and changed attitudes toward habilitation, perhaps not as far as we wish. Nonetheless, I don't think that there is a thinking professional around who would say that early intervention can be ignored. Indeed, the best time to start working with a child is when you first discover that something's going wrong. In fact, the best time to screen is at birth so that you can intervene and minimize the impact of the disability. In the process of putting together programs for early intervention, people in special education and in the habilitation service areas have become individuals who truly live and work through the holistic approach. Holism is a concept that a human being is not a series of discrete parts but that the summation and interaction of the parts create an individual who must be attended to as a unit. As intelligent professionals we can no longer only treat a child's ears, deal with a child's language, work with a child's mobility, or deal with the child's cognition to the exclusion of the rest of that human being. Indeed, people in your fields often are the frontrunners in educating other people to that fact.

There was an audiologist, a woman whom I had the privilege of hearing address a meeting of otolaryngologists, who tried to explain this holistic concept. She had been given about 10 minutes for the presentation with 5 minutes for questions and answers.

This chapter is an edited transcript of Kenneth Moses's presentation at the ASHA National University Affiliated Facilities Conference held at Gallaudet College on May 12–14, 1982, as part of training activities partially funded by Administration on Developmental Disabilities Grant No. 90DD0005/01.

This format fits the medical model; if you can't say it in 15 minutes, it can't be important. Well, this person did it wonderfully. She said, very simply, "The next time a set of ears walks into your office, see what is between them. You will notice that something is carrying the ears. Please consider that something more than an 'ear carrier.' It might indeed have some influence on some decisions you might make, surgically, medically, etc. We call this the child. In considering that, and the interactions thereof, you might want to listen to what's going on with the rest of that ear carrier before making your decisions."

I thought it was a unique and clever way of driving the point home. My assumption is that such a point does not have to be driven home to you. I have to extend it a bit, though, and say that the next time a child walks in with a set of impaired ears, a developmental disability, a cognitive problem, the combination of hearing impairment/developmental disabilities—please note that there might be one or two other people hanging around the "ear carrier." At least one or two other people, I think, who might be part of the issue, and whom you might want to consider in your treatment program. They are sometimes called parents.

To separate parents from the child is as conceptually fallacious as to separate the child's ears from the rest of the child. There's one unit—the child. If your facility has an attitude and a stance that the parents are a separate unit, and most places have such an attitude, you will do things that treat the parents and child as though they are divisible. You will set up treatment for the child, you will set up structures for the child, and only then you will work with the parents to facilitate the work with the child. If you understand that parents and child are one unit, then child habilitation automatically implies inclusion of the parents. Inclusion of parents as a unit means that you structurally have to do very different things within your setting than if you conceptualize treatment of the child with parents helping you—or, more honestly, treatment of the child while trying to keep parents from disrupting the treatment. We are talking about an attitudinal structure. If you are going to include the parents as part of the unit, you've got to know a lot about who and what each parent is and what the interaction between parent and child is about.

I do a lot of workshops on the emotional development of impaired children and adults; that is, how impairment impacts emotional development. Do you want to know the single, strongest element that impacts development? The attitude of the parent towards the child, which is affected by the impact on the parent of having an impaired child. Parents change their normal, spontaneous child-rearing practices because of the emotional impact of having an impaired child. That is the primary debilitating force that inhibits the emotional development of impaired children. What does this imply? You've got to deal with the parent in terms of the emotional impact of having an impaired child, not because it's a nice thing to do, but because it's central to child habilitation. How many of you have built parent counseling, parent education, and parent training into your programs?

Note that I distinguish between parent education, parent counseling, and parent training. These are three distinct issues that oftentimes are mixed together. Typically when I ask professionals what you do now in your parent counseling programs, what you emphasize, who does the counseling, with what goals and structure, I get this answer:

Our social worker and social-worker students do the counseling in our program, and it's offered as a crisis arises.

A program that offers counseling only when a crisis is identified is a pathology-oriented program; that is, you have to present a symptom to be treated. In other words, it is not a prevention program; it is a treatment program for some type of mental illness or stress already present, identifiable as pathology, and in need of treatment. Most parent programs in the counseling area are pathology- and crisis-oriented.

The next question I ask is, How many professionals have had direct training in the area of parent counseling? How many of you deal with parents who are displaying various characteristics of being under emotional stress? You see, if prevention is going to occur, it will start with you. Once you bring in the social worker, psychologist, or psychiatrist, you are bringing in a pathology model. Imagine yourself in the circumstances of having an impaired child, and all of a sudden you are sent down the hall to see a social worker.

Crazy-making Circumstances

You—the special educator, audiologist, speech/language pathologist—are the ones who deal firsthand with the people who are under stress in a circumstance that is most appropriately dealt with by you rather than by psychologists, social workers, or psychiatrists. You are the people who can take a truly holistic approach in the treatment of the child and deal with the emotional impact upon parents of having an impaired child within a nonpathology-oriented environment.

A friend of mine talked to me recently about getting a very despicable diagnosis. What was the main problem she was feeling? The professional's insensitivity, lack of relating, and lack of understanding her life situation beyond simply offering the diagnosis and treatment recommendations. That circumstance to me is a "crazy maker." That approach causes more mental illness than a cadre of social workers, psychologists, and psychiarists can cure.

In my opinion, most parents of impaired children are healthy people in an unhealthy circumstance. People in a "crazy-making" circumstance, not crazy people! What are the "symptoms" of being a parent of an impaired child? What are the difficult things you face every day, and could any of your reactions to these things be diagnosed as "symptoms" that could require a psychologist, social worker, or psychiatrist? Are reactions to trauma really symptoms?

Most parents are frustrated to the point of tears, but most professionals aren't trained to deal with tears. What do you do when parents cry? I've seen all sorts of techniques. I have seen diagnostic sessions with three or four professionals in the room who have a tacit agreement that, if a parent cried, they would turn to each other and have a little chat until the parent pulled it together. Another disturbing technique that I've seen is: "They need their privacy, so we'll all make believe that they are in another room crying and then, when they're done, we'll talk to them again."

What else do you encounter besides crying parents? Tired parents. People who are tired, depleted, and burned out. "I can't deal with it any more. For God's sake, don't ask me to do anything else. I can't handle it," they say. And angry parents. One of the definitions of depression is anger turned inward, and that's probably how we got the formal sign for anger (the hand turned inward toward the face). Parents who are angry at the professional can scare you and get you to act out. Whenever I have parents that are angry, invariably they are the ones to whom I forget to return phone calls. They are also often the ones that don't follow through, yet they call back to catch us at not following through. When I hear, "Mrs. Jones is on the line," I hope it isn't one of the angry parents. They are scary. They can be very abusive, very insulting, and very confrontive about the services that we are offering.

Another "symptom" is evidenced in the parent that separates from the child's problems and says, "Here's my child. Please fix him." It's an interesting form of dependency, isn't it? Sort of like, "I can't handle it, but you're designated as a professional, licensed by the state, and have wonderful credentials hanging on your wall, so you must know a lot. Because my child is impaired, he or she is your responsibility."

Another type is the nonemotional, intellectual parent. A stereotypic example is, "Verna and I are both grad-u-ates of a very fine eastern university, and we know how to deal with these problems." How do you touch these parents? How do you teach them?

Overenthusiastic parents—the professional parent of the impaired child—is another type of symptom. The "I'm giving up my whole life and willing to devote my life to language acquisition" parent. The parents who get so involved that they frighten you. They frighten you with the expectation, the implicit expectation that you'll do the same, so that they can call you at eleven at night if they have some questions.

Denying parents are probably the singularly most frustrating parents according to most professionals. I'm not just talking about denying an initial diagnosis; I'm talking about denying throughout the child's development. They also exhibit all sorts of magical behavior. "I don't have to do anything," they say. "This doesn't have to change my life. I'll just live with the kid, and you'll fix it."

Then there is the overly protective parent. I have a very simple definition of overprotection: when a parent does not permit a child to do something that he or she obviously can do.

How about the parents who spend 24 hours a day, 7 days a week with one afflicted child to the detriment of everyone around them, including themselves? "The gravity of the cross I bear." They wrap the child around themselves and march off into the sunset.

Also, there are many apathetic parents. In fact, a lot of professionals will come to me and say, "We would like to start a parent group in our setting because we've got a lot of apathetic parents. We know you're an expert on the theory of how to start a parent group. We tried two or three times, we sent out 138 flyers, we had follow-up phone calls, and seven people showed up at the first meeting, four the second, and we didn't even dare to call a third meeting out of embarrassment." How can we get apathetic parents involved? Provide poor service, and be arrogant about it; then you will get the finest parent organization you've ever seen in your life. What I am implying, of course, is that parent organizations are not formed by professionals; they are formed by parents out of parents' needs. If there is no need, you will not get a parents' organization started. If you are not meeting the needs of parents, or if you are not tuned in to what parents want, they won't show up; neither would you.

Some of our professional staff have a hard time handling parents who really do adjust to their child's handicap. I love that concept. I got called in to see a family with a bunch of kids. I can't really remember how many, but a gaggle of kids. It was a very, very religious, self-contained family; you almost had a feeling of the Waltons in this group. They had a very impaired Down's syndrome child who was entering a program. A social worker met with the family, and this family indicated no discomfort whatsoever about having this child. The staff was so convinced that there was some type of astounding pathological denial, that I was called in to consult in the case.

I asked to go into the home with the social worker, so we made a home visit. I want you to know that I never wanted more in my life to be a child in a family than in this family. This mother was stirring a pot of spaghetti while she was nursing the youngest one, doing math homework with the one over here, and watching how the other children got washed, which must be a nightly routine. They had a big double sink in the basement—the gray, deep double sinks—one filled with soapy water, the other clear. All of these kids stood in a row, naked. I just wanted to take my clothes off and get washed and nurtured. This was a family for whom the impact of the loss was not there. There was no loss. They loved children! They loved to take care of children. My guess is that when they started to approach the empty nest, they would get foster children, or they would adopt children. These people lived for nurturing children. Therefore, an impaired child was just like all the rest of them. A little different, that's all. And, truly, there was no pathology.

Two other groups of parents that are also very difficult to deal with are retarded parents with normal children and parents of institutionalized adults who, over a period of many years, have given up their family identity. Then someone tries to reunite the parents with their institutionalized child. Families get caught in the dragnet of de-institutionalization into the community—by physicians, ministers, teachers, and friends. After their fighting the concept of institutionalization, often keeping the child for five, seven, nine years; after our having to get heavier and heavier-handed with them to finally let go of the child, to institutionalize; after their going through years of bereavement around institutionalization, then ultimately separating—finally the family members have put their lives back together. Their kid's now 27 or 32 or whatever; he or she has been in the institution 10 or 15 years. Then the dragnet comes. Someone tells the family there's a new concept called deinstitutionalization—reintegration into the community. Wouldn't you like your kid back? Such parents say, "Excuse me? Are you talking to me? You can't be talking to me." They are terrified, confused, and furious.

How to help retarded parents of nonimpaired children is similarly very, very difficult. It is one of those issues that really needs attention, that needs a team approach. But I won't directly deal with that problem here. It is a very particular and special problem that requires indepth attention and discussion.

What do you do with all of these families, what do you do when people are despondent or crying, or when people are overprotective, or when people are behaving in a fashion that manifests denial? I've been watching you as I go across the country doing workshops; I've peeked into your diagnostic sessions and into your feedbacks and into your parent meetings, and I know what you do. You stare at your fingers, stare at the ceiling, and hope it will go away soon. Or, if you're an aggressive person who likes measurable results, you go right up against it. You're going to tell them the right way to live and how to fix things, how to do this and face that and how to be proper about it.

But these parents are so much better at resisting you than you are at breaking through. It's just amazing, how difficult it is.

The Process of Grieving

I'd like to give you a theoretical concept with some recommendations. First, I worked long and hard getting together a definition of grieving, and I've changed it as I go along. Here's where it is at this moment. See how it fits you. Grieving—*i, n, g*—is a gerund form. Not grief. You can't say, I have grieved or I have had a bad grief period. No, it is lifelong; once this change occurs, it's for life: That is what produces our character. Grieving is a process, not a product. It's a process whereby a person separates from a significant lost dream, a fantasy, or a projection into the future. I think this is an important definition because the first thing it does, among other things, is to get you away from being too concrete about grief. Do you know what I mean? "Well, Mrs. Jones, I understand that you're rather upset about Joey's hearing impairment, but I have to tell you, relative to other children, Joey's hearing impairment is really not that substantial. Now, we have very good equipment, and new ways to amplify sound, and we can deal with these things. There's really not that much to be upset about."

My father died the 13th of March after a very long and arduous disease. He died 12 days before his 78th birthday, and I am still very much in the midst of grieving. I am far from beyond the acute pained state. So you have a chance to hear someone who is in an acute grief state. I loved him very much. I struggled in every way possible for him to be comfortable, to be cured, to be near me. It was impossible; he was in California and then in Massachusetts in a nursing home, which is the last thing I wanted. But it had to be done. I had no options left; I had tried them all. And when he died, he wanted to die. I didn't see him when he died. I had said my goodbyes, and I had done some good grief work with him.

He had invited me to California to talk about dying. He was very sick, but his mind was clear right to the end. So he started talking with me about the division of property, about where all the things were, about what he wanted said at his funeral, and what traditions he needed to have carried out. He went through everything about dying. It was incredible. We did all of our unfinished business, and he told me something to be said at his funeral. All he wanted said at his funeral was, "I leave this world with no bad feelings towards anybody." What was very powerful was his emphasis on who was left behind, not upon him. Anyway, we worked for a day and a half, talking about his dying. Finally, he was finished and I was finished, and then we cried. We laughed and we argued a little and we did what we had to do.

After we were all done, I said, "Listen, Dad, have you finished everything you've got to talk about in terms of dying?" He thought a while and said, "Yeah." So I said, "Well, now I know what to do in case you die. But what if you live?"

He cracked up at that point, as I did. It may be a little grotesque for you to deal with but, for us, it was wonderful. It was the best grief intervention I've ever made. Because he responded, "Oh, I hadn't thought about what am I going to do if I live!" So we started to talk about what he was going to do, including that afternoon, every minute he had left of his life.

My brother saw him at 4:30; he died at 9:30. That morning he'd been complaining incessantly about pain and about how lousy the place was. He was irascible and irritable, difficult to talk with and suffering. That afternoon, he was fine; perfectly fine. My brother came and said, "Do you want anything?"

"No."

"How do you feel?"

"Fine."

"Do you want to talk?"

"No."

"Well, you said you wanted a haircut this week. And I can give you a shave, too, if you want. Do you want that?"

My father said, "Yeah." So my brother gave him a haircut and shave. And my father said something that was totally uncharacteristic of him in the last number of years: "I want some after-shave lotion."

"Excuse me?" said my brother.

"I want some after-shave lotion."

"Oh, okay." So my brother went down to the car, drove to the drugstore, bought a bottle of after-shave lotion, drove back, went back upstairs, and applied that after-shave lotion.

"You want anything else?" said my brother.

"No."

"Do you want me to stay?"

"No."

At 7:30 that night he slipped into a light coma, and at 9:30 he died. He did not have pneumonia, he did not have a stroke, he did not have a heart attack. He just died. A close friend of mine, a therapist, listened to that story, and said, "I think I know what he was doing with the after-shave." I couldn't see what the after-shave could mean. She said, "He went out young and healthy and attractive; that's how he went." That's how I'll think of it, true or not.

A lot of people came up to me and said, "You know, Ken, what's to grieve? Your father was a wonderful man. He lived a full life. He was old. He was terribly sick. He wasn't going to get better. He wanted to die, and he died on his own terms. You haven't lost anything." Those people were too concrete; they were looking too concretely. No one ever asked me, "What did you lose when your father died?" Had they asked, I would have said, "I don't know. But I feel a lot of pain, and I'm working on it to figure out what I've lost; it's taken me this long to start to define it."

You don't know what the parents of an impaired child have lost until they tell you. What were their dreams for that child? It's not in the concreteness of the impairment.

Parents have dreams for who or what their child is supposed to be for them. The impairment is a great spoiler, and it triggers a grief response. The same is true with death, or with divorce, or with being fired, or with a separation. There are dreams we have for this life. And the people, the ideals, the concepts that we attach to, tightly, profoundly, from inside, are the mainstream of what makes us human and alive, and what connects us to life. When that breaks, when we lose that, we get despondent, depressed, life loses its meaning.

Our love attaches us to people, and parents attach to their children in utero. Both parents do. In the expecting of the child, they project themselves onto the child, and they generate dreams of who that child is supposed to be. The disability shatters those dreams. There are parents who have a child with the mildest learning disability, a minor problem compared to the kids that you see, but whose lives are destroyed because their dream was to be perfect. And where did that come from? Maybe that came from parents who said, "There's only one way to survive in this world, only one way to be loved, only one way to be okay. Be perfect!" Maybe they almost made it until they got that one kid who has a learning disability. And that world crashed down on them. Their entire life, that's all. So sitting there saying, "Mrs. Jones, this is nothing to be so upset about. It's just a little learning disability. What's the big deal?" Hey, you don't know what they've lost. That's why the definition of grieving is so important.

Grieving is the process whereby a person separates from a significant dream, fantasy, or projection into the future. We're talking about love, investment, and attachment, the mainstream of life. Our children speak for that. How does the grieving process work? How do we separate from the dream? We probably know the checklist since we all know something about grieving. Many of you have read Elizabeth Kubler-Ross's book, *On Death and Dying,* and perhaps some of the articles that followed it. Unfortunately, a lot of people have the idea that grieving is like a checklist that you move through. "Listen, Mrs. Jones, you've sustained a substantive loss; therefore, I advise that you move yourself through denial, anxiety, guilt, depression, anger; because I've read that until you do you can't grieve. So now would be as good a time as any to start." Sometimes clinicians and teachers get so concrete and simplistic it frightens me. Grieving is not moving through a checklist of feelings. Incidentally, they're not stages because stages are epigenetic—one, two, three, four, and you can't do two until you've done one. Grieving is a process of feeling in a very loose order. The order is irrelevant anyway, because it's very fluid. People can feel two feelings at the same time; sometimes, three. Overachievers attempt all five in one day.

Grieving, as a series of feeling states, moves a person through a philosophic, attitudinal struggle of how to deal with the undealable, how to shift your feelings and attitudes. Let's consider denial. Denial is the single most reported problem in clinics, hospitals, and diagnostic settings, because people who are denying don't do what you want them to do. They don't get the hearing aid. They don't do the auditory training. They don't learn sign language. They don't work on the cognitive exercises or whatever it is you want them to do. They don't show up for appointments, or they cancel. They drive you crazy. At least, that's my experience.

The anxiety of parents scares you because it also makes you anxious. It's catching. An anxious parent can make a professional very anxious. You say, "My God, she's right. She can't handle it. So I don't trust her with him." In contrast, we tend to skirt around depression. We call it despondency, or lack of investment, or something like that. Parents get depressed as part of normal grieving. Also, they get angry. And there's one feeling we failed to mention. I can't believe people like you, with your commitment and investment in parents, people who are supposedly caring people would forget this one—an imbedded message, guilt.

A Conceptual Framework

These are the feelings that I believe you'll be bucking every day, and that are central to child habilitation. We are prone to diagnose these feeling states and call them pathology. They are prone to distance us from parents. But you may respond, "I don't know what to do with them." I now would like to offer a conceptual framework that might give you some support.

Denial. No one is prepared for bad news. To be prepared, you would have to obsessively and compulsively live your entire life while preparing for that news. With your luck, you'd encounter one of those you hadn't gotten to yet. No one can emotionally or conceptionally prepare for the awful things that can happen to human beings. More importantly, you can't think about it too much and still live your life freely. You couldn't breathe the air, eat food with additives, drink coffee, drink booze, drive cars without seatbelts, tailgate, or cross streets.

There's much jeopardy around us. Anything can happen to anybody. So how is it you move around so freely? How is it that you do cross streets and you do smoke and you do eat food with additives and you do drink, etc.? You're in denial, my friends. Perpetual denial. Do you know how denial sounds? "It can't happen to me." Now, if you don't call that denial, no one does. Incidentally, there's always somebody in a group who says, "I'm on an ovo-lacto vegetarian diet, and we grow the food ourselves, and we make our own cheese, have our own cows. I don't drive a car. I ride a bicycle—with a helmet. I don't smoke. I don't drink. I don't drink coffee. I don't eat food with additives, and we have an air cleaner." If such a person is reading this, I would ask, "Do you touch public doorknobs?" If so, you are in jeopardy. And there's no way to hide from it; there's no way to fool yourself. So we do many of these things every day. Otherwise, we couldn't function. So what happens when something terrible happens? You are totally unprepared to deal with it. And what happens if you feel the full impact of something that you're totally unprepared to deal with? Total psychological collapse.

Denial buys the time that permits the person to find the inner strength, the ego strength, and the external supports to deal with the "undealable." What are the external supports? For parents, they are the friends they can really rely upon, the professionals that they need to learn about and consult, the new language that they have to learn about their child's disability, the techniques, the laws, the issues of special education, the issues of medication, etc. Once you have that knowledge, the support of the people, and the sense that there is a strength within you that can deal with this even though at the time you thought there wasn't, then you can let it sink in. That awareness has tremendous implications on how you do diagnostics and how you do ongoing habilitation for the child/parent unit. Denial buys the time. It's necessary, it's healthy, it's important. Yet, you need to work with the child at the same time. Dealing with parental denial in a constructive way is part of your responsibility in dealing with the child. If you don't, you alienate the parent. Then what have you got?

Anxiety also serves a positive use. How can it be positive? We imply in our culture that anxiety is negative, pathological, and even of organic origin. Who reading this does not know about the medication, Valium? I've never had people say, "I don't know what Valium is." Now, I'm aware that every one reading this has encountered Valium because of lower back pain. I know that none of you took it for anxiety. It was for something else. But there are some people who take Valium when they get nervous, and they think that is reasonable. They have a philosophic stance that says nervousness, or anxiety, is a biochemical problem. I've got too many "whatevers" jumping around in my system, so I'll put in some "whatothers" to bring it down, and we'll have treated the problem.

Well, I have this rather controversial thought. It may be apropos to be anxious when, for instance, you've just been told that you have an impaired child. When every corner of your life will be changed, when demands are going to be put upon you against your will that you don't believe that you can meet, when all that you value is put in jeopardy. Do you think it might be apropos to get anxious, and do you think, further, that it's a biochemical problem which should be treated with Valium, or booze, or even progressive muscle relaxation? ("I note that you are a Type A personality, an anxious person, Mrs. Smith, particularly since we spoke about your child. We're going to teach you how to relax. We're going to start with your feet and toes. All right, tense up those toes. Now let's relax.") I had a friend who once went to a workshop on relaxation. She said, "When they started at my feet, I said, 'My God, they're starting at my feet. By the time they get to my head, I'm going to be psychotic! They're starting at the wrong end.' If they don't start at the top and work down, forget it!"

I'm prone to believe that anxiety mobilizes the person, mobilizes the energy to face this enormous life-threatening change, and focuses the energy so the person can cope. Which means, stop trying to calm parents. That's not helpful. ("Mrs. Jones, there's nothing to get excited or agitated about. Why don't you just calm yourself down, and we'll talk.") You know, now you've got an anxious person who feels like a failure on top of it. ("I'm anxious and I can't calm down. They asked me to. You know, it's part of my treatment, I should calm down.") Yet, what if anxiety is needed to mobilize the energy to produce change? Then it means something else.

Depression. Is depression really anger turned inward? Anger about what? Parents of an impaired child get depressed in the service of grieving over the loss of a dream that they associate with the child. There are four words that I'm going to give you (looking them up in the dictionary won't help you one bit): *Competence. Capability. Value. Potency.* What is it to be competent? A capable professional? A valuable human being? A strong person? Could we come up with a unified definition of these four terms so that everybody would say, "We all know what that is, and we're solid on it." Not only couldn't you come up with a unified statement, but the statement you believe today, you yourself might not believe even tomorrow. A 14-year-old would say, "Competent professionals are people who do their jobs with no mistakes." Simple. That's competence. Competence is not making any mistakes. That's what the 14-year-old would say. That's why adolescence is so awful. In contrast, a 40-year-old person might say, "Competence is when you learn from your mistakes." A 60-year-old might say something altogether different.

Whatever definition the person has of competence, capability, value, and strength, it gets challenged when there's a substantive loss. What does the parent say? How can I be a competent parent when I can't fix this? How capable a human being am I when this is throwing me off and I can't seem to hold everything together? Of what value am I if I can't even produce a normal kid? How limited is my potency, my strength as a man or a woman, when this is hurting me so deeply, affecting me so profoundly? People who are depressed are reevaluating their definitions of competence, capability, value, and potency. Parents rework their definitions by coming from the negative side, by interacting with other people, and by saying, "I am an incompetent, incapable, valueless, weak person." A person who is depressed, therefore, does not need a mood elevator, does not need an elbow, does not need a cheer-up, and does not need to hear, "Things are not as bad as you think." What *is* needed is a sensitive other human being to sit and permit the person to verbalize and to struggle with these very personal difficult-to-make definitions.

Guilt. Parents of impaired kids feel and manifest guilt while grieving over the loss of a dream. This issue really bothers our scientific and intellectual sectors. We can get very upset with guilt, because we figure it's very superstitious, stupid, ignorant, and we know that intelligent, intact people don't feel guilt. That's more primitive. Right? Hogwash. We simply cannot accept that our lives are meaningless, that our impact on life is meaningless. To put it another way, you can say to a guilt-ridden parent, "Mr. Smith, the fact that you had an affair prior to conceiving this child has nothing to do with the fact that he has Down's syndrome. Down's syndrome is not influenced by such things. Down's syndrome is a peculiar crossover of chromosomes." We can be scientific about this. Because we know what causes Down's syndrome, don't we? We're pretty sure that we know what makes the chromosome cross over, don't we? We don't? Well, we're pretty sure it's not an affair that does it, aren't we? I think you feel solid about that, don't you? I would hope so!

When we say to a parent, "It's not your fault," here's the answer you could get from a bright and philosophical parent: "Well, if it's not my fault, then I have a question for you. Why should I be humane, or caring, or sensitive, or legal, or ethical, or moral? Why should I be ambitious, committed, or invested because nothing means anything, right? What you're saying is, 'Whether I am or am not any of those things, this stuff just happens.' Is that right? Nothing means anything, is that what you're trying to tell me? The impact of the person I am, the way I've lived, the things I do, and things I don't do have no meaning. Is that correct? Is that what you're trying to tell me?" You say, "Well, no; not exactly. I just mean that this is a discrete error." "Oh, really? How does that work? How can it work that who I am, what I do, the way I behave, the way I live, what I feel, what I think, is totally irrelevant to something so central and important to me. How is it? How do I incorporate that?"

The guilt-ridden person is struggling with his or her meaning, impact, significance in life. There are no easy ways, no easy words to comfort this person. One has to go inside and struggle with guilt and find some significant other person who can listen and relate to the struggle. This is normal and necessary for healthy people; it is not a manifestation of pathology.

There are different ways that guilt shows. There is the parent who says, "I caused my child's handicap; I can tell you how." That person has a story. And some of them are real doozies. How do you deal with people who have kids with fetal alcohol syndrome? What do you do with that parent who walks in and says, "I did it; I did it. The doctor told me not to drink, you know, I mean, well, I got nervous and I always drink, and I didn't think it would matter, and so I drank anyway, and I caused my child's handicap. By the very diagnosis of my child, obviously I did it." What do you say to this parent? I think that what 98 percent of the professionals do is deny the feeling. But denial puts you in a jam and makes interaction very uncomfortable. And a lot of parents are sensitive enough that they'll pick something up. They're expecting something. When parents walk into a clinic with a child diagnosed as having fetal alcohol syndrome, they know that the professionals they'll meet are child advocates and invested in children. And they walk in with a kid who's impaired because of them.

There are other disabilities that are directly created by parents. "I was drinking too much, and I got into a car. They told me I was drinking too much, but I didn't care. We got into the car, we had a car accident, and now my kid's a quadraplegic. I did it." That's a direct "I did it."

Guilt and Denial

The philosophic stance that's been helpful for me and which may be helpful for you is this: There are many points in our lives when we are maladaptive in struggling with something that's difficult for us to deal with, such as difficulties about work, difficulties in our marriage, various difficulties. Then we act out. All of us do things that are dangerous, stupid, and inappropriate at different points in our lives. Some of us get caught. In the case of an impaired child, the question I always like to ask myself and answer once again is: Have I ever met a parent who intended to impair a child?

I've worked with child abusers. I've worked with one of the most horrible cases in the Chicago area, ever. It was child abuse. The mother went into a psychotic state, and when her 2-year-old messed her pants the third time in a row, because she had diarrhea, the mother went berserk, filled the bathtub with scalding hot water, stripped the clothes off the child, and dropped the child in the tub. Ninety percent of the child's body was burned, just a circle of the face untouched. This child was the most severely burned child in the burn unit ever to have survived. I worked with the family. I liked the mother. She's a very nice person, but she had lost it.

Have you lost it sometime? Have you broken something, or gotten physical, or stormed out of the house? Have you done something that you really didn't want to do? Have you been so churned up and so maladapted that, in trying to change something that you couldn't tolerate, you'd do anything?

Did this mother intend to almost destroy her child? She had terrible remorse, awful remorse. I've never met a parent who intended to impair his or her child.

So, when I'm sitting with a parent of a fetal alcohol syndrome child, or anything else like that, I need to quickly remind myself that I've done stupid things too. I don't know why some people get caught and some don't. This woman got caught in a real, awful, hurtful way that affected another human being; but she and the child are still a unit. Each child still needs a parent, and the parent needs that child, for both of them to grow; and my job is human growth. And that's how I deal with these situations, and maybe that can help you. That's one way of dealing with the parent who feels he or she caused a child's handicap.

The second way of manifesting guilt is, "This is punishment for something terrible I have done, thought, or felt. It's a comeuppance for my attitude and actions." Or, the third way, "Good things happen to good people, and bad things happen to bad people." And that's the end of the story. "I'm guilty and ashamed that it happened to me, and that's all there is to it." You don't have to have a big discussion. "I must be bad because it happened to me." End of discussion.

Anger. We have an internalized sense of justice, what we think is fair, right, and proper in this life; not law, but what we think is fair and proper and balanced. When you have an impaired child, inevitably that sense of justice is challenged. It just feels so unfair, and there are parents who say, "Why me? This is wrong. This is unfair. I don't deserve this." When something violates our sense of fairness or justice, we get angry, and we look around for somebody who's going to get it. I'm fairly sophisticated about walking into doors; apparently I do more of it than most people. So if I walk into a door, the first thing I do is do in the door. That goes without saying. You know, I'm walking along, and I'm reading something, and once again, boom. I walk into the den door. The stupid door. You know, I stand there, and then a wonderful, creative thought comes to me. I say, "Who was in the den last?" I'm going to get it out. I'm going to find a way to get it out.

Parents of impaired kids feel their sense of fairness or justice violated. Who violated it? If we get angry at a door, then surely we can find someone or something to get angry at over an impaired child. Parents generally get angry at the impaired child, but most of them have been taught that that's too horrible even to speculate about, so they displace the anger. Guess upon whom—spouses, brothers and sisters of the impaired kid, professionals. Then upon other family members or their best friend who's insensitive or who has a kid the same age. The anger just flows; yet it is serving a purpose. To come out of a crisis on your feet, you have to redefine your sense of justice and fairness. You have to learn how to look at your impaired child and still feel that the world is basically fair and just and okay and safe to live in, that it's worth investing yourself in a thinking fashion. That takes some work.

Grieving, as the process of separating from a significant lost dream, fantasy, or projection into the future, is an internal struggle; but grieving also requires a significant other person to help you in the struggle, to listen to you, to accept your feelings as they are, to acknowledge the legitimacy of your struggle. When you have all these feelings, feelings that a large portion of the culture might designate as pathological, you need someone to validate the feelings as healthy, normal, and indeed even necessary.

How do we do this now on a clinical level? How can we move attitudes to a different level? I would like to address denial, first in terms of intervention and then in terms of structures that can be set up within programs to address these issues in a non-pathological fashion.

Denial permeates the treatment process. Every time there's a new demand made, that demand implies another required change in the parent's life. Every time there is further diagnosis, or a requirement to change behavior around the child's disability, you're going to encounter denial. So you will need some techniques to deal with it. The major one, which has to do with your overall attitude, is that denial is positive and must be accepted as legitimate. Don't try to confront it directly or you'll lose. You may be pushing because you think it's good habilitation to get a hearing aid on a child, but when the parents are denying, they're fighting for their lives. They are saying, "I cannot yet accept that this has happened."

There are four levels of denial. You can trace them developmentally, but that's incidental. Simply recognize that there are four different types of denial that people manifest. You will see them, not only in the areas of dealing with the parents of impaired kids, but in yourself whenever you try to deal with something that's difficult. The first and most obvious is the denial of fact. "Disability? What disability?" You are working with a child who, as best you can determine, has not yet figured out that the sounds made with the mouth might have something to do with communication. Yet the parent is telling you that at home the kid uses a 50-word vocabulary. This is a good example of denial of fact.

Next is denial of implication, which also includes extent and permanence. This form of denial is illustrated by the parent who basically says, "I accept that he's hearing impaired, but he doesn't need to go into a special program. I accept that he's a slower learner than most kids, but that just means it'll just take him a little longer to learn everything that everyone else learns."

Denial of implication is also denial of consequences. "So, I've got an impaired kid, so what? What's the big deal? It's not going to change my life. We're not living in the dark ages, you know. I mean, a hundred years ago, did they have specialists like you folks? Of course not. Why, we have legislation that gives people the right to integrate into society and to have the least restrictive environment possible, and there are handicapped parking spaces all over the place, and new medical breakthroughs, and attitudes have changed all over the place. So what's the big deal?" That's denial of consequence.

The last is denial of feeling. "Yes, I have an impaired child. Yes, it's awful. Yes, it's difficult. Yes, it's permanent. Yes, it's going to be a big struggle. But it doesn't matter. It just doesn't upset me. I'm just that kind of person, you know what I mean? I don't know what there is to get so upset about. And you keep looking at me like I should be upset that I have a child like this. Are you waiting for me to cry or something? I don't know why people make such a big deal about this." This represents severance from feeling. It's the continuity in the way human beings interact with the world and with change. There are three simple components: you feel something; you think something; and then you act. Jumble that sequence around and you've got trouble. To figure you can act before you think often gets you into trouble. It usually then goes: act, feel, and think. When people get into a denial struggle they jumble that order. They don't permit the order to work.

For you to get a habilitation program off the ground with the child or parent, you need some systems in your diagnostic structure, or in your ongoing treatment structure, to deal with denial. First, recognize denial and have an attitude of acceptance. There is a different type of intervention for each level of denial, and this has strong implications for your skills and what you can do. To address denial of fact, continually, relentlessly, verbally, and through writing, accumulate facts and then sensitively and gently present to the parent those facts as you know them. Continue even though they are telling you that they don't want to hear them and don't understand them. Here is where your sensitivity, your humor, your sense of how human beings deal with the "undealable" comes in. Don't distort the facts. Don't soften them. I always love it when clinicians and teachers ask me, "How do you tell people bad news? What's the best way to tell them so that it won't upset them?" It's absurd!

The Facts, Please

My favorite joke about unpleasant facts deals with the Marine sergeant who gets a telegram at morning muster that one of his men's father had died—Frank Smith's father. All right, so, at the end of muster, he says, "Smith, step front and center. Your father's dead." A lieutenant standing by the side says, "Oh, my God! Oh, my God!" He pulls the sergeant aside, and he says, "Sergeant, you can't do that. You can't just pull a guy out of line and say, 'Your father died,' just like that. You've got to have some sensitivity. You've got to share bad news with a little finesse, a little sensitivity. You know what I mean?" Four months later, Jones's mother dies. The sergeant gets a telegram. At the end of morning muster, he stands in front of the men and shouts. He says, "All men with surviving mothers, one step forward. Not so fast, Jones." Maybe it softened it for him, I don't know. Like I say, we get like that. We get real funny. We deal with people like they're crazy.

How do I tell this mother, who already had a diagnosis for her child of retardation or some other developmental disability, that now we've found a hearing impairment? Oh, God. How am I going to tell these parents? You walk in like someone should throw a net over you. You're acting really weird. "Comfortable? Want some coffee? That's a pretty dress. Pretty dress. I remember an aunt once had a dress like that." And in your head, "Oh God, I hope they just guess it and save themselves. Somebody ought to help me with this. Where's the psychologist when you need him?" That doesn't help.

Be simple, succinct, and clear. Forget all the verbiage. Forget all the test data. Just deal with the facts: "We've done the testing. Your child has a serious hearing loss." If, indeed, the diagnosis is deafness, "Your child is deaf." Stop. Don't go over the audiogram or explain how we test hearing or discuss speech frequencies or. . . . Forget it. Special education and amplification? Forget it. They don't want to hear it. At that moment, they're likely at the level of denial of fact. Politely make your next appointment when they have enough time to gain some internal strength and external support to start to deal with it. Unless of course, they ask you for more; then share more information. But this business of dumping all the details on people often is just to handle our own anxiety. We then get irritated with them, and we call them "deniers" when they come back and they don't remember any of the details. Please, keep putting yourself in the position of the parent who cannot accept bad news at this point. You've got to do some work to prepare the system for it. Denial of fact is dealt with by sharing facts openly.

Sometimes one needs to take a familiar circumstance and say to the parent, "Okay, during the day, when the doorbell rings and the dog gets up and runs to the door and the brother or sister runs, well, what does Billy do?"

"Well, Billy's not very sociable, so Billy doesn't care who's at the door."

"I see. So Billy doesn't get up and go to the door?"

"Well, no. It has nothing to do . . . I mean, he hears fine; it has everything to do with the fact that he's just . . . he never was a very social kid. In the beginning, when I would come up to the crib, he'd never smile for me or anything; he was just like that."

"I see, I see. Does Billy like to eat? Does he like food?"

"Oh, yeah. He's kind of a chowhound."

"Do you ever let Billy lick the bowl when you're making cookies or whipped cream or something like that?"

"Yeah."

"Does Billy come in the kitchen when you turn on the beater?"

What you're doing is just gradually introducing fact after fact for the parent to keep evaluating as the diagnosis very gradually starts to sink in. Continue until there are too many facts to maintain denial of fact. It takes a lot of skill and time, and I'm sure you think that you've got better things to do. Very gently and creatively present the facts in ways the parents can understand. Not your facts from instruments, from tests, and from observations. Who cares? They'll get back by saying, "I know someone who graduated from your school. As a matter of fact, I think it was a cum laude. He was recently arrested for fraudulent behavior and fined severely for improper and unprofessional stuff." A lot of parents are suspicious of people who graduate from a university. So get them to deal with the facts, but the facts from their vantage point.

Denial of implication often is best dealt with by exposure to similarly disabled individuals. For example, professionals who work with parents of hearing-impaired kids can arrange discussions with panels of deaf adults or exposure to individual deaf adults. Please, don't bring out all of the glowing successes—the presidents of companies, the architects, and the Ph.D.s. Bring ordinary people like the parents themselves so they can see the inherent implications. Also, there are audiotapes and records available which simulate various degrees of hearing loss. Such recordings are very useful when discussing the implications of an impairment. If you've ever used such materials with a parent, you have seen their denial cracking. You have to be very gentle and be prepared to give them more information that's constructive and habilitative as the denial starts coming down. They may understand the audiogram and have the hearing aid on the kid, but they may still be denying the implications. "That's just a high frequency hearing loss. So what? You know, so you can't hear birds. So what?" All of a sudden they realize: "Oh, my God!"

With denial of consequence, parents also are denying feelings. You have to encourage the parent to talk in a very self-centered way about feelings—my feelings; what's happened to my life; what's so hard about it; what hurts; what's been lost; what's been disrupted; how the marriage, how the work are going.

Let me just give you a structure of three strategies that I have found useful for families experiencing denial, anxiety, and all the other grieving states. While the three parts obviously overlap, I think they should be kept conceptually separate; they deal with different programs, and I think they should go in order.

Number one is parent education. These programs, incidentally, should not be voluntary or required; they should be part of the program just like six-month evaluations are part of your program. Parent education involves giving information. It should be step one because you're most likely dealing with denying parents. A lot of denying parents will deny the facts and their implication. So you want them to have information. Here's where you have different professionals come to talk with parents each week. They have a once-a-week meeting for whatever number of weeks you want—8 weeks, 12 weeks, etc. They may come in on Wednesdays while their child is in the program, or they may come in the evening. During such meetings, the audiologist and the speech/ language pathologist come in to discuss hearing loss and communication, the psychologist comes in and talks about emotional development, the physician comes in and talks about medical implications, and the lawyer comes in and talks about advocacy. You provide all of the information. Every single one of the speakers should have printed handouts. Let parents take these home, because when they are frankly denying, they're not going to hear it. If they take materials home, later on they'll sneak a peek.

Second is parent groups (I don't like to call them counseling groups because that implies pathology). Here parents can share their feelings on having an impaired child. The ideal group, frankly, is run by a paraprofessional parent, thereby wiping clean the implication of pathology. Your psychologist, social worker, or psychiatrist should be a consultant to whom? All of you. Consultant to. And if you identify a parent who is pathological, there's your referral resource. But this parent group is oriented to feelings of the parents. No discussion about kids. If the parent comes in and says, "I don't understand how one hearing aid does this and the other one does that and . . . ," a good response by the person running that group is, "You seem concerned about your ability to handle your kid's problems." It is not, "Oh, well, the behind-the-ear model is. . . ." That's not what that group is for.

The parent group is second because it implies that the denial of fact will have moved to the denial of feelings, and that you are pushing into anxiety and then all the other feelings which you want to be able to talk about in an 8- to 12-week period of time. Your goal is that, in the parent education process, you will have broken through enough so that parents can now experience and share those feelings openly.

Third is parent training, and don't start this earlier. This is when you train your parents to become active members in the habilitation process. This is when you train parents to do language stimulation. You teach them sign language. You teach them auditory training. Whatever it is, whatever the philosophy. Without the first two steps, however, parents can't do this. It's like asking a person to swim before that person has defined the need to swim. "Swim? I'm ten thousand miles away from water. Why should I learn how to swim?"

So the recommended sequence is parent education, then parent groups focusing on the feelings, and, finally, parent training. This conceptual framework begins with the assumption that parents and children are inseparable and that professionals and parents are most commonly separated by the emotional states that parents exhibit when they are grieving over a dream shattered by having an impaired child. To the extent that you can accept the legitimacy, reasonableness, and indeed the habilitative element of the grieving itself, your attitudes will change. With that change, you can start to put together a holistic program that helps parents while working cooperatively with the child.

Part III

Profiling Potential: Tools of the Team

Chapter 7

The Pediatrician's Role in Early Identification

Ronald S. Fischler

When a child is referred for a comprehensive developmental evaluation, someone—the pediatrician, family physician, teacher, or family—has suspected that a problem exists. Parents may have heard conflicting information from previous physicians, other professionals, friends, or relatives; as a result, they typically have a number of fears. Most families want answers to these questions: (1) Is there a problem? (2) What is the nature of the problem—its name or diagnostic "label," severity, and extent? (3) What caused it and was it preventable? (4) What can we expect in the future? (5) What is the best treatment? (6) What do we need to do?

The physician's role involves characterizing the problems, formulating a medical diagnosis, determining the cause, looking for medically or surgically treatable conditions, and identifying conditions with genetic implications that can be prevented in subsequent offspring. In addition, the physician searches for associated medical complications, assesses the family's understanding and adjustment to their handicapped child, and participates in interdisciplinary treatment and follow-up (Table 1).

Table 1. Role of the Developmental Pediatrician in Interdisciplinary Assessment

1. Establishing a medical diagnosis.

2. Conducting a search for cause, particularly for conditions that are medically or surgically treatable or have genetic implications.

3. Evaluating the child's general health status, with attention to detecting the presence of preventable or treatable complications.

4. Ascertaining the family's understanding and adjustment to caring for the handicapped child.

5. Participating in interdisciplinary efforts aimed at optimizing the outcome for the child and his or her family, utilizing available medical and nonmedical treatment modalities in the community.

6. Following up the child's health and developmental status, the family's adjustment, and the appropriateness of treatment, in conjunction with other members of the interdisciplinary team.

Over the past 10 to 20 years, there have been numerous significant medical advances that positively affect handicapped children and their families. These include improved curative health services, such as neonatal intensive care units that now enable many premature infants to survive. While the outlook for the majority of such infants is excellent, a significant number have permanent residual handicaps. In addition, medical treatment for many chronic and previously fatal diseases, such as spina bifida, cystic fibrosis, and cancer, has improved and has resulted in prolonged survival, although some of these children have persistent handicaps.

Improvements in preventative health services have also occurred. Immunizations for mumps, rubella, polio, measles, and other childhood diseases have markedly reduced their frequency and thus prevented their handicapping effects on children. The discovery of Rh-immune globulin has resulted in a marked reduction of kernicterus due to Rh incompatibility of the newborn, a condition which often leads to sensorineural hearing loss and athetoid cerebral palsy. Such treatable metabolic diseases as phenylketonuria (PKU) and hypothyroidism are now routinely screened for at birth before the manifestations are evident, leading to early treatment and the prevention of later handicaps.

Advances in clinical genetics enable many conditions to be identified before pregnancy in potential carriers of genetic diseases or in early pregnancy by amniocentesis. Genetic counseling based on the results of such studies assists families in making informed choices in order to reduce the number of children born with serious genetic handicaps. The recent development of sophisticated ultrasound imaging permits detection of a number of major birth defects, and, in a few cases, has even led to treatment in utero (Frigoletto et al., 1982).

Improvements in rehabilitation services have also occurred. Some of these involve medical advances, such as restorative, orthopedic, plastic, ENT, and urological surgical procedures. Other advances include new hearing devices, educational interventions beginning in infancy, and improved understanding of how children with handicaps and their families cope. Over the past decade, such legal mandates as the Education for All Handicapped Children Act (Public Law 94-142) have created a continuum of services in most communities that include early screening, diagnostic procedures, and an array of treatment services and social supports, so that most handicapped children can be cared for at home, attend public school, and receive modern interventions to help them compensate for handicaps and improve their lives and their family's adjustment. In 1982, representatives from four major professional organizations (the American Speech-Language-Hearing Association, American Academy of Pediatrics, American Academy of Otolaryngology, and the American Nurses Association) developed an expanded position statement to identify infants at risk for hearing impairment. This is another example of improvements in preventative and rehabilitative management of the individual at risk for developmental disability (see Appendix to this chapter).

In order to combine highly specialized assessment and interventions with a holistic concern for the family, multidisciplinary diagnostic teams have formed. As a result, a new category of physician has emerged, the developmental pediatrician, specially trained to deal with developmental and behavior problems.

This chapter will present an overview of medical factors in the assessment of hearing-impaired developmentally disabled children. The goal is to present the essence of a modern medical approach in the context of an interdisciplinary model. For greater depth and detail on individual disorders, which are beyond the scope of this chapter, the reader is referred to recently published references and texts (Bergsma, 1973; Jaffe, 1977; Konigsmark & Gorlin, 1976; Smith, 1978).

Types, Frequency, and Causes of Childhood Hearing Impairment and Disabilities

A vast number of conditions may cause childhood disabilities with hearing impairment. It has been estimated over a 15-year period that more than 30 percent of the hearing-impaired population has other disabilities as well; current data (see Chapter 3) reflect the heterogeneity of the population of hearing-impaired developmentally disabled children (Gentile & McCarthy, 1973; Gordon et al., 1982).

In defining both the nature and cause of an individual child's disability, the physician seeks to ascertain when the condition had its onset. Conditions that arise during pregnancy are grouped into *prenatal causes.* Those that arise due to insults during labor and delivery are termed *perinatal;* and those that develop after birth, *postnatal. Congenital* handicaps are those present at birth (thus encompassing the prenatal and perinatal periods).

Childhood handicaps including hearing impairment are also grouped by whether the etiology has genetic or nongenetic basis. Genetic conditions arise in the prenatal period and account for approximately 30 to 40 percent of cases, nongenetic conditions for approximately 30 percent, and conditions of unknown etiology (termed *idiopathic*) for approximately 30 percent (Northern & Downs, 1978; see Table 2).

Table 2. Timing and Causes of Childhood Disabilities with Hearing Impairment

Prenatal onset (approximately 40 percent of cases)	Postnatal onset (approximately 10 percent of cases)
Genetic syndromes	Trauma — accidental/child abuse
Intrauterine infections	Infections
Teratogens	Tumors
Maternal illnesses	
	Idiopathic (unknown cause; approximately 30 percent of cases)
Perinatal onset (approximately 20 percent of cases)	
Birth trauma	
Anoxia/asphyxia	
Kernicterus	
Infections	
Prematurity	

Ascertaining the cause or etiology of childhood handicap is important for several reasons. First, a small but significant number of conditions are medically or surgically treatable or correctable. Second, conditions that are genetically determined may be preventable in subsequent offspring by techniques of prenatal diagnosis and genetic counseling with selective termination of pregnancy when fetuses are affected. Third, the search for etiology also aids families in their adjustment to caring for their handicapped child. Even if a specific etiology cannot be found, many causes can be ruled out, which may help to relieve families of guilt. Knowing the diagnosis and etiology also may yield information on associated complications and on prognosis. Because of the variability of most conditions, statements of prognosis are usually estimates. Thus, caution must be exercised, and early prediction must be modified after follow-up of each child's progress during treatment.

Prenatal Causes of Childhood Disabilities and Hearing Impairment

Genetic Syndromes. Genetic syndromes make up most but not all conditions having their onset in the prenatal period. A syndrome is a grouping of particular signs and symptoms into a recognizable pattern. Approximately 3 to 5 percent of all newborn infants have one or more major birth defects (congenital malformations). Most of these are genetic in origin, but some arise because of congenital infections or toxic exposures, others are from unknown causes. Genetic causes of profound hearing impairment occur in 1 of every 2,000 live births and account for approximately 50 percent of cases of profound childhood hearing losses (Konigsmark & Gorlin, 1976). Most genetic hearing loss is sensorineural rather than conductive.

Accurate diagnosis of a genetic cause of hearing loss and related handicaps is important in order to provide the family with information on recurrence risk in subsequent offspring and to determine whether prenatal diagnosis is available. Prenatal diagnosis may involve *amniocentesis,* which means the removal, at 16 to 20 weeks' gestation, of a small amount of amniotic fluid that bathes the fetus. Special tests are then performed to determine whether the fetus is affected by a specific genetic abnormality. Hundreds of genetic conditions can now be diagnosed in this manner, with the number rising each year, although very few causes of hearing loss can be diagnosed prenatally at present. Parents who learn that their fetus is affected may opt to terminate the pregnancy. The goal of genetic counseling is to provide accurate information to families affected by genetic conditions so that they may make informed decisions concerning their reproduction. Facts must be stated in terms that the family can understand, and counselors must take care not to impose their values. Families with handicapped children often experience a mourning process in their adjustment to caring for their disabled child (see Chapter 6); those families with children having genetic abnormalities have been noted to feel particularly guilty (Jackson & Schimke, 1978). Whether this is also true for parents who are themselves disabled is yet to be explored.

Genetic causes are subdivided into three categories with differing inheritance risks: single mutant gene disorders, chromosomal abnormalities, and multifactorial genetic disorders (Table 3).

Table 3. Genetic Syndromes: Categories and Examples

Single Mutant Gene Disorders	Chromosomal Abnormalities
Autosomal Dominant	Trisomy 13
Alport's syndrome	No. 18 Long Arm Deletion syndrome
Waardenburg's syndrome	Down's syndrome (Trisomy 21)
Treacher Collins' syndrome	
Deafness alone	**Multifactorial (Polygenic) Disorders**
Autosomal Recessive	Cleft lip/palate
Pendred's syndrome	Spina bifida
Usher's syndrome	
Hurler's syndrome	
Deafness alone	
X-Linked	
Hunter's syndrome	
Deafness alone	

As a brief review, it should be kept in mind that genes are composed of DNA and are arranged on chromosomes, which are contained in every living cell of the body. Human chromosomes consist of 23 pairs (46 all together) including two sex chromosomes, the X and Y. Children receive one of each pair of chromosomes from the mother and one from the father. Males receive, in addition, the Y chromosome from the father and the X from the mother. Females receive one X chromosome from each parent.

Single Mutant Gene Disorders. Single mutant gene disorders account for approximately 80 percent of genetic abnormalities. Well over one thousand single mutant genes have been identified, the number rising each year. The patterns of inheritance of single gene disorders were described by Mendel and follow autosomal dominant, autosomal recessive, or X-linked inheritance patterns (Jackson & Schimke, 1979).

A dominant condition requires that only one gene in the pair be heterozygous, with one abnormal gene and one normal gene. Variability in the severity of a dominantly inherited condition is frequent and is referred to as varying *penetrance.* Autosomal dominant conditions are passed on to 50 percent of the offspring. The family history will reveal either that the disorder is present in one parent or that it is not present at all in the family, which indicates that the gene represents a new spontaneous mutation. In such cases, the parents have no increased recurrence risk for subsequent children, but the affected child will pass the disorder on to 50 percent of his or her offspring. An example of an autosomal dominant condition is Alport's syndrome (hereditary deafness with nephritis). Dominant causes of childhood deafness account for approximately 10 percent of cases of profound childhood hearing impairment (Jaffe, 1977; Konigsmark & Gorlin, 1976).

A recessive condition requires both genes of the pair to be abnormal, a homozygous state. Both parents are carriers (heterozygous) and generally have no symptoms. Each contributes an abnormal gene to the affected child. Autosomal recessive inheritance patterns imply that 50 percent of the offspring will be carriers (like the parents), 25 percent will be affected, and 25 percent will be normal. Recessive conditions are generally more severe than dominantly inherited ones, and they account for approximately 40 percent of profound childhood hearing loss (Jaffe, 1977). This pattern of inheritance clusters in siblings with apparently normal parents and is much more likely to occur in the offspring of matings between blood relatives (consanguineous matings). For some recessive conditions, such as sickle cell anemia or Tay-Sachs disease, it is possible to detect carriers by blood tests. Prenatal diagnosis is also available for a number of these conditions. Because so many different recessive conditions may cause hearing loss, marriage between two deaf individuals does not necessarily result in a high risk that their offspring will also be deaf. Other examples of recessive conditions include Usher's syndrome (congenital deafness and retinitis pigmentosa) and Pendred's syndrome (hearing loss and goiter).

X-linked (sex-linked) conditions are inherited on the X chromosome and may follow a dominant or recessive inheritance pattern. X-linked dominant conditions are rare and affect both males and females. Most X-linked disorders are recessive; females with two X chromosomes are thus heterozygous and appear normal but carry the abnormal gene; males with only one X chromosome are affected by the disorder. A carrier female passes the gene to 50 percent of her sons, who manifest the disorder, and to 50 percent of her daughters, who become carriers like herself. In X-linked conditions there is a lack of male-to-male transmission and a "skipping" of generations. X-linked disorders account for approximately 3 percent of severe childhood deafness (Jaffe, 1977). Hunter's syndrome, which includes skeletal abnormalities, is an example of a mucopolysaccharidosis syndrome with X-linked inheritance.

Chromosomal Abnormalities. A second type of genetic disorder occurs as the result of abnormalities in small or large segments of the chromosomes, each of which contains many genes. Abnormalities of chromosomes may occur either during meiosis, the process of cell division resulting in the formation of germ cells (egg or sperm), or during mitosis, the cell division that occurs in the fertilized egg or embryo. During these delicate cell reproductive processes, chromosomes may be broken, deleted, duplicated, or rearranged. Recent advances in clinical genetics have made it possible to use special staining techniques (banding) to examine individual chromosomes from blood, skin, or amniotic fluid under the microscope and to display them as karyotypes. The number and configurations of chromosomes define specific disorders. Chromosomal abnormalities occur in about 1 of every 200 live births; the commonest is trisomy 21 (Down's syndrome), which involves an extra number 21 chromosome. In general, chromosomal abnormalities result in multiple congenital malformations evident at birth. While both genetic causes and nongenetic causes (such as congenital infections or toxic exposures) can also produce multiple malformations, the presence of the malformations ordinarily signals the need to examine the chromosomes.

The inheritance risk of chromosomal disorders increases with parental age and depends on whether the parents' chromosomes are normal. Parents with a "balanced translocation" configuration in their chromosomes may have a 15 to 100 percent risk that subsequent children will be affected; parents with normal chromosomes may have only 1 to 3 percent recurrence risk (Jackson & Schimke, 1979). Since chromosomes from the fetus may be obtained by amniocentesis, prenatal diagnosis affords accurate prediction of whether the fetus has a chromosomal abnormality or not. Amniocentesis is routinely offered to all mothers over 35 years old and to families who have had a child affected with a chromosomal abnormality.

Multifactorial (Polygenic) Inheritance Patterns. Many defects are not inherited in the patterns described so far, but cluster more frequently in certain families than in the general population. It is postulated that multiple genes contribute to causing such abnormalities. Recurrence risk is relatively low (3 to 5 percent) but increases with the number of affected individuals in the family (Jackson & Schimke, 1979). Cleft lip and palate, spina bifida, and congenital heart disease are examples of disorders with polygenic inheritance patterns.

Toxins/Drugs/X-Ray Exposure/Maternal Disease. Certain drugs ingested by the mother during pregnancy have been associated with birth defects, including hearing loss. The most widely known of these drugs is Thalidomide, associated with limb and ear deformities. Antibiotics of the aminoglycoside group (Kanamycin, Gentamycin, Neomycin, Streptomycin) have caused ototoxicity to mothers and sensorineural hearing loss in their infants, although this is rarely reported. Moderate to heavy alcohol use during pregnancy may cause multiple malformations, growth deficiency, and retardation, although hearing loss has not been reported as a sequela.

Exposure to X rays or radioactive materials during early pregnancy has resulted in microcephaly and congenital malformations, although hearing loss has not been specifically described. Environmental toxins, such as lead or mercury, are associated with birth defects but not specifically hearing loss.

Such maternal metabolic illness as PKU or thyroid disorders may adversely affect the fetus. Offspring of mothers with PKU are nearly always retarded. Offspring of diabetic mothers show a greater number of congenital malformations. Other maternal diseases or medicines used to treat them may have adverse effects on a developing fetus. Diseases that compromise blood flow to the placenta (placental abruption, toxemia) may result in fetal brain damage.

Intrauterine Infections. Certain infections of the mother that occur at critical times during pregnancy may cross the placental barrier and invade fetal tissues. The fetal brain, liver, cochlea, and numerous other organ systems may be adversely affected, resulting in malformations, growth deficiency, or malfunction. All of these infections produce a broad spectrum of signs and symptoms. Some are clinically recognizable at birth, others may produce nonspecific multiple malformations. The diagnosis of intrauterine infection is determined by culturing the offending organism or detecting specific antibodies in the infant's blood. As a group, congenital infections are an important cause of childhood malformations and hearing impairment. Recent medical advances have brought several of them under control. These infections are commonly denoted by the acronym STORCH: Syphilis, Toxoplasmosis, Rubella, Cytomegalovirus, and Herpes Simplex.

Congenital syphilis is a rare cause of malformations today. Caused by a spirochete, syphilis in the mother invades fetal tissues during the second and third trimester and produces low grade infection that progresses quietly over years until it is detected. Clinical manifestations of congenital syphilis in the newborn period include nasal discharge, rash, anemia, jaundice, and bone defects. In late childhood, saddle nose, abnormal teeth, saber-shaped shins, and perforated palate may appear along with sensorineural deafness, vestibular dysfunction, mental retardation, and other neurological findings. Treatment with penicillin, ideally of the mother during pregnancy, prevents the development of these manifestations. All mothers who receive prenatal care are screened for syphilis with a blood test during pregnancy.

Congenital toxoplasmosis infects the mother during the first or second trimester with the protozoan *toxoplasma gondii* and may produce a flu-like syndrome with invasion of the fetus causing meningitis, hepatitis, and chorioretinitis. The newborn may show a skin rash, jaundice, seizures, calcification noted on skull X ray, small head, blindness, deafness, mental retardation, spasticity, and convulsions. The diagnosis rests on clinical suspicion and on specific blood tests. Treatment with sulfa antibiotics may alter the course of this disease. Avoidance by pregnant mothers of raw meat and roaming cats may prevent contact with the disease.

Congenital rubella is a once common viral infection occurring in epidemics and producing malformations in the fetus when the mother is infected during the first or second trimester. As recently as the 1960s epidemic, 10 to 20 thousand children were born with congenital rubella syndrome, which accounted for approximately 10 percent of congenital hearing loss. Since the advent of the rubella vaccine (now given routinely at 15 months), the number of cases has fallen dramatically. Mothers with rubella may experience a rash and fever or may be entirely without symptoms. Affected infants show a variety of defects, including malformations of the heart (50 percent), cataracts or glaucoma (40 percent), mental retardation, microcephaly (40 percent), sensorineural hearing loss, autism, and growth deficiency. Newborns may show a transient skin rash and jaundice. The diagnosis is usually made by obtaining serial antibody measurements from mothers and infants. All mothers are routinely screened for rubella antibody during pregnancy.

Cytomegalovirus is a ubiquitous agent that produces no symptoms in the majority of infected individuals but may produce congenital malformations and hearing loss when the mother and fetus are infected during early pregnancy. Approximately 20 percent of pregnant mothers and 1 percent of newborns harbor the virus. Fortunately, only 5 percent of infected infants develop symptomatic manifestations, which resemble those of congenital rubella and toxoplasmosis. These include rash, hepatitis, meningoencephalitis with intracranial calcifications, sensorineural hearing loss, and chorioretinitis. Long-term residua include hearing loss, blindness, mental retardation, microcephaly, spasticity, seizures, growth deficiency, and a variety of other malformations. For infants who acquire the virus at or after birth, the outcome is usually benign, although some reports of progressive deafness, learning disability, and other neurologic manifestations have appeared. At present there is no known effective treatment or preventative strategy. There is a risk of recurrence in subsequent offspring, but, fortunately, the risk is low.

Herpes simplex virus infections (either type 1–oral or type 2–genital) generally produce skin ulcers in the mothers. Direct contact during passage through the birth canal or after birth may infect the fetus and produce an overwhelming and usually fatal infection. Survivors generally have major neurologic sequelae. Delivery by caesarean section for mothers who have active infections appears to prevent the neonatal disease. The use of new antiviral medications offers some promise in the treatment of this devastating disease.

Perinatal Causes

Birth Trauma and Prematurity. Perinatal causes of childhood handicap include birth trauma and diseases of the neonate that result in damage to the brain or such other structures as the cochlea or middle ear structures.

A number of conditions can deprive the fetus of oxygenated blood during the course of labor and delivery, long enough for permanent brain damage to occur (three to six minutes). These include premature separations (abruptions) of the placenta, toxemia, and compression of the umbilical cord. Difficult forceps deliveries can result in skull fractures, with damage to the brain and middle ear structures. Distressed full-term infants may aspirate at birth and develop a severe pneumonia (meconium aspiration). Premature infants with immature lungs may develop respiratory distress syndrome (hyaline membrane disease), and some of them develop complications, including brain hemorrhage, chronic lung disease, and blindness due to toxicity from oxygen on immature eyes (a condition known as retrolental fibroplasia or, more recently, as retinopathy of prematurity).

Severe jaundice, the accumulation of the pigment bilirubin in the bloodstream, may result in brain damage called kernicterus. Symptoms include irritability, abnormal posturing, a shrill cry, sensorineural impairment, and later mental retardation with athetoid cerebral palsy. In the past, kernicterus occurred principally as the result of Rh incompatibility. The advent of Rh-immune globulin (Rhogam) and the development of phototherapy, with close monitoring of blood bilirubin levels, has resulted in the near disappearance of this form of kernicterus. Today, kernicterus is seen primarily in critically ill premature infants and appears to bear no relationship to bilirubin levels, making prevention difficult. In the past, there was considerable controversy as to whether bilirubin levels in the high normal range (less than 20) could cause learning disabilities and hearing loss. At present there appears to be little support for this belief (Levine & Maisels, 1983).

Premature infants have a greater likelihood of suffering complications than full-term infants (Behrman & Vaughan, 1983), and the risk is inversely related to size and gestational age (Table 4, page 110). With the advent of computerized tomographic (CT; noninvasive techniques of examining brain anatomy) and ultrasound scanning, it is evident that as many as 40 percent of premature infants suffer cerebral hemorrhage (often without evident symptoms), and there is considerable variability in prognosis. Some children even with severe hemorrhage may have a normal outcome.

Infections and Ototoxic Antibiotics. Infections of the newborn, particularly bacterial meningitis caused by Group B streptococcus or E. coli, continue to be associated

Table 4. Outcome for Premature Infants 1975-79

Birth Weight *(grams)*	Gestational Age *(weeks)*	Mortality (%)	Survivor Handicapped (%)
750-1000	26-29	80	20-55
1000-1500	29-32	20	19
1500	32	10	12

with high rates of neurologic sequelae including sensorineural hearing loss. In addition, antibiotics of the aminoglycoside group (Kanamycin, Gentamycin) are known to be ototoxic. However, with careful monitoring of blood levels, ototoxicity is rarely seen. As discussed previously, neonatal herpes simplex can cause a devastating infection of newborns with high mortality and severe neurologic residua in most survivors.

Postnatal Causes

Trauma continues to be a leading cause of childhood morbidity and mortality. Injuries may be accidental and involve motor vehicles or serious falls. Near-drowning is also a common cause of childhood brain damage resulting in chronic handicap. Non-accidental trauma from child abuse may involve violent shaking or direct blunt trauma to the head. With basilar skull fracture, direct injury to the cochlea may occur, leading to sensorineural deafness. It is hoped that efforts to educate the public on home and water safety, use of car seats for babies, and parenting skills will reduce the number of these preventable causes of childhood handicaps.

Infections, particularly bacterial meningitis caused by hemophilus influenza, neisseria meningitis, and pneumococcus, lead to permanent neurologic residua in approximately one-third of cases and to sudden sensorineural hearing loss in approximately 5 to 10 percent. Viral encephalitis may also lead to brain damage and hearing loss. Mumps during childhood is probably the most common infectious cause of acquired hearing loss. Although mumps is generally a benign illness, it may lead to unilateral sensorineural hearing loss in approximately 5 percent of cases and, rarely, to bilateral loss. Since the advent of the mumps vaccine (given routinely at 15 months), this infection is now rare.

Tumors of the brain or brainstem are rare but may cause progressive loss of mental and motor function, behavioral changes, seizures, headache, vomiting, paralysis, and hearing loss when they involve areas of the brain involved in hearing.

Loud noise, although not a cause of multiple handicaps, may induce transient or permanent sensorineural hearing loss. It may occur after one-time exposure but is more likely to occur after chronic exposure. Concern has been raised about the risk to infants in incubators who experience relatively loud background noise for days, weeks, or months (Bess, Peek, & Chapman, 1979). At the present time, however, it does not appear that this is a clinically significant cause of acquired hearing impairment.

In the past, episodes of high fever (as occurred with scarlet fever) were thought to be ototoxic; at present, most fevers that result with common illnesses are not considered hazardous. Fevers greater than 108°F (42°C) are apt to be associated with neurological sequelae including hearing loss. Fever may be indicative of an underlying neurological infection, such as meningitis or encephalitis, that sometimes may not be clinically recognized.

Medically Treatable Complications

In addition to making a specific diagnosis and conducting a search for cause, the physician is also concerned with assessing general health status and detecting any medically treatable complications. While the list of potential complications is long and depends on the specific underlying condition, the most common complications are listed in Table 5.

Table 5. Common Medically Treatable Complications in Disabled Children

Nutritional problems—failure to thrive (undernutrition); obesity; vitamin/mineral deficiencies

Vision problems—strabismus, refractive errors, cataracts

Hearing problems—otitis media

Dental problems, feeding problems

Seizures

Heart problem (if congenital heart disease present)

Asthma

Aspiration pneumonia

Reflux esophagitis

Constipation

Scoliosis

Joint contractures and deformities

Kidney malformation (especially in conjunction with abnormalities of external ears)

Acute otitis media is the most common infection during childhood. More than two-thirds of all children experience at least one episode by age five. Otitis media is most common in the first two years of life, and episodes decrease in most children as they grow older. Approximately 20 percent of children experience a recurrent course with frequent episodes every few weeks or months and are often referred to as "otitis prone" (Paradise, 1980). Episodes are caused by bacterial infection (and to a much lesser extent by viruses) and usually follow viral upper respiratory infections. Bacteria such as pneumococcus, hemophilus influenza, and streptococcus are the usual offenders and produce symptoms of ear pain, irritability, fever, and a self-limited illness lasting several days. Otitis media may rarely cause such severe complications as meningitis and mastoiditis.

Approximately 30 percent of children are found to have middle ear fluid following a bout of otitis media or on routine examination. Such children have serous otitis media, which, unlike acute otitis media, generally causes no symptoms. In the past, it was thought that this fluid was sterile; however, it is now clear that bacteria are present approximately half the time, although it is not clear whether serous otitis is an infectious problem (Paradise, 1980). Allergy is also thought to play a role, as are abnormal function of the Eustachian tube and possible blockage by enlarged adenoids. Children who drink from a bottle while supine are also thought to be at higher risk for both acute otitis and serous otitis. Serous otitis media resolves spontaneously in one month (60 percent of the cases) but may persist for periods longer than four months (5 percent of the cases). Some surveys reveal serous fluid and Type B or C tympanograms in nearly 30 percent of randomly studied children (Bluestone et al., 1983). Decongestants and antihistamines, while frequently prescribed, have not been shown to be of benefit, although antibiotics may speed resolution (Paradise, 1980).

In recent years, considerable controversy has surrounded the significance of serous otitis and recurrent otitis media. Although rare, these conditions may lead to complications such as cholesteatoma (a benign tumor of the middle ear) or chronic perforation of the eardrum (chronic otitis media). Much more commonly, fluid in the middle ear space is associated with borderline normal, mild, or moderate conductive hearing loss, and a number of studies have suggested that this degree of hearing loss may impair language development and lead to learning difficulties in some children (Paradise, 1981). Some authors suggest that these effects may be greater in children with handicaps or in children from understimulating environments than in healthy children from stimulating environments. Although those studies have been criticized (Paradise, 1981; Ventry, 1980), for those individuals with permanent sensorineural hearing impairment, the additional loss due to middle ear complications can have detrimental effect on hearing aid usage as well as on language learning and academic performance.

For children with recurrent bouts of acute otitis media, avoidance of bottle propping and the use of low dose continuous antibiotic have been of benefit in reducing numbers of attacks. As mentioned earlier, decongestants and antihistamines have not been beneficial (O'Shea et al., 1982). In the light of current uncertainty, it appears prudent that normal children with normal language development be followed medically and audiologically. Children who are at high risk for language problems should be aggressively managed with early ENT referral for consideration of ventilating tubes and/or adenoidectomy. These include children with recurrent otitis media who do not improve with prophylactic antibiotics; children with persistent serous otitis and language delay, moderate hearing loss, or visual or mental handicaps; and children from understimulating environments.

Conduct of the Medical Assessment

Preparation for Evaluation. To make the most productive use of professional time in the conduct of the interdisciplinary evaluation, it is prudent to have an administrative assistant or member of the diagnostic team serve as case manager and collect relevant data on the child to be assessed prior to the evaluation. Such data should first include a statement of parent questions and concerns, obtained by telephone interview and by a comprehensive questionnaire completed by the parents (Cadol, 1981). In some circumstances, the parent will need assistance from a parent advocate, for example, a social worker or administrative assistant, to complete this questionnaire. The questionnaire should cover family demography, parent concerns, medical history, social history, family history, and a list of previous health, educational, and rehabilitation service providers. Second, questions, concerns, and observations by the referring person should be obtained by telephone interview. Third, past birth and medical records and records from any intervention programs or previous assessments should be obtained.

These data are compiled in the case file and summarized on a one-page case abstract, which is made available to all members of the diagnostic team in advance of the evaluation and is discussed at a brief (15-minute) staffing to plan the evaluation strategies. Specialized tests or consultations are scheduled as part of the evaluation. Experience has shown that the need for such consultations or tests can be anticipated in advance in most cases. It is also helpful to have some "free time" available between the evaluation and the time of staffing, so that unforeseen tests or consultations, such as brainstem audiometry, can be scheduled. It is most desirable to have all tests completed by the time of staffing and parent conference; however, certain test results, such as those from chromosome or amino acid studies, may not be available for days or weeks, necessitating a follow-up parent conference.

Clinical History. After reviewing the case abstract, past medical records, and parent questionnaire, the physician schedules 60 to 90 minutes to interview the parents and child and perform the physical examination (Table 6, page 114). The session should be unhurried, uninterrupted, and conducted in a friendly and supportive manner, as the parents and child are often anxious during the evaluation. When children are able to contribute, they should be asked what they understand about the problem and what they would like to find out.

In taking the medical history, the physician is concerned with the facts surrounding the pregnancy, labor, delivery, newborn course, and subsequent health, growth, and development. He or she is also concerned with how the parents have come to understand the child's problems. In taking the developmental history, the physician asks about developmental milestones and seeks to learn when the problem was first detected and whether development has proceeded steadily or whether there has been a loss of previously acquired functions (regression). Slow, steady progress suggests a static or nonprogressive process, which will be the case in most situations, while regression points to a progressive process, such as a degenerative disease or brain tumor.

The physician also asks about sleep and behavior problems and looks for clues concerning difficulties in the parent-child interaction. Use of such open-ended questions as "What kind of baby was he/she?" may yield valuable information on early parent perceptions and infant temperament. "What do you think about his/her development?" may expose parental worries and fears of mental retardation. These can be followed up by asking the parents to define what they mean by mental retardation.

In the review of systems, the physician asks about each organ system in orderly sequence to establish the presence of associated health problems or complications. For example, staring spells, sudden falls, and repetitive movements may suggest a previously unsuspected seizure disorder. Documentation of medications, hospitalizations, surgical procedures, allergies, and immunizations complete this section of the medical history.

Table 6. Medical Assessment and Report (SOAP Format)

SUBJECTIVE

Medical History

Chief complaint—reason for evaluation, parent/child concerns

Present and past medical history
Pregnancy, birth, newborn problems
Childhood illnesses, hospitalizations, surgery
Medications, allergies, immunizations

Developmental history
Milestones, onset, parent perceptions of child
Rate of learning, special programs, behavior problems

Review of systems
Head, eyes, ears, mouth, lungs, heart, bowels, kidneys, bones/joints, seizures, nutrition

Family History

Significant illnesses in siblings, parents, and extended family: birth defects, mental retardation, seizures, miscarriages, stillbirths, deaths

Social History

Family demographics, understanding of child's problems, coping mechanisms

OBJECTIVE

Physical Examination

Growth—height, weight, head circumference

General appearance—unusual proportions, ill?

Head, neck, ears, mouth, chest, lungs, heart

Abdomen, back, genitals, extremities

Neurological examination
Mental status, communications, interactions with parents/examiner
Cranial nerves, sensory function, balance, tremor
Motor function—symmetry, strength, muscle bulk and tone
Reflexes—tendon, protective, primitive

Laboratory Tests and Medical Specialty Consultations

ASSESSMENT—problem list
PLAN—recommendations

The family history should begin with screening questions concerning the presence of significant diseases in parents, siblings, grandparents, and other close family members. In particular, information on spontaneous abortions, stillbirths, childhood deaths, handicaps, and early onset hearing loss in other family members is sought. Finally, asking whether or not the parents are blood relatives may suggest the possibility of recessively inherited disorders. If answers to any of these screening questions are positive, a full genetic pedigree should be performed to assess inheritance patterns.

Physical Examination. After completing the interview (which ordinarily takes 80 percent of the allotted time), the physician performs the physical examination. By this time, the physician should have been able to put the child at ease, offering toys and interacting with the child during the clinical interview. In performing the examination, the least threatening or uncomfortable procedures are done first, leaving the ear, throat, rectal, and genital examinations for last. At the outset, the child's growth is plotted on norm-referenced growth grids for height, weight, and head circumference. A small head often reflects poor brain growth due to prior damage. Eighty-five percent of children with microcephaly (head circumference less than third percentile) are mentally retarded (Martin, 1970). A large or enlarging head suggests the possibility of hydrocephalus. Patterns of growth and body proportions may suggest such specific metabolic disorders as hypothyroidism or certain types of hereditary dwarfism.

The physician next forms an impression of the child's overall appearance: Does he/she look well or sick? Well nourished or undernourished? Proportionate or mis-proportioned? Normal facial features resembling the parents or unusual appearing facies which suggest a syndrome arising in the prenatal period? The presence of congenital anomalies is sought in a number of body parts, including the skin and the head; size, shape, and position of the ears and eyes; nasal features; and hairline. The hands, fingers and palmar creases, and feet are common sites of minor congenital anomalies, as are abnormalities of chest shape, presence of heart murmur, and abnormalities of teeth and palate. The presence of three or more congenital anomalies strongly suggests a syndrome of prenatal onset (Smith, 1978).

The abdomen is examined with attention to enlargement of the liver and spleen, as seen with certain storage diseases (mucopolysaccharidoses or Tay-Sachs disease). The extremities may show evidence of joint contractures, as seen with cerebral palsy, and the back is examined for curvature (scoliosis). The eyes are screened for the presence of cataracts or retinal lesions (chorioretinitis), as seen with intrauterine infection, and vision screening is performed using picture cards (or the Snellen Test in older, cooperative children). The alignment of the eyes is also screened to rule out strabismus. (For more information on vision problems with hearing-impaired developmentally disabled children, see Chapter 9). The eardrums are visualized and eardrum mobility assessed by pneumatic otoscopy for the presence of middle ear fluid or retraction due to excessive negative pressure, as seen with serous otitis media.

The neurologic examination includes attention to mental alertness and communication skills as well as symmetry of motor function. Asymmetry, with a clear hand preference before age two, suggests neurologic injury to the nonpreferred side. Tremor may suggest cerebellar injury. Muscle tone may be increased (spasticity) or decreased (hypotonia). Muscle strength and bulk are also assessed. Reflex testing includes deep tendon reflexes (such as the knee jerk), protective reflexes (parachute), and primitive reflexes (such as the Moro or asymmetric tonic neck reflex) that normally disappear after infancy. Persistence of primitive reflexes in older children occurs with cerebral palsy.

Laboratory Tests. While performing the history and physical examination, the physician begins to form clinical hypotheses as to the nature of the problem, associated complications, and likely etiology. The choice of laboratory and X-ray studies should be based on a logical conceptualization of the problem, rather than a "shotgun" approach.

Tests to confirm or rule out medically treatable conditions and those with genetic implications are most important. The list of possible tests is vast, as are the conditions that cause childhood handicaps with hearing impairment. Some authors recommend "routine" urine amino acids and thyroid screening for all handicapped children (Gabel & Erickson, 1980). An EEG may be helpful if seizures are suspected; a CT scan if hydrocephalus, brain tumor, or degenerative disease is suspected; and chromosome and antibody studies for intrauterine infections (STORCH) if multiple congenital abnormalities are found. A urine screen for mucopolysaccarides may be helpful if the child's appearance suggests this type of disorder. Family audiograms and urinalysis are important if Alport's syndrome is suspected.

Medical Specialty Consultation. In addition to specific laboratory tests, the physician performing the medical assessment as part of the diagnostic team must know when to ask for consultative assistance. This will vary depending on the physician's training and experience. In general, hearing-impaired developmentally disabled children with conductive hearing loss, ear anomalies, or recurrent or persistent serous otitis media should probably be seen by an otolaryngologist to rule out medically treatable causes of hearing loss. An ophthalmologist may provide diagnostic information (since many conditions may have associated eye findings) and may help preserve optimal vision. Children with congenital abnormalities or a positive genetic family history should be seen by a geneticist or dysmorphologist to aid in syndrome identification and genetic counseling; children with significant orthopedic abnormalities, by a pediatric orthopedist; and children with progressive neurologic findings, by a pediatric neurologist. It is ideal to schedule all of these consultations during the interdisciplinary evaluation process and to provide feedback to parents once the case is staffed and the findings synthesized and prioritized. Otherwise, parents are likely to be confused and overwhelmed by the myriad of findings, specialty jargon, and possibly conflicting recommendations.

Staffing/Report Writing. Following the medical evaluation and medical specialty consultation, the physician communicates verbally with the consultants and composes his/her thoughts, using appropriate reference texts and atlases of genetic syndromes as needed (Bergsma, 1973). In writing the report, clinical findings are listed following the customary format for medical report writing, including the chief complaint, present and past medical history, review of systems, family history, social history, and physical examination (Table 6). The assessment should include a discussion of the major hypotheses and list the pertinent findings in problem-oriented format (Weed, 1969). Recommendations should generally be deferred until the case is staffed. All treatment recommendations are listed and priorities determined in the overall interdisciplinary case evaluation summary. At the staff conference, the physician summarizes principal findings, clinical conclusions, and recommendations; asks and answers questions and engages in discussion with other team members; and plans the approach to presenting diagnostic findings to the family, based on assessment of the family's understanding, educational level, and stage of adjustment. (See Chapter 6 on working with families of hearing-impaired developmentally disabled children.)

In most assessments of hearing-impaired developmentally disabled children, the physician will be a key participant in the parent conference. Depending on the findings and on the particular team, other participants will include the psychologist, audiologist, speech/language pathologist, and/or educator. At the conclusion of the staffing, those selected to present the findings to the family should meet briefly and clarify what findings will be presented, who will present them, and how. It is often helpful to have one of the participants play the role of parent advocate and pay particular attention to the parent's verbal and nonverbal cues that indicate confusion or understanding. The parent conference ordinarily takes 45 to 60 minutes and may require one or two sessions, depending on the particular case. Those conducting the parent conference should be familiar with the findings and with the family and be skilled in helping families understand complex and often emotionally troubling news. Findings should be presented clearly and sensitively, avoiding jargon while setting a pace appropriate for the family. Spurious details should be omitted; these are not remembered and only cloud the important information. The family should be encouraged to participate actively. Goals of the parent conference are to help parents understand what is wrong, what caused the problem, its severity and prognosis, and what can be done to help (Martin, 1981).

Parental understanding can be assessed by the nature of the questions asked and by nonverbal and verbal emotional responses. Parent conferences are therapeutic in that they cause families to move from a stage of bewilderment about whether a problem exists to a realization and a clearer understanding of the nature of the problem and a readiness to accept treatment. At the conclusion of the parent conference, roles should be clarified and the follow-up interval determined. Sometimes follow-up with a member of the team may occur as soon as one week after the conference, particularly when the amount of information or the parent's emotional responses are overwhelming. Typically, follow-up with a member of the team occurs in four to six weeks to assess early family adjustment and to ensure that treatment has begun. Reevaluation of progress and prognosis will usually occur in 6 to 12 months.

Conclusion

The physician involved in interdisciplinary assessment of the hearing-impaired developmentally disabled child functions both as a generalist (within a field of medical subspecialists and nonmedical specialists) and as a specialist (with respect to practicing pediatricians and family physicians, who rely on him or her to assist them in the assessment of complex childhood developmental problems). In the past, physicians were poorly trained to perform these functions. In recent years, however, a number of university-affiliated facilities have established graduate fellowship training programs for pediatricians. Graduates, who regard themselves as "developmental pediatricians," have distributed themselves to most urban areas. In addition, new texts and journals have appeared, and issues concerning disabling conditions are given greater attention in pediatric journals. Training programs have also been developed and implemented for medical students, residents in pediatrics and family practice, and practicing physicians, to better acquaint them with the unique needs of the handicapped population. They also learn about working closely with professionals from such fields as speech and hearing sciences, education, psychology, and rehabilitation (Guralnick & Richardson, 1980).

References

Behrman, R., & Vaughan, V. (1983). *Nelson's textbook of pediatrics* (pp. 351–352). Philadelphia: W. B. Saunders.

Bergsma, D. (Ed.). (1973). *Birth defects: Atlas and compendium.* Baltimore: A. R. Liss.

Bess, F., Peek, B., & Chapman, J. (1979). Further observations on noise levels in infant incubators. *Pediatrics, 63,* 100–106.

Bluestone, C., et al. (1983). Workshop on effects of otitis media on the child. *Pediatrics, 71,* 639–652.

Cadol, R. (1981). Medical history and physical examination. In W. Frankenburg, S. M. Thornton, & M. E. Cohrs (Eds.), *Pediatric developmental diagnosis.* New York: Thieme-Stratton.

Frigoletto, F., Birnholz, J., & Greave, M. (1982). Antenatal treatment of hydrocephalus by ventriculoamniotic shunting. *JAMA, 19,* 2496–2498.

Gabel, S., & Erickson, M. (Eds.). (1980). *Child development and developmental disabilities.* Boston: Little, Brown.

Gentile, A.,& McCarthy, B. (1973, November). *Additional handicapping conditions among hearing impaired students* (Series D, No. 14). Washington, DC: Gallaudet College Office of Demographic Studies.

Gordon, S., Appell, M., & Cooper, E. (1982). Medical issues in overall management of the severely handicapped hearing impaired child. In B. Campbell & V. Baldwin (Eds.), *Severely handicapped/hearing impaired students.* Baltimore: Brookes.

Guralnick, M., & Richardson, H. (1980). *Pediatric education and the needs of exceptional children.* Baltimore: University Park Press.

Jackson, L., & Schimke, R. (1979). *Clinical genetics: A source book for physicians.* New York: Wiley.

Jaffe, B. (Ed.). (1977). *Hearing loss in children: A comprehensive text.* Baltimore: University Park Press.

Konigsmark, B., & Gorlin, R. (1976). *Genetic and metabolic deafness.* Philadelphia: W. B. Saunders.

Levine, R. L., & Maisels, M. J. (Eds.). (1983). *Hyperbilirubinemia in the newborn: Report of the Eighty-fifth Ross Conference on Pediatric Research.* Columbus: Ross Laboratories.

Martin, H. (1970). Microcephaly and mental retardation. *American Journal of Diseases of Children, 119,* 128–131.

Martin, H. (1981). Parent conferences. In W. Frankenburg, S. M. Thornton, & M. E. Cohrs (Eds.), *Pediatric development diagnosis.* New York: Thieme-Stratton.

Northern, J., & Downs, M. (1978). *Hearing in children.* Baltimore: Williams and Wilkins.

O'Shea, J., Langenbrunner, D., McClosky, D., Pezzullo, J., & Reyes, J. (1982). Childhood serous otitis media. *Clinical Pediatrics, 21,* 150–153.

Paradise, J. (1980). Otitis media in infants and children. *Pediatrics, 65,* 917–943.

Paradise, J. (1981). Otitis media during early life: How hazardous to development? A critical review of the evidence. *Pediatrics, 68,* 869–873.

Smith, D. (1978). *Recognizable patterns of human malformations.* Philadelphia: W. B. Saunders.

Ventry, I. (1980). Effects of conductive hearing loss: Fact or fiction? *Journal of Speech and Hearing Disorders, 45,* 143–156.

Weed, L. L. (1969). *Medical records, medical education, and patient care.* Cleveland: Case University Press.

Appendix
Joint Committee on Infant Hearing Position Statement

The following expanded position statement of the Joint Committee on Infant Hearing was adopted by the Legislative Council of ASHA in November 1981. Representatives of the member organizations who prepared this statement include: American Speech-Language-Hearing Association—Arthur Dahle, Sanford Gerber, Laszlo Stein, Evelyn Cherow, ex officio, and Martha Rubin, Chair; Marion Downs and George Mencher, consultants; American Academy of Otolaryngology—Head and Neck Surgery—Ralph Naunton and Kenneth Grundfast; American Academy of Pediatrics—Robert Hall and Jean Lockhart; and the American Nurses Association—Violet Katz.

Early detection of hearing impairment in the affected infant is important for medical treatment and subsequent educational intervention to assure development of communication skills.

In 1973, the Joint Committee on Infant Hearing Screening recommended identifying infants at risk for hearing impairment by means of five criteria and suggested follow-up audiological evaluation of these infants until accurate assessments of hearing could be made. Since the incidence of moderate to profound hearing loss in the at-risk infant group is 2.5–5.0 percent, audiologic testing of this group is warranted. Acoustic testing of all newborn infants has a high incidence of false positive and false negative results and is not universally recommended.

Recent research suggests the need for expansion and clarification of the 1973 criteria. This 1982 statement expands the risk criteria and makes recommendations for the evaluation and treatment of the hearing-impaired infant.

I. Identification

  A. Risk criteria

    The factors that identify those infants who are AT RISK for having hearing impairment include the following:

From *Asha, 24*(12), 1017–1018. Copyright 1982 by American Speech-Language-Hearing Association. Reprinted by permission.

1. A family history of childhood hearing impairment.
2. Congenital perinatal infection (e.g., cytomegalovirus, rubella, herpes, toxoplasmosis, syphilis).
3. Anatomic malformations involving the head or neck (e.g., dysmorphic appearance including syndromal and nonsyndromal abnormalities, overt or submucous cleft palate, morphologic abnormalities of the pinna).
4. Birth weight less than 1500 grams.
5. Hyperbilirubinemia at level exceeding indications for exchange transfusion.
6. Bacterial meningitis, especially H. influenza.
7. Severe asphyxia which may include infants with Apgar scores of 0–3 who fail to institute spontaneous respiration by 10 minutes and those with hypotonia persisting to two hours of age.

B. Screening procedures

The hearing of infants who manifest any item on the list of risk criteria should be screened, preferably under supervision of an audiologist, optimally by three months of age, but not later than six months of age. The initial screening should include the observation of behavioral or electrophysiological response to sound.* If consistent electrophysiological or behavioral responses are detected at appropriate sound levels, then the screening process will be considered complete except in those cases where there is a probability of a progressive hearing loss, e.g., family history of delayed onset, degenerative disease, or intra-uterine infections. If results of an initial screening of an infant manifesting any risk criteria are equivocal, then the infant should be referred for diagnostic testing.

II. Diagnosis for Infants Failing Screening

A. Diagnostic evaluation of an infant under six months of age

1. General physical examination and history including:
   a. Examination of the head and neck
   b. Otoscopy and otomicroscopy
   c. Identification of relevant physical abnormalities
   d. Laboratory tests such as urinalysis and diagnostic tests for perinatal infections
2. Comprehensive audiological evaluation:
   a. Behavioral history
   b. Behavioral observation audiometry
   c. Testing of auditory evoked potentials, if indicated

B. After the age of six months, the following are also recommended:

1. Communication skills evaluation
2. Acoustic immittance measurements (impedance measurements)
3. Selected tests of development

III. Management of the Hearing-Impaired Infant

Habilitation of the hearing-impaired infant may begin while the diagnostic evaluation is in progress. The Committee recommends, however, that whenever possible the diagnostic process should be completed and habilitation begun by the age of six months. Services to the hearing-impaired infant under six months of age include:

---

*This Committee has no recommendations at this time regarding any specific device.

A. Medical management

    1. Reevaluation

    2. Treatment

    3. Genetic evaluation and counseling when indicated

B. Audiologic management

    1. Ongoing audiological assessment

    2. Selection of hearing aid(s)

    3. Family counseling

C. Psychoeducational management

    1. Formulation of an individualized education plan

    2. Information about the implications of hearing impairment

After the age of six months, the hearing-impaired infant becomes easier to manage in a habilitation plan, but s/he will require the services listed above.

Appendix Bibliography

Early Intervention

Ling, D. (1981). Early speech development. In G. T. Mencher & S. E. Gerber (Eds.), *Early management of hearing loss* (pp. 319–335). New York: Grune and Stratton.

McFarland, W. H., & Simmons, B. (1980). The importance of early intervention. *Pediatric Annals, 13*–23.

Skinner, M. (1978). The hearing of speech during language acquisition. *Otolaryngologic Clinics of North America, II*(3), 631–650.

Identification of Hearing Impairment in Infants

Bess, F. H. (1977). *Childhood deafness.* New York: Grune and Stratton.

Greenstein, J. M., Greenstein, B. B., McConville, K., & Stellini, L. (1976). *Mother-infant communication and language acquisition in deaf infants.* New York: Lexington School for the Deaf.

Northern, J., & Downs, M. (1978). *Hearing in children.* Baltimore: Williams and Wilkins.

Diagnosis and Management

Gerber, S. E., & Mencher, G. T. (1978). *Early diagnosis of hearing loss.* New York: Grune and Stratton.

Mencher, G. T., & Gerber, S. E. (1981). *Early management of hearing loss.* New York: Grune and Stratton.

Simmons, F. B. (1980). Diagnosis and rehabilitation of deaf newborns: Part II. *Asha, 22,* 475–479.

Evoked Potential Audiometry

Despland, P., & Galambos, R. (1980). The auditory brainstem response as a useful diagnostic tool in the intensive care nursery. *Pediatric Research, 14,* 154–158.

Galambos, C., & Galambos, R. (1979). Brainstem evoked response audiometry in newborn hearing screening. *Archives of Otolaryngology, 87,* 86–90.

Starr, A., Amlie, R. N., Martin, W. H., & Sanders, S. (1977). Development of auditory function in newborn infants revealed by auditory brainstem potentials. *Pediatrics, 60,* 831–839.

Chapter 8

The State of the Art in Audiologic Evaluation and Management

Brad W. Friedrich

Historically, evaluation of the auditory status of developmentally disabled individuals has constituted one of the major challenges confronting audiologists. Techniques presently exist which allow the audiologist to ascertain the auditory status of the large majority of children with developmental disabilities and multihandicapping conditions, regardless of age or the nature of the handicaps. Nonetheless, the assessment of developmentally disabled individuals continues to be problematic. Professionals other than audiologists sometimes assume that early identification of hearing impairment is not possible. In other instances, the early assessment of auditory status is not judged critical to the comprehensive evaluation of developmentally disabled children for purposes of establishing early intervention programs.

Hearing impairment has often assumed a position of secondary importance in the educational and communicative management of the developmentally disabled. Furthermore, children may be labeled untestable because of perceived difficulties in audiological testing that are attributed to such factors as age, behavior, and the mere presence of developmentally handicapping conditions. In many instances, test results may be equivocal and incomplete, precluding the formulation of accurate and useful clinical impressions regarding auditory status. The inevitable consequence has been a delay in the identification of persons with communicatively and educationally handicapping hearing impairments and in the implementation of appropriate management and habilitative services.

The problem appears to be one of lack of proper referral and application of existing audiological procedures rather than the nonavailability of appropriate test procedures. Difficulties encountered in the evaluation of the auditory status of developmentally disabled children typically reflect a lack of consideration of developmental, neuromotor, and behavioral factors that exert significant influences on the assessment of these children.

The purpose of this chapter is to address special considerations in the audiological evaluation of developmentally disabled children. The manner in which these developmental, neuromotor, and behavioral factors may compromise the administration of existing clinical assessment procedures and the interpretation of audiological data will come under particular scrutiny. It is hoped that, by identifying these factors and highlighting some mechanisms for their control, the audiologist may meet the challenge of identifying hearing-impaired developmentally disabled children at the earliest possible age and describing hearing impairments in a manner sufficient to permit the implementation of appropriate intervention.

The Interdisciplinary Model

Before proceeding to a consideration of audiological assessment, an overview of the audiologist's role in the evaluation and management of hearing-impaired developmentally disabled children in the context of the interdisciplinary service model is in order. The audiologist has not always assumed a proper or prominent role in the interdisciplinary evaluation and management process. A number of factors have undoubtedly contributed to this problem, including the difficulties audiologists have encountered in the past in the assessment of hearing impairment in the developmentally disabled population as well as the audiologist's traditional association with the medical environment for the delivery of services. As a result, academic programs have not always emphasized the training of audiologists to recognize and assess the impact of peripheral hearing impairment upon communicative and academic performance and achievement. In clinical and educational environments, the audiologist has often served in an adjunct role in the development of intervention and management strategies both at the time of initial identification of a child's handicaps and during follow-up (Kenworthy, 1982).

The audiologist traditionally has focused principle attention on the evaluation of auditory function; the selection, application, and evaluation of amplification systems; and the provision of counseling services regarding the nature of the hearing impairment and its implications for the development of communicative behaviors. The mandates of federal and state legislative bodies and regulating agencies have helped focus the audiologist's attention on education and habilitation to a greater extent. Audiologists are now employed by educational systems in greater numbers although their role has remained limited in many instances (Garstecki, 1978). Nevertheless, audiologists, regardless of work environment, must be prepared to interact in a more positive and direct manner with those involved in the educational process. The audiologist is the principle professional responsible for the clinical assessment of auditory function. Clinical data acquired by the audiologist are integral to educational, communicative, and vocational planning. Predictive relationships exist between clinical data and a child's actual communicative and educational performance. However, additional factors related to a child's developmental status, behavior, and learning environments interact with the sensory deficit and ultimately determine achievement. Consequently, the audiologist's direct involvement in the ongoing assessment of performance and progress outside the clinical environment is also required.

Obviously, the audiologist who is responsible for the care of hearing-impaired developmentally disabled children cannot work in isolation. As with the evaluation of all hearing-impaired individuals, determination of the adequacy of a developmentally disabled child's hearing for development of linguistic skills and communication constitutes the prime goal of the audiological evaluation. Yet, input from a number of disciplines is critical if a child's hearing loss is to be understood in the context of abilities in all spheres of development. The audiologist must join the interdisciplinary team in determining the relative impact of a child's disabilities on development, particularly the development of communicative abilities.

In addition, the interdisciplinary model has proven to have particular relevance to the audiologist since it provides the framework for the application of principles of child development crucial to the evaluation of hearing in children with handicaps. In practice, the interdisciplinary team members provide the developmental information instrumental to the successful evaluation of a child. For example, knowledge of a child's cognitive, communicative, and neuromotor status is vital to the selection and administration of test procedures, management of the child and behavior-shaping in the test environment, and the interpretation of audiological data. Similarly, while the audiologist can devise a program of intervention specific to a child's hearing impairment and based solely upon knowledge of the audiological factors related to that impairment, the program is likely to be more appropriate and successful if the child's impairment is viewed in the developmental framework.

Audiological Assessment

A variety of behavioral and electrophysiological assessment procedures are available for the evaluation of auditory function. The effective utilization of these procedures with difficult-to-test pediatric populations is highly dependent upon careful consideration and control of procedural and subject variables that reflect the developmental, neuromotor, and behavioral status of these children. The limitations on response measurement imposed by these factors may otherwise compromise the audiological evaluation. In addition, the ability of the audiologist to describe adequately the auditory status of hearing-impaired developmentally disabled children is dependent upon the careful integration of data from the entire test battery.

Thorough descriptions of the procedures that comprise the audiological test battery are readily available in the literature. Consequently, the intent of this discussion is to review special considerations in the application of these procedures to the developmentally disabled. Particular emphasis will be placed upon behavioral techniques for the assessment of auditory sensitivity. Behavioral procedures are viewed by this author as providing the most useful impression of a child's auditory status when applied appropriately and supplemented by electrophysiological procedures as necessary. Limitations inherent in existing electrophysiological procedures and the tendency of many audiologists and referral sources to question the validity of behavioral testing suggest the need for this emphasis.

Table 1 presents a protocol for the audiological evaluation of developmentally disabled children. While this discussion will concentrate on assessment procedures, the importance of a thorough developmental case history obtained through parent interview and record review cannot be overstated. The case history should provide the audiologist with a picture of a child's status in developmental spheres other than hearing, speech, and language. Information regarding a child's cognitive, motor, social, emotional, and behavioral status as well as medical and educational background is necessary. In this manner, the case history provides a solid framework for audiological evaluation and management. While a variety of case history forms and questionnaires are available,

Table 1. Audiological Evaluation Protocol for Developmentally Disabled Children

A. Developmental case history

B. Developmental screening (as necessary)

C. Audiological assessment

   1. Behavioral assessment of auditory sensitivity

   2. Electrophysiological measurements (including auditory brainstem response testing and acoustic immittance measurements)

   3. Auditory discrimination abilities (including speech recognition tests)

   4. Other diagnostic procedures

   5. Clinical observation of child's performance and behavior

D. Interpretation of audiological data and information

E. Interdisciplinary team review

F. Formulation of initial audiological management plan

G. Counseling and feedback to caregivers

clinicians are urged to exercise caution in the use of forms that detail specific questions to be asked in a parent interview. Skilled clinicians will be able to respond best to parental concerns, needs, and requests if they keep the general content areas in mind and are not compelled to secure background information in a specified order or manner. In addition, the interdisciplinary model often will not require the audiologist to obtain detailed historical information if that information is already available through the work of other team members. However, a clinician must ensure that adequate information is obtained at the time of the audiological evaluation to give proper direction to audiological testing and initial counseling.

Behavioral Assessment of Auditory Sensitivity

The behavioral measurement of auditory function in hearing-impaired developmentally disabled individuals requires careful consideration of stimulus selection and calibration. Stimulus selection is guided by the need to (1) utilize stimuli that are specifiable both electroacoustically and psychoacoustically, (2) maximize the audiologist's ability to elicit and observe responses, and (3) obtain sufficient frequency-specific data to delineate peripheral sensitivity for the frequency range that is most critical for purposes of communication.

Conventional pure tone and speech stimuli are available for monaural testing via earphones, and calibration is accomplished readily in accordance with standards and measurement procedures specified by the American National Standards Institute (ANSI 3.6-1969). However, sound field measurements are frequently required for the assessment of difficult-to-test individuals who do not tolerate earphones or fail to provide repeatable responses in the earphone testing condition. Speech stimuli, frequency-modulated (warble) tones, and narrow-band noise stimuli are most useful for purposes of assessing sensitivity via loudspeaker presentation in the sound field. Noisemakers and environmental sounds have been favored by some individuals; however, they lack sufficient frequency-specificity and introduce additional problems for both electro-acoustic and psychoacoustic calibration. The availability of both narrow-band noise and frequency-modulated signals (warble tones) to acquire frequency-specific information allows stimulus type to be changed during test sessions and helps counteract habituation to test signals. In addition, some listeners appear to respond more consistently and at lower intensity levels to one of the stimulus types or the other (Sanders & Josey, 1970).

Unfortunately, no standard reference values are available which specify intensity levels corresponding to normal threshold for stimuli delivered in the sound field. The findings of several studies (Dirks, Stream, & Wilson, 1972; Stream & Dirks, 1974; Tillman, Johnson, & Olsen, 1966) have suggested that sound field testing introduces several variables into the measurement of sensitivity which do not require consideration with earphone testing. For example, the azimuth at which a loudspeaker is placed influences threshold measurements. Furthermore, a threshold advantage accrues to the binaural listening condition relative to monaural listening conditions and varies as a function of azimuth. These variables are often overlooked both in the calibration of sound fields and in the interpretation of clinical data. Thus, a careful analysis of each sound field used for behavioral measurements of auditory function is mandatory to determine appropriate reference sound pressure levels for all test signals. Morgan, Dirks, and Bower (1979) have proposed a useful procedure to accomplish this task.

The interpretation of audiological data obtained utilizing behavioral measurements of sensitivity is complicated for very young and developmentally handicapped children because of difficulties associated with the psychoacoustic calibration of test stimuli. Children in the early stages of development fail to provide responses at their true threshold levels utilizing either behavioral observation or visual reinforcement testing paradigms. Children at these developmental levels apparently lack the requisite cognitive, attentional, and auditory experiences to respond to the least intense signals actually audible to them. Whether this is specific to the testing paradigm, the sensory modality under test, or a combination of these factors has not been determined. Furthermore, it seems reasonable to conjecture that the speech and frequency-specific stimuli utilized in most clinical environments today lack the salience necessary for the infant to respond at threshold.

The intensities of auditory signals used for evaluation purposes typically are refer-enced to average threshold for normal adult listeners. Since infants and low-functioning children are not expected to provide responses at levels corresponding to true threshold, the lowest intensities at which they respond are referred to as minimum response levels. Thus, minimum response levels do not reflect a loss in auditory sensitivity; they reflect the decreased responsiveness to auditory stimuli expected of children at lower develop-mental levels. The interpretation of the minimum response levels at which an infant responds during clinical testing has rested upon comparisons with the minimal signal intensity levels required to elicit responses from normally developing children of a comparable age with normal hearing. Judgments for developmentally handicapped children must be based upon careful consideration of the individual child's developmental age rather than chronological age. However, the audiologist should be wary of operating under the assumption that a handicapped child will provide responses in a manner exactly analogous to the normal child whose chronological age corresponds to the handicapped child's developmental age.

Research on Response Levels

Unfortunately, only a limited number of investigations (Hoversten & Moncur, 1969; Matkin, 1977; Northern & Downs, 1978; Thompson & Weber, 1974; Wilson & Moore, 1978; Wilson, Moore, & Thompson, 1976) have provided data which attempt to specify the intensity levels at which normal infants may be expected to provide either behavioral or visually reinforced head turn responses to auditory signals. As a result, existing developmental data are incomplete and imprecise for purposes of drawing definitive conclusions regarding a child's peripheral auditory sensitivity.

Many audiologists rely upon data summarized from other sources and presented by Northern and Downs (1978) to make judgments regarding the appropriateness of a child's responses and, hence, auditory sensitivity. However, the data are pertinent only to the use of behavioral observation procedures, and the parameters of the test stimuli for which data are presented are not specified by Northern and Downs. In addition, the data fail to reflect either the frequency-specificity or the various types of auditory stimuli used in clinical facilities today.

A number of investigators (Hoversten & Moncur, 1969; Matkin, 1977; Thompson & Weber, 1974; Wilson & Moore, 1978; Wilson, Moore, & Thompson, 1976) have explored minimum response levels for different auditory stimuli using behavioral observation and visual reinforcement procedures. Wilson and his colleagues elicited responses from infants ages 6–18 months at intensity levels only slightly higher than those required to elicit threshold responses from adults in the same listening situation. In addition, the range of responses for the Visual Reinforcement Audiometry (VRA) procedure was considerably less than for Behavioral Observation Audiometry (BOA), approximating the range of responses observed for adults. Thus, Wilson and his colleagues suggest that near threshold responses can be obtained from infants as young as six months of age utilizing the VRA paradigm. Matkin reported average minimum response levels for his subjects at higher intensity levels when VRA was used in a clinical setting. While normal infants may indeed provide responses near threshold, Matkin's finding is more consistent with clinical experience which suggests that a wider range of minimum response levels should actually be considered developmentally appropriate. The findings of Wilson and his colleagues undoubtedly reflect, at least in part, a homogeneous group of research subjects characterized by higher socioeconomic and parental educational backgrounds. Greater variability in response levels should be expected with the more heterogeneous patient populations encountered in active clinical practices.

While the aforementioned studies have provided some useful data upon which to base clinical judgments regarding auditory sensitivity, only a very few investigators have concerned themselves specifically with the application of behavioral observation and visual reinforcement procedures to developmentally disabled and multihandicapped children. Greenberg, Wilson, Moore, and Thompson (1978) and Thompson, Wilson, and Moore (1979) have demonstrated that VRA is appropriate for use with Down's syndrome and other developmentally delayed children. They contended that children must be functioning at a developmental age of 10–12 months if the procedure is to be used successfully. More recently, it has been suggested that youngsters with cognitive, neuromotor, or a combination of deficits and functioning at levels as low as six months of age can be conditioned successfully (Thompson & Folsom, 1981; Friedrich, Resnick, Bookstein, & Balfour, 1982). The conditioning process may be more complex and lengthy and the maintenance of conditioning bonds during a test session more variable. However, it appears that a high percentage of youngsters functioning at 6–8 months of age are conditionable and capable of providing consistent minimum response levels.

Friedrich et al. (1982) reported minimum response level data based upon the research reviewed above and clinical experience over a five-year period with both normal and developmentally disabled children. Figure 1 depicts for frequency-specific stimuli the intensity range of responses considered to be appropriate for children at various developmental age levels. Several points demand underscoring:

1. Minimum response levels obtained while utilizing BOA can be expected to approach true threshold as a child approaches a six-month level of development.

2. Responses obtained using BOA can be expected to be established at intensity levels above true threshold at all developmental levels.

3. A significant percentage of children developmentally as young as six months of age can be expected to provide reliable conditioned responses with the VRA procedure, suggesting that attempts should be made to condition children functioning at that level.

4. The VRA, when appropriate, can be expected to yield better minimum response levels than BOA at developmental levels of six months of age and older.

5. Developmentally handicapped children may provide responses at or near threshold regardless of developmental level when the VRA paradigm is used. However, a greater range in response levels may be expected at the lower developmental age ranges.

Figure 2 provides similar information for speech awareness responses. In general, minimum response levels for speech are established at better intensity levels than those for either narrow-band noise stimuli or warble tones, undoubtedly reflecting the greater salience of speech stimuli for young children. Differences tend to be minimized between the BOA and VRA procedures, and speech awareness responses at or near threshold can be expected with both procedures at developmental levels above six months. However, a broad-band speech stimulus obviously has limited value in ascertaining a child's exact auditory status. Elicitation of a response to a broad-band signal at an intensity level within normal limits suggests only that hearing sensitivity is normal for a portion of the frequency range characteristic of that signal. Thus, the low frequency components of

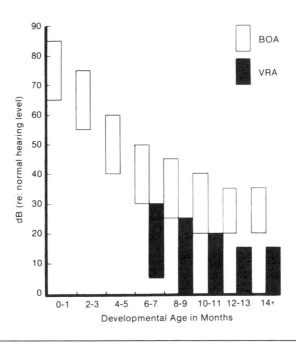

Figure 1. Minimum response levels expected at various developmental age levels for frequency-specific stimuli (narrow-band noise stimuli and frequency-modulated tones).

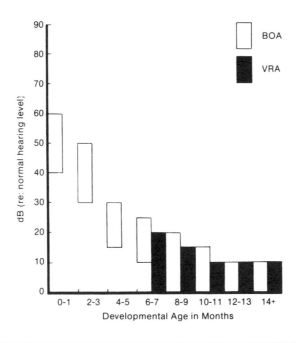

Figure 2. Minimum response levels expected at various developmental age levels for speech awareness.

speech may be sufficient to elicit a normal speech awareness response from a child with a communicatively significant hearing impairment in the high frequencies only.

Pediatric Test Procedures

Behavioral pediatric test procedures routinely used in clinical facilities today are distinguished primarily by the response modes and reinforcers they incorporate. Consequently, the selection of a test procedure for use with a given child is dependent in large part upon determination of an appropriate response mode. Conditioned Play Audiometry (CPA), Tangible Reinforcement Operant Conditioning Audiometry (TROCA), and Visual Reinforcement Audiometry (VRA) are standard tools in the pediatric test battery for the assessment of peripheral auditory sensitivity and are based upon operant conditioning principles. Both CPA and TROCA require volitional motor responses. Utilizing CPA, a child is conditioned via instruction or demonstration to complete a specific play activity (e.g., dropping blocks in a bucket) in response to presentation of an auditory signal. The TROCA requires that a child depress a button or bar which in turn triggers a dispensing device to provide a tangible reinforcer (e.g., an edible reinforcer or token) to the child. The VRA procedure, on the other hand, capitalizes upon a child's head turn response to auditory stimulation. The child is conditioned to turn his or her head toward an attractive visual reinforcer (e.g., animated toys or lights) upon presentation of a test stimulus. This technique does not require the same type of volitional motor response as the other procedures and has been demonstrated to be successful with children as young as six months of age.

For younger infants, the audiologist must rely upon the use of Behavioral Observation Audiometry (BOA). Formal conditioning or shaping of response behavior is not attempted during BOA. Instead, the audiologist observes changes in a child's behavior and activity upon presentation of test stimuli. An infant's behavioral responses can take any of a number of forms and are often subtle, requiring the observations of experienced examiners. With the exception of TROCA, these techniques have been devised utilizing normally developing children. While there is a dearth of literature addressing their specific application to developmentally disabled children, clinical experience suggests that they have achieved widespread application to children characterized as difficult to test.

The response mode associated with a given technique must be within the developmentally disabled child's cognitive and physical capabilities. Furthermore, the response mode must be associated with reinforcement that assists the audiologist in minimizing a child's habituation to the test signal and task. Lloyd and his colleagues (Lloyd, 1966, 1977; Lloyd, Spradlin, & Reid, 1968) have given particular attention to the importance of response modes and reinforcement in the assessment of sensitivity for frequency-specific stimuli utilizing operant procedures. The type and schedule of reinforcement should be selected to sustain a child's attention, interest, and cooperation for a period of time sufficient to maximize the amount of data obtained as well as the reliability of that data. Furthermore, the reinforcement should not be so interesting or elaborate as to interfere with the test task itself. Indeed, Lloyd et al. (1968) identified the selection and administration of reinforcement as the critical factors in the development of TROCA with a severely-to-profoundly handicapped population in an institutional setting. Martin and Coombes (1976) described development of a tangibly reinforced procedure for establishing speech reception thresholds in young children. Weaver, Wardell, and Martin (1979) verified the appropriateness of the technique and apparatus for use with young mentally retarded children. The procedure incorporated a device in the form of a clown which dispensed reinforcers when body parts, corresponding to 1 bisyllabic and 11 monosyllabic words used as test stimuli, were correctly depressed.

All too often, however, pediatric test procedures are selected and applied with little systematic regard for the developmental status of children. A child's developmental level rather than chronological age should be preeminent in the selection and administration of test procedures. This emphasis is critical if realistic expectations are to be set regarding a child's behavior, attention, and task performance in the test environment.

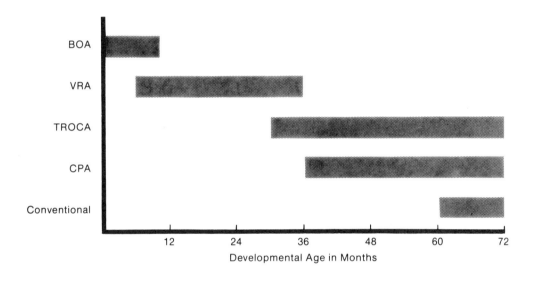

Figure 3. Guideline for the selection of pediatric behavioral procedures for the assessment of auditory sensitivity.

Figure 3 presents a guideline for the selection of pediatric audiological procedures. It indicates developmental age ranges for which the various assessment procedures are appropriate. Use of such a guideline and the interpretation of data are predicated upon accurate identification of a child's level of development. The audiologist need not assume responsibility for the formal assessment of a child's developmental status and, specifically, cognitive abilities. Formal cognitive assessment involves examination of a child's abilities in a variety of component skill areas. The interpretation of those results is dependent upon an examiner's ability to identify and analyze interactions among the skills observed and relate the findings not only to a child's current level of functioning but to potential for development as well.

Cognitive profiles may reflect a consistent level of performance across all skill areas, or they may be characterized by a scattering of abilities among skill areas. The latter profile often complicates the determination of a child's true level of intellectual function since scattered skills may reflect learning which has occurred rotely or through intensive training (e.g., completion of a form board, matching skills, and so forth). These abilities frequently reflect a child's ability to accomplish tasks that, while of some functional use, do not actually reflect higher levels of reasoning or problem-solving behavior. In the presence of a variable cognitive profile, the likelihood of encountering success with a particular response mode will be heightened if it is selected in accordance with a child's best abilities in areas that reflect more complex intellectual functioning, regardless of whether they are language- or nonlanguage-mediated abilities. The scattered, or splintered, skills often tend to overestimate a child's overall level of function and prove less useful in predicting the successful application of a particular technique.

In general, the audiologist may base decisions regarding test selection and data interpretation upon information from one or more of the following sources: (1) a thorough developmental case history which ascertains both the course and the rate of the child's development as well as current level of development; (2) parental estimations of level of function; (3) review of appropriate diagnostic and treatment reports, when available, from other clinical disciplines and educational programs; (4) administration of selected developmental screening procedures; and (5) clinical observations of the child's behavior.

Delineation of a child's neuromotor function is necessary to determine if a physical disability exists that may preclude or interfere with the use of a response mode judged to be appropriate to a child's cognitive capabilities. Physical limitations associated with mental retardation may also interfere with a child's ability to provide specific conditioned motor responses to auditory stimulation. Such manifestations of physical disability as extraneous or involuntary movements and the persistence of primitive reflexes associated with cerebral palsy may be responsible for a child's inability to provide consistent conditioned responses. Primitive reflexes, for example, are elicited in response to the position and movement of a child's body in space and reflect the control of central nervous system centers in the cerebellum, basal ganglia, and other brainstem structures during infancy. They disappear as higher brain centers assume control and provide for the maintenance of postures and the generation of complex and coordinated movements.

One reflex is of more than passing interest to the audiologist because it may be interpreted as a response or elicited when a child turns his/her head to a visual reinforcer, resulting in a protracted evaluation and limited data. The asymmetrical tonic neck reflex (ATNR) is elicited in infants by turning the head to one side. The infant assumes a "fencing" position, with the extremities extended on the side toward which the infant's head faces and flexed on the opposite side. This reflex is readily elicited in infants until it is suppressed by higher brain centers at about five months of age. In children with neuromotor dysfunction, the ATNR may persist and never disappear. It may also reemerge in children who have suffered motor disability secondary to traumatic head injury. The persistence of this primitive reflex may then interfere with normal posturing and movement. Unlike the normal infant, the impaired child may encounter enormous difficulty breaking out of the reflex pattern. Consequently, it may interfere significantly with the audiological evaluation.

Developmental Age Levels

While the concept of developmental age level is useful for purposes of test procedure and response mode selection, the assumption cannot be made that the developmentally disabled child will respond in a manner exactly parallel to the normally developing youngster at the corresponding level. Thus, even when the selection of CPA or VRA appears sound on the basis of a child's cognitive and motoric status, testing may be complicated. Specifically, the repeatability of responses upon successive stimulus presentations may be highly variable during a test session. Uncooperative behavior or fluctuations in activity level related to a child's level of cognitive function or physical disability may obscure responses, and response strength may be reduced. Furthermore, the speed and efficiency of responses, including recovery from response, may be compromised while response latency may be increased and more variable. Fatigue and habituation to test signals and response tasks may be more rapid.

In other words, neither a mentally retarded 3-year-old child functioning at a 1-year-old level nor a normally intelligent 5-year-old with severe neuromotor involvement secondary to choreoathetoid cerebral palsy is expected to provide responses in a manner consistent with those of a normal youngster at either the same developmental or chronological age. Nor are the specific behaviors and difficulties encountered predictable to a high degree. As a consequence, procedures must be employed to minimize the potential measurement problems associated with a child's specific developmental and behavioral status.

Utilization of a specific prestimulus observation period allows the audiologist to monitor a child's level of activity and behavior state prior to presentation of each test stimulus. The observation period provides a basis for the comparison of prestimulus and poststimulus activity to assist in the detection of change in behavior or activity which signifies that a response has occurred. Moreover, the prestimulus period permits the audiologist to accommodate himself or herself to the individual attributes and response characteristics of the patient. This also permits the audiologist to deliver test signals at times judged to be optimal for the elicitation of observable responses, particularly when BOA is utilized. Variations in interstimulus intervals will help reduce both habituation and fatigue as well as the occurrence of false/positive responses associated with regular test signal intervals.

Utilization of two experienced examiners is not possible in all facilities; however, it does permit continuous monitoring and shaping of a child's behavior during a test session and assists in minimizing the potential detrimental effects of observer bias. By engaging a child's interest and attention with developmentally appropriate play activities, an examiner attempts to sustain a consistent low level of activity against which responses may be discerned most easily. Special consideration must be given to the choice of play materials, presentation of materials, expected responses, and control of the environment (Bendet, 1976). Activities that sustain a child's interest and facilitate suitable activity at a 12-month level of development will not necessarily be suitable at the 2-year level. This principle is particularly important for behavioral observation and visual reinforcement procedures.

Observer bias has been reported to be high when Behavioral Observation Audiometry is utilized for testing infants (Langford, Bench, & Wilson, 1975; Ling, Ling, & Doering, 1970; Moncur, 1968; and Weber, 1969). More recently, Gans and Flexer (1982) assessed observer bias in the judgment of responses from severely-to-profoundly multihandicapped children and suggested, as did Weber, that bias can be minimized if observers are denied knowledge of stimulus events. Response judgment also can be facilitated if the agreement of two examiners is required before a response is identified as present for any single stimulus presentation. Generation of a record of all stimulus presentations and response judgments assists in the determination of thresholds or minimum response levels while providing evidence of response variability for any individual child.

The importance of properly positioning a child in accordance with his/her cognitive and motor abilities cannot be overestimated. It contributes to a reduction in extraneous and involuntary movements that might otherwise interfere with behavioral testing. It also contributes to a child's comfort, improving the likelihood of maintaining interest and cooperation for the duration of a test session. The goals of proper positioning are (1) to stabilize the child's body position, particularly the trunk, in a seated upright position; (2) to optimize the child's range of motion in the upper extremities; (3) to facilitate head and neck control; and (4) to maintain the child's body and head in a mid-line, forward-facing position. In many instances, proper positioning is achieved through the use of adaptive equipment specifically designed for the individual child. In other instances, the specific guidance of physical and occupational therapists is necessary to optimize a child's position for assessment.

Proper positioning permits a child, within the limits of his/her capabilities, to participate actively in an evaluation session and engage in those play activities designed to shape behavior during testing. More importantly, the child with choreoathetoid involvement may gain enough control over use of the upper extremities to complete play audiometric response tasks consistently. Similarly, the low functioning youngster whose head control is poor may be able to demonstrate sufficient head and neck control to provide consistent head turn responses to visual reinforcers when properly positioned and supported.

The need for audiologists to maintain an attitude of flexibility is the principle prerequisite for the assessment of children characterized as difficult to test. Indeed, the audiologist must remain flexible to meet the specific needs of children who present different developmental and behavioral profiles. However, this author's experience has suggested that the audiological evaluation benefits from adherence to well-defined test protocols. Effective protocols optimize response identification, minimize a child's fatigue and habituation to both test stimuli and test tasks, increase the repeatability of threshold estimates and minimum response levels, and decrease the time required to establish response levels while improving the likelihood of obtaining sufficient behavioral data to allow a child's auditory status to be defined as completely as possible.

Test protocols provide a framework for the initiation of testing, behavioral conditioning, and adaptive selection of the type, frequency, and intensity of successive test stimuli. For example, prior to the actual measurement of responses, a preparatory testing phase permits the examiner to verify the appropriateness of a selected response mode, including reinforcer, and to ascertain any unforeseen difficulties related to a child's behavior and his or her cognitive and motor status. A preparatory phase also permits examiners to determine those changes in a child's activity and behavior that constitute true responses to auditory stimulation utilizing BOA. Similarly, following elicitation of an initial behavioral response, conditioning bonds can be established between an auditory stimulus and the reinforcer at a level clearly audible to the child. Specific criteria to indicate that a child is conditioned should be met before formal testing is commenced.

In some instances, a physically handicapped child's degree of motor involvement may render cognitively appropriate procedures inadequate for purposes of assessing auditory sensitivity. Assessment is particularly frustrating when cognitive abilities are normal or at a level which otherwise does not preclude comprehensive evaluation. Therefore, alternate response modes may need to be determined for individual children (Friedrich, 1980). For example, a child may be able to indicate a response with an eye movement or exhibit sufficient control over movement of a certain body part to provide a repeatable response mode. In other instances, special response transducers available with electronic communication devices may be adapted and used in conjunction with audiometric equipment much as push buttons have been used with adults to signal responses. Their effective use depends upon selection of an appropriate transducer and determination of a compatible motor activity. Communication devices (such as manual communication boards, electronic communication systems, and speech synthesizers) also can be adapted for the administration of speech audiometric measures to nonvocal children who cannot provide reliable pointing responses or verbal responses. The use of such equipment is highly dependent upon the ingenuity of the examiners. However, certain audiological procedures should not be omitted from an evaluation simply because a physical disability requires a more innovative approach.

Assessment of Speech Discrimination Abilities

Tests of auditory discrimination that attempt to assess how well a listener understands spoken messages at suprathreshold levels have been a significant component of the audiological test battery for many years. A variety of test materials have been developed to evaluate the effects of peripheral auditory dysfunction on the processing of spoken messages. In addition, information gleaned from these tests has been used in the selection of hearing aids and the development of therapeutic goals. Although few audiologists would dispute that useful data are provided by these tests, controversy has centered on whether commonly used clinical measures accurately reflect or predict communicative efficiency.

Three tests for children appear to have gained widespread acceptance in clinical audiological facilities today: (1) Phonetically-Balanced Kindergarten (PBK-50) word lists (Haskins, 1949); (2) Word Intelligibility by Picture Identification (WIPI) Test (Ross & Lerman, 1970); and (3) Northwestern University–Children's Perception of Speech (NU-CHIPS) Test (Elliott & Katz, 1980). To a large extent, the development of these tests has been based upon the desire to maintain features of commonly used "adult" speech recognition tests while accommodating linguistic and response mode considerations which preclude their use with children. Consequently, they incorporate, as test stimuli, monosyllabic nouns that are presumed to be within the vocabularies of young children and attempt with varying degrees of success to maintain a degree of phonetic balance comparable to the adult materials and representative of the English language. The WIPI and NU-CHIPS tests are closed-set procedures that require the identification of pictures representing the test words, while the PBK-50 test is open set and requires a verbal response.

The linguistic and response mode considerations addressed in the development of these materials must also be addressed in the selection, administration, and interpretation of these tests with the developmentally disabled. The audiologist must be prepared again to select a test appropriate to both the physical and cognitive capabilities of the listener. The special considerations addressed in the preceding section are relevant to the use of speech recognition tests as well. However, communicative abilities assume special prominence in the utilization of these measures.

Steps must be taken to ensure that word items in a given speech recognition test are within a child's receptive vocabulary. Unless a test is selected in accordance with this principle, error responses may be interpreted as reflecting a discrimination deficit when, in fact, the test word may be unfamiliar. A number of authors have commented on the appropriateness of the various speech recognition tests for children at different levels of receptive vocabulary development. Sanderson-Leepa and Rintelmann (1976) investigated the WIPI and PBK-50 tests and suggested that they are appropriate beginning at ages 3½ and 5½ years, respectively. Matkin (1981) has advocated use of these tests at ages 4 and 6 years. Elliott and Katz (1980) concentrated particular attention on the selection of word items in the development of the NU-CHIPS test, attempting to identify both stimulus and foil items which would be within the receptive vocabularies of most 3-year-olds. On the basis of this literature, a guideline for the selection of pediatric speech recognition tests is presented in Table 2. The Peabody Picture Vocabulary Test has proven valuable for determining a child's receptive vocabulary age.

Table 2. Guideline for Selection of Pediatric Speech Recognition Tests

Procedure	Receptive Vocabulary Age (years)
PBK-50	5½-12
WIPI	3½-6
NU-CHIPS	3-6
Informal	(3

When receptive vocabulary level precludes the use of formal speech discrimination tests, Matkin (1981) suggested that informal assessment may provide useful information regarding discrimination abilities and assist in the delineation of ear differences and the evaluation of hearing aids. The audiologist may assess, for example, the identification of familiar words represented by pictures or toy objects, differentiation of words with varying stress patterns (Erber & Alencewicz, 1976), or verbal imitation of consonant/

vowel combinations. However, a child's performance must be interpreted cautiously since it may not reflect later performance with formal test procedures or actual peripheral speech discrimination capabilities. Instead, such informal tools may serve principally to provide information regarding a child's current level of auditory behavior development. Similarly, Finitzo-Hieber, Gerling, Matkin, and Cherow-Skalka (1980) investigated the use of familiar environmental sounds as an alternative to speech stimuli for assessing auditory discrimination abilities in children with limited verbal abilities. Their Sound Effects Recognition Test (SERT) incorporates a closed-set format with a picture-pointing response.

A listener's expressive speech and language skills are no less important than receptive vocabulary level in the selection of speech recognition test procedures since utterances must be intelligible if verbal responses are to be used. Incorrect responses may be attributed to discrimination deficits when, in fact, they reflect errors in articulation. They may reflect a specific articulation disorder or the listener's developmental or chronological age. In such instances, a picture-pointing response may be required even though the child is cognitively capable of verbal repetition.

Test developers have succeeded in the identification of monosyllabic words found in the receptive vocabularies of young children. Their success has commonly been viewed as eliminating errors associated with the use of unfamiliar words if tests are selected on the basis of receptive vocabulary age. However, a number of studies (Elliott, Connors, Kille, Levin, Ball, & Katz, 1979; Elliott & Katz, 1980; Sanderson-Leepa & Rintelmann, 1976; Schwartz & Goldman, 1974) have suggested that the speech recognition performance of normally developing children with normal hearing will improve as a function of age. These age-related effects are of special concern because they may reflect the ability of subjects at higher levels of development to achieve semantic closure more easily, relying upon fewer acoustic cues for word identification (Elliott & Katz, 1980; Resnick, 1982). This raises the question of utilizing monosyllabic words to assess phonetic discrimination deficits related to peripheral hearing impairment. More importantly, use of these materials may be particularly problematic for the assessment of children whose linguistic experience has been compromised by hearing impairment, mental retardation, auditory processing disorders, and so forth. The impact of cognitive functioning on the performance of children on speech recognition tests is not well understood. Thus, while useful information can be obtained from the administration of existing pediatric speech recognition tests to hearing-impaired developmentally disabled children, caution must be exercised in drawing conclusions that performance deficits reflect solely peripheral discrimination problems.

Acoustic Immittance Measurements

Acoustic immittance measurements constitute an objective means of assessing certain aspects of function of the auditory mechanism, particularly the integrity of the middle ear system. They are a valuable tool in the identification and diagnosis of both auditory pathology and hearing impairment in children and difficult-to-test patients for whom middle ear problems are prevalent and often difficult to assess while utilizing behavioral assessment tools. Acoustic immittance measurements provide information regarding the mobility of the tympanic membrane/middle ear system, middle ear pressure, the status of the auditory ossicles, eustachian tube function, and the neural pathways underlying the stapedial muscle (acoustic) reflex.

A detailed review of the principles of acoustic immittance measurements and their clinical applications is beyond the scope of this discussion. Comprehensive reviews are readily available (Feldman & Wilber, 1976), as are reviews that examine the administration and interpretation of acoustic immittance measurements with pediatric populations (Lamb & Dunckel, 1976; Northern & Downs, 1978).

To summarize, the acoustic immittance battery consists of three principle measurements: tympanometry, static compliance, and acoustic reflex measurements. Clinical judgments are based most soundly upon a consideration of the results of all three measurement procedures in combination. They are enhanced further when interpreted in conjunction with other audiometric data. Tympanometry is the measurement of the compliance of the tympanic membrane when air pressure is varied systematically in the external auditory canal. Maximum tympanic membrane compliance is observed when the air pressure in the ear canal is equivalent to the air pressure in the middle ear cavity. Thus, tympanometry provides an indirect measure of middle ear pressure. The procedure also assesses the mobility of the tympanic membrane/middle ear system. Mobility is reduced when the middle ear cavity is fluid-filled, but may be increased in the presence of a discontinuity of the ossicles. Static compliance is assessed with the system at rest and reflects a comparison of compliance at atmospheric pressure and with the tympanic membrane held in a rigid position.

Static compliance measurements are affected by such factors as age, sex, and pathology. Consequently, static compliance values are highly variable and alone are of limited use in the differentiation of normal and pathological ears. They are of value only when considered in combination with other data. Acoustic reflex measurements capitalize upon the contraction of the stapedius muscle in response to auditory stimulation at high intensity levels. The contraction of the muscle exerts a pull on the ossicular chain which in turn produces a momentary reduction in the compliance of the tympanic membrane. It is the reduction in compliance that is measured. An acoustic reflex threshold for a signal is established by determining the lowest intensity level producing a reflex.

Several investigators have reported the use of acoustic immittance procedures with developmentally disabled individuals for both screening and diagnostic purposes, citing high rates of success in obtaining measurements and the contribution of the data to the determination of auditory status (Bashore, 1976; Borus, 1972; Fulton & Lamb, 1972; Fulton & Lloyd, 1968, 1969; Lamb, 1975; Lamb & Norris, 1969, 1970; Ruth & Niswander, 1976). Procedures and principles of interpretation associated with the application of acoustic immittance measures to adults and nonhandicapped children are essentially the same for developmentally disabled individuals. Nonetheless, the measurements possess particular advantages for this population. First, they assist in the identification and diagnosis of middle ear dysfunction when behavioral assessment techniques are unsuccessful or stop short of adequately defining a problem. This is especially critical because middle ear problems are more prevalent among severely developmentally disabled individuals (Bruns, Cram, & Rogers, 1978; Fulton & Lamb, 1972; Keith, Murphy, & Martin, 1976). The value of the procedures is heightened for developmentally disabled individuals with severe peripheral hearing impairments, because assessment of auditory sensitivity alone may fail to identify a conductive hearing loss superimposed upon a sensorineural impairment. In such instances, aggressive management of middle ear problems medically and audiologically is necessary to stabilize a child's hearing and optimize the use of amplification and the reception of auditory information.

Acoustic reflex measurements have been used to estimate peripheral auditory sensitivity in infants and difficult-to-test patients. Specific procedures that involve the determination of acoustic reflex thresholds for both pure tone and noise band stimuli have been proposed by a number of investigators (e.g., Jerger, Burney, Mauldin, & Crump, 1974; Niemeyer & Sesterhenn, 1974). The procedures are based upon the principle that reflex thresholds for pure tones typically are established at intensity levels higher than those for noise bands in intact auditory systems. For sensorineural losses of cochlear origin, the difference in the threshold levels for the two signal types changes in a reasonably systematic manner as a function of degree of impairment. The difference typically decreases as the degree of hearing impairment becomes greater. Unfortunately, when hearing impairments are defined categorically (e.g., mild-moderate), only moderately accurate predictions have been reported. Jerger et al. (1974), in an extensive study, reported that prediction is poorer for severe hearing impairments. Accuracy is better for individuals with normal sensitivity or mild impairments. This has been borne out by Ruth and Niswander (1976), who suggested that the procedure is useful in providing objective evidence of normal hearing in multihandicapped children. Jerger et al. also suggested the potential utility of the procedure for prediction of audiometric configuration when reflex thresholds for low-pass and high-pass filtered noise bands are compared.

Thus, attempts to predict hearing impairment precisely on the basis of acoustic reflex measurements have been futile. Basing clinical impressions on the procedure for purposes of audiological management, including the selection of amplification, is dangerous. Acoustic reflex threshold data utilized in this manner achieve value only when considered in combination with other findings. They can assist in the confirmation of clinical impressions and, in some instances, may focus attention on inconsistencies in data which suggest the need for additional evaluations to ascertain a child's hearing.

Electrophysiological Assessment Procedures

Investigators have long sought to develop a procedure for difficult-to-test patients which is objective, does not require patient cooperation, and can be applied clinically in a cost-effective manner without posing undue risk to the patient. As a consequence, a number of procedures that attempt to measure physiological responses to auditory stimulation have been studied to determine their clinical utility. These have included measurement of the conditioned galvanic skin response to pure tones initially paired with electrical shocks to elicit autonomic changes in skin resistance (Hardy & Pauls, 1952; Spradlin, Locke, & Fulton, 1969); changes in heart rate response (Gerber, Mulac, & Swain, 1976; Schulman, Smith, Weisinger, & Fay, 1970); changes in respiration rate (Bradford, 1975; Hayes & Jerger, 1978; Poole, Goetzinger, & Rousey, 1966); and inhibition of the auropalpebral reflex (Reiter, Goetzinger, & Press, 1981). For a variety of reasons, none of these procedures has achieved widespread use with difficult-to-test patients. However, for the past 20 years continuous attention has focused on the measurement of electrical activity from the auditory system as a means of objectively determining a child's auditory status.

Electrical potentials from the auditory system have small amplitudes and stable temporal relationships to eliciting stimuli. The development of electrophysiological procedures for the detection of these potentials coincided with the advent of small laboratory computers in the early 1960s. This equipment permits electrical activity from the auditory system to be summed and averaged for multiple stimulus presentations, effectively "canceling out" random ongoing neurological activity while enhancing the signal-to-noise ratio and the observation of the time-locked small magnitude potentials.

Numerous investigators have concerned themselves with the study of evoked potentials generated at sites extending from the cochlea of the inner ear to the cortex. The potentials typically have been categorized according to latency of occurrence after stimulation and presumed site of origin. A number of references are available which comprehensively review the potentials and the procedures developed to measure them both experimentally and clinically (Davis, 1976; Skinner & Glattke, 1977).

Initial attempts to develop a clinically useful evoked potential procedure concentrated on the measurement of cortical, or late, evoked potentials. They are relatively large amplitude responses elicitable by pure tones at intensity levels approximating behavioral threshold. However, these twin advantages have been countered by high variability in amplitude, latency, and waveform configuration. The cortical potentials are influenced by a host of factors, including age, state of arousal, sedation, and central nervous system pathology. As a result, the identification of cortical responses has proven to be especially difficult for developmentally disabled children, and their measurement has achieved only limited clinical application today.

Electrocochleography (ECoG) measures electrical activity from the cochlea and the auditory nerve more directly. As a result, ECoG has much to recommend it as a clinical procedure; it provides a direct assessment of peripheral function and has proven to be highly reliable and sensitive to behavioral threshold, particularly above 2,000 Hz. In addition, the measurement of the cochlear and auditory nerve potentials is confounded by fewer subject variables. Electrocochleography, however, requires the placement of an electrode at the promontory of the cochlea in the middle ear cavity. This necessitates a surgical procedure which has limited the routine and cost-effective application of ECoG in clinical facilities.

Over the past decade, the auditory brainstem response (ABR), or early evoked potentials, has received intensive investigation. Principal attention will be focused on ABR testing because it is the one evoked potential procedure which has achieved widespread clinical use today. The ABR procedure constitutes an objective, reliable, and noninvasive approach for assessment of neural activity in the auditory nervous system at subthalamic levels. The auditory brainstem response is not influenced by states of arousal, sedation, or attention and can be recorded with electrodes placed on the surface of the skin. The professional literature is replete with descriptions of ABR testing procedures and studies of their applications to various patient populations for purposes of both audiological and neurological assessment.

For all evoked potential measurements, averaging computers sample electrical activity present at the site of surface electrodes for a specified period of time. Because the

ABR is of very small magnitude, the electrical activity must be amplified, usually by a factor of 50,000–100,000, and averaged for multiple stimulus presentations, typically 1,024–2,048. The electrical activity is also filtered by the amplifier over a frequency range approximating 100–3,000 Hz, because the early evoked potentials constitute a "fast response waveform."

The ABR waveform is multiphasic and characterized by several discernible peaks and valleys (see Figure 4). The wave peaks are numbered in accordance with their order of occurrence. Wave V is typically the most prominent peak and often the only peak easily identified at lower stimulus intensities. The auditory brainstem response typically occurs within the first eight seconds following stimulus onset. The latency of the individual waves is inversely related to intensity while the amplitude of the waves is directly related. Wave latencies are also related to a child's chronological age. The latency of wave V progressively shortens until its adult value is reached by 15–18 months. Waves I–IV sequentially reach adult values at earlier ages. This apparently reflects the myelinization of auditory neurons, a process which begins at the periphery of the auditory system in infants.

A number of researchers have suggested that the individual waves may reflect neural activity at successively higher points in the auditory system; however, considerable questions remain regarding the exact sites of origin. Wave I does appear, however, to be related temporally to the auditory nerve action potential. The measurement of individual wave peaks is influenced by a variety of factors, including electrode placement site and rate of stimulus presentation. The detection of earlier waves tends to be enhanced, for example, by slower rates of presentation.

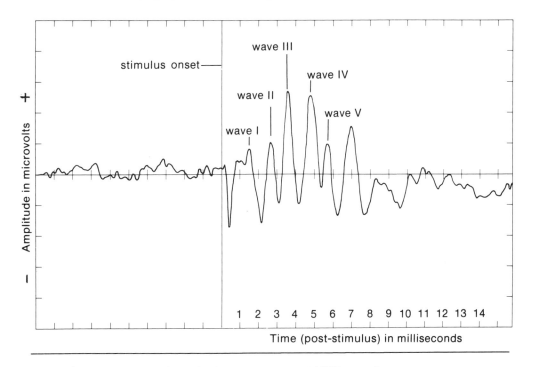

Figure 4. A "normal" auditory brainstem response (ABR) waveform.

ABR Limitations

Elicitation of the auditory brainstem response is dependent upon the use of abrupt-onset signals which produce synchronous neural discharges in the auditory system. Consequently, click stimuli are typically used in clinical testing. The responses to clicks characteristically reflect the response of the cochlea in the higher frequency region (2,000–4,000 Hz). Thus, the ABR procedure provides only limited frequency-specific information. Short duration "tone pips" have not proven to be sufficiently sensitive for purposes of providing more detailed frequency-specific information. Furthermore, the intensities of clicks are typically limited by earphones to a maximum of approximately 85–90 dBnHL, restricting the audiologist's ability to define with certainty the presence of significant residual hearing.

Several investigators recently have discussed the specific application of the ABR procedure to determine the peripheral auditory sensitivity of neurologically impaired and multihandicapped children. Jerger, Hayes, and Jordan (1980) and Shimizu (1981) reported difficulties observing auditory brainstem responses in children with central nervous system involvement and suggested that the procedure may be of limited use with these children. Worthington and Peters (1980) reported on four patients with central nervous system pathology whose ABRs were either absent or definable only at high stimulus levels, even though they possessed normal or near normal peripheral auditory sensitivity as measured with behavioral techniques. Salamy, Mendelson, Tooley, and Chaplin (1980) reported a reduction in the amplitude of individual waves of the ABR for infants judged to be at high risk for central nervous system involvement.

Resnick, Friedrich, Smyke, and Heinz (1980) observed typical ABR waveforms in only a small number of neurologically impaired and developmentally disabled children. They concurred that the presence of central nervous system involvement as well as increases or changes in motor and neurological activity in developmentally disabled children, even when sedated, may complicate the identification and interpretation of auditory brainstem responses and contribute to increased response variability within test sessions. Yet, they also reported a greater success rate in the determination of the peripheral auditory sensitivity of their patients than reported by Jerger et al. and Shimizu. Resnick et al. attributed their success in overcoming some of these difficulties to the utilization of equipment and procedures designed to enhance the sensitivity and reliability of ABR measurements. Among other approaches, they urged recording prestimulus as well as poststimulus activity to provide a basis of comparison for response judgments. They also stressed the need for careful consideration of conditions of artifact rejection during testing to minimize negative effects associated with increased motor and neurological activity which may obscure responses.

Resnick et al. also suggested that exclusive reliance on wave latency measures is inadequate for purposes of interpreting ABR data audiologically. For example, the latency of wave V, the most prominent wave in the ABR, obtained at several intensities is often the basis for judgments regarding sensitivity. Wave V typically is prolonged in the presence of peripheral hearing impairment. Yet, wave V also may be prolonged due to central nervous system pathology while earlier waves, particularly wave I, are not so affected. This results in a lengthening of the normal time interval between waves I and V. Thus, procedures and test protocols designed to enhance the detection of wave I, the most peripheral component of the ABR, are crucial to decisions regarding sensitivity. Determination of wave I latency permits the audiologist to identify the wave I–V interval and any prolongation in wave V latency due to factors other than peripheral hearing impairment. Wave V latency values might otherwise lead to erroneous conclusions about sensitivity. Other procedures to enhance ABR interpretation with developmentally disabled children have been described in detail by Resnick and her colleagues (Friedrich et al., 1982; Resnick, Friedrich, Heinz, & Talkin, 1981).

The findings of these investigators collectively suggest that the use of standard procedures for the acquisition and analysis of ABR data is inadequate for differentiation of the effects of peripheral auditory dysfunction and central nervous system dysfunction in developmentally disabled youngsters. These difficulties, in combination with limitations associated with the frequency-specificity of data and maximum available stimulus intensity, suggest that considerable caution needs to be exercised in the interpretation of ABR data. In short, ABR testing does not constitute a single complete procedure for the determination of auditory status in difficult-to-test individuals. Consequently, the decision to complete ABR testing should not be based simply upon a child's age or the presence of developing handicapping conditions. Referrals should be based upon (1) behavioral data which suggest but do not define the nature of a potential hearing impairment, (2) inconsistencies in audiometric data which fail to rule out hearing impairment, and (3) the failure of developmentally appropriate behavioral test procedures to yield reliable data regarding a child's auditory status.

Hearing Aid Selection and Evaluation

The selection and evaluation of wearable amplification for children has been a subject of special concern to audiologists for many years, particularly as increasing numbers of hearing-impaired children have been identified at younger ages and judged to be candidates for hearing aid use. In many instances, audiologists have adopted approaches and procedures used with adults and either applied them directly or modified them for use with older children. Alternative approaches are required, however, for infants and younger children. As discussed earlier in this section, these approaches are generally appropriate for hearing-impaired developmentally disabled youngsters as well when selected and utilized on the basis of a child's developmental status. However, special considerations are necessary for the application of amplification devices and formulation of realistic goals for hearing aid use by the hearing-impaired developmentally disabled population. Unfortunately, a body of literature that addresses hearing aid selection and evaluation for the developmentally disabled is virtually nonexistent. Indeed, Matkin (1977) pointed out that only limited clinical research has been conducted regarding the pediatric population in general.

For hearing-impaired children, general agreement exists that amplification should be provided as early as possible to foster development and use of residual hearing. Early amplification is believed to minimize the potential effects of sensory deprivation associated with hearing impairment, enhance the development of language and communication skills (regardless of educational philosophy or communication approach), and facilitate psychosocial and cognitive development. Despite this fact, amplification frequently has been withheld or delayed for the developmentally disabled, particularly when cognitive or physical disabilities are severe. This situation apparently reflects, at least in part, difficulties associated with the accurate identification of hearing impairment, problems encountered in the formal selection and evaluation of devices, and judgments that disabilities are so severe as to preclude the use of an amplification device or render its use meaningless. However, no significant literature exists to support the latter viewpoint, and, as we have seen, the large majority of developmentally disabled youngsters can be evaluated effectively.

The application of hearing aids to developmentally disabled children has been compromised by other factors as well, including (1) the difficulties associated with the acceptance of instruments by children, (2) the low priority attached to the use of hearing aids by some parents and educators as well as other professionals, and (3) the failure to provide consistent and systematic programs of training in the proper use and care of amplification devices. These problems have persisted despite the existence of programs (McCoy & Lloyd, 1967; Moore, Miltenberger, & Barber, 1969) and curricula (Hyde & Engle, 1977; Potocki & Miller, 1980) that address hearing aid use and adjustment for developmentally disabled youngsters. These programs, and indeed the efforts of most audiologists, focus on training parents, teachers, and other caregivers to assume responsibility for placing hearing aids on individuals and caring for them. Tucker and Berry (1980) reported success in the development of a behavioral training program designed to give severely handicapped institutionalized students independence in putting on their own hearing aids in several different environments. Thus, it is short-sighted to deny amplification categorically without investigation of its potential use with individual listeners.

The problems associated with hearing aid use seem to be predominantly related to goal-setting. Goals must be established that are appropriate and reasonable in terms of a child's developmental and behavioral as well as auditory status. Depending upon the potential of the individual for cognitive and physical development, specific goals of hearing aid use might include the following: (1) to improve receptive speech and language skills; (2) to improve expressive speech and language skills; (3) to facilitate use of alternate modes of communication (manual communication, communication boards and devices); (4) to facilitate vocational potential; (5) to facilitate development of self-care skills, functional life skills, and other activities of daily living; (6) to provide sound awareness and signal-warning information; and (7) to facilitate control and management of behavior. Obviously, the use of amplification will be critical to the child with academic potential. Goals for hearing aid use will parallel those typically established with normally developing youngsters. However, neither a normal rate of development nor achievement of the same levels of performance should be expected, particularly when cognitive abilities are limited.

The selection and evaluation of an amplification system involves several distinct steps: (1) preselection, (2) clinical evaluation, (3) trial period of use, and (4) follow-up hearing aid performance assessment. Preselection refers to the selection of hearing aids for clinical trial and formal evaluation based upon audiological findings, review of the electroacoustical characteristics of aids, and clinical experience (Matkin, 1981). The preselection process is considered by this author to be an especially crucial step in the application of hearing aids to developmentally disabled individuals. In some instances, an initial recommendation may need to be based solely on preselection considerations if a child's developmental and behavioral status precludes formal clinical assessment of aided performance at the time of selection. In other instances, of course, the preselection process is a prelude to formal clinical evaluation of the appropriateness of one or more instruments.

Preselection Decisions

During the preselection process, preliminary decisions are reached concerning (1) type of hearing aid (body-type, ear level, in-the-ear); (2) arrangement (monaural, binaural, pseudobinaural, or y-cord); (3) frequency response (gain characteristics and frequency range); and (4) maximum output or SSPL 90 (including type of output limiting system). These considerations have been addressed at length by other authors (Matkin, 1981; Ross & Tomassetti, 1980) and do not require detailed scrutiny here. However, several points need to be highlighted regarding preselection for hearing-impaired developmentally disabled individuals. First, body-type aids frequently have been selected to meet the gain requirements of individuals with severe-to-profound hearing impairments, facilitate manipulation of hearing aid control switches by caregivers, and avoid problems associated with keeping instruments on young children. Recent developments in hearing aid technology have led to the increased marketing of ear-level instruments which now meet the needs of most impairments regardless of degree. Furthermore, they are flexible electroacoustically and provide amplification which extends into the higher frequencies judged to be critical for speech discrimination. When coupled with properly fitting earmolds to minimize external feedback problems, they can meet the needs of those with severe-to-profound impairments.

This author has encountered considerable success in the use of ear-level instruments with developmentally disabled children 18 months and older. Body-type aids are now reserved primarily for infants and children whose status affects their acceptance of amplification or compromises significantly a caregiver's ability to manage the other types of aids. It is important to note that behavioral modification approaches have facilitated the acceptance of instruments by some children with significant behavioral problems, including self-stimulatory behavior.

In general, those considerations that enter into the selection and adjustment of the frequency response and other amplification characteristics of an aid for adults and normally developing children are applicable to hearing-impaired developmentally disabled persons. The central goal remains one of optimizing auditory input and facilitating the reception and understanding of spoken language. Yet, assessment of tolerance levels for intense auditory signals to determine the appropriate maximum output of a hearing aid is often difficult with individuals at lower levels of development. As a consequence, particular caution needs to be exercised in setting the saturation sound pressure level (SSPL 90) of a hearing aid to avoid potential risks associated with overamplification, including temporary or permanent threshold shifts and the rejection of amplification. Audiologists need to be aware that the sound pressure level generated by a hearing aid in a child's external ear canal may be increased as a consequence of the smaller size of the canal. Thus, it seldom seems advisable to set an instrument to an

SSPL 90 in excess of 125 dB SPL. This underscores the point that audiologists must remain cognizant of theoretical principles underlying the use of amplification with children when test procedures do not yield specific data and the child is unable to report subjective reactions.

Following preselection, the clinical evaluation of a hearing-impaired listener's performance with amplification assists the audiologist in determining the appropriateness of a particular instrument and the selection of one aid from among several in a comparative hearing aid evaluation. Of equal importance, however, is the fact that the evaluation should provide data which permit the audiologist to judge the specific benefits of hearing aid use for a given patient. The data should assist the audiologist and other professionals in the identification of realistic goals for intervention as they pertain to the use of residual hearing. The data should also prove useful for purposes of counseling family members and others regarding the potential limitations and advantages of hearing aid use.

The goal of any hearing aid evaluation is to select an instrument and/or adjust it to provide the wearer access to the widest possible portion of the average speech spectrum (at normal conversational levels) at a usable sensation level and comfortable listening level. This is deemed appropriate to optimize a hearing-impaired listener's reception and understanding of spoken language. It is important to note that sound energy which contributes significantly to the perception and discrimination of speech messages is present through at least 6,000 Hz and is not confined to the 500–2,000 Hz region which traditionally, but inaccurately, has been labeled the "speech frequencies."

As noted above, a variety of test procedures are available to assist the audiologist in hearing aid selection. However, conventional measures of speech recognition performance, loudness tolerance, and comfortable listening levels usually are not possible with nonverbal, low-functioning individuals. Consequently, a number of investigators have described procedures that permit the audiologist to estimate the sensation levels at which portions of the average speech spectrum are received when aided (Byrne & Fifield, 1974; Byrne & Tonisson, 1976; Gengel, Pascoe, & Shore, 1971; Pascoe, 1975). These procedures involve the measurement of aided thresholds for frequency-specific stimuli. The sensation levels at which various portions of the average speech spectrum are received are determined through a comparison of aided thresholds at various frequencies to the intensity levels corresponding to respective frequency bands of speech signals. A comparison of unaided and aided thresholds also permits the determination of the functional gain of an instrument, a measurement which reflects the interaction between an aid and the real ear.

Subsequent to selection, a hearing aid customarily is issued for an initial trial period. This period is considered especially critical for the developmentally disabled child to monitor acceptance and adjustment to amplification. Ideally, the audiologist should assume responsibility for direct issuance of the amplification system and supervision of the trial period. During this period, input from family members and educators as well as other professional personnel involved in the child's program contributes to final decisions regarding modifications and adjustments of the system, schedule for use, and the formulation of realistic goals for hearing aid use. Finally, a performance assessment should be completed prior to the end of the trial period. This should include an electroacoustical analysis of the hearing aid to ensure that it is functioning in accordance with manufacturer's specifications. Formal clinical evaluation of the child's aided performance also should be completed to help reach final decisions regarding modifications and adjustments and to verify the appropriateness of the child's perform- ance with amplification. These data should assist the audiologist in providing caregivers a final orientation to hearing aid use and in setting initial goals.

Summary

The audiologist has a central and ongoing role to play in the evaluation and management of hearing-impaired developmentally disabled children. The inter- disciplinary process is vital to the completion of the audiological evaluation itself as well as to determination of the communicative, developmental, and educational significance of a child's hearing impairment in the presence of additional handicaps. The audiologist has a battery of behavioral and electrophysiological test procedures that permits assess- ment of the auditory status of the large majority of hearing-impaired developmentally disabled children regardless of age or accompanying handicaps. Reliance upon electro- physiological procedures, and ABR testing in particular, as the sole means of establish- ing auditory status is discouraged. Instead, the integration of data from a number of carefully selected procedures is viewed as providing the most reliable and useful impres- sion of a child's auditory status. Furthermore, both behavioral and electrophysiological procedures must be selected, administered, and interpreted in accordance with a careful consideration of a child's cognitive, neuromotor, and behavioral status.

These considerations are necessary if appropriate programs of intervention, includ- ing the use of amplification, are to be established. Thus, decision making within the framework of an interdisciplinary model is optimal for the audiologist to contribute to the special habilitative needs of hearing-impaired developmentally disabled children.

References

American National Standards Institute. (1970). Specifications for audiometers (ANSI S3.6-1969). New York: Author.

Bashore, S. R. (1976). The use of tympanometry for screening developmentally disturbed children. *Audiology and Hearing Education, 2,* 35–40.

Bendet, R. M. (1976). Evaluating hearing of the low-developmental-level child. *Asha, 18,* 407–414.

Borus, J. (1972). Acoustic impedance measurements with hard of hearing mentally retarded children. *Journal of Mental Deficiency Research, 16,* 196–202.

Bradford, L. (1975). Respiration audiometry. In L. Bradford (Ed.), *Physiological measures of the audio-vestibular system.* New York: Academic Press.

Bruns, J. M., Cram, J. T., & Rogers, G. J. (1978). Impedance and otoscopy screening of multiply handicapped children in schools. *Language, Speech and Hearing Services in Schools, 10,* 54–58.

Byrne, D., & Fifield, D. (1974). Evaluation of hearing aid fittings for infants. *British Journal of Audiology, 8,* 47–54.

Byrne, D., & Tonisson, W. (1976). Selecting the gain of hearing aids for persons with sensorineural hearing impairments. *Scandinavian Audiology, 5,* 51–59.

Davis, H. (1976). Principles of electric response audiometry. *Annals of Otology, Rhinology and Laryngology, 85* (Suppl. 28), (3, Pt. 3).

Dirks, D. D., Stream, R. W., & Wilson, R. H. (1972). Speech audiometry: Earphone and sound field. *Journal of Speech and Hearing Disorders, 37,* 162–176.

Elliott, L. L., Connors, S., Kille, E., Levin, S., Ball, K., & Katz, D. (1979). Children's understanding of monosyllabic nouns in quiet and in noise. *Journal of the Acoustical Society of America, 66,* 12–21.

Elliott, L. L., & Katz, D. R. (1980). *Development of a new children's test of speech discrimination.* St. Louis: Auditec.

Erber, N. P., & Alencewicz, C. M. (1976). Audiologic evaluation of deaf children. *Journal of Speech and Hearing Disorders, 41,* 256–266.

Feldman, A. S., & Wilber, L. A. (1976). *Acoustic impedance and admittance: The measurement of middle ear function.* Baltimore: Williams and Wilkins.

Finitzo-Hieber, T., Gerling, I. J., Matkin, N. D., & Cherow-Skalka, E. (1980). A sound effects recognition test for the pediatric audiological evaluation. *Ear and Hearing, 1,* 271–280.

Friedrich, B. W. (1980). Clinical evaluation of hearing in developmentally disabled children. In L. J. Bradford and F. N. Martin (Eds.), *Audiology, 5,* 8.

Friedrich, B. W., Resnick, S. B., Bookstein, E. W., & Balfour, P. B. (1982). Behavioral and electrophysiological evaluation of auditory function in multi-handicapped children. Mini-seminar presented at the Convention of the American Speech-Language-Hearing Association, Toronto, Ontario, Canada.

Fulton, R. T., & Lamb, L. E. (1972). Acoustic impedance and tympanometry with the retarded: A normative study. *Audiology, 11,* 199–208.

Fulton, R. T., & Lloyd, L. L. (1968). Hearing impairment in a population of children with Down's syndrome. *American Journal of Mental Deficiency, 73,* 298–302.

Fulton, R. T., & Lloyd, L. L. (Eds.). (1969). *Audiometry for the retarded.* Baltimore: Williams and Wilkins.

Gans, D. P., & Flexer, C. (1982). Observer bias in the hearing testing of profoundly involved multiply handicapped children. *Ear and Hearing, 3,* 309–313.

Garstecki, D. (1978). Survey of school audiologists. *Asha, 20,* 291–296.

Gengel, B. W., Pascoe, D., & Shore, I. (1971). A frequency-response procedure for evaluating and selecting hearing aids for severely hearing-impaired children. *Journal of Speech and Hearing Disorders, 36,* 341–353.

Gerber, S. E., Mulac, A., & Swain, B. J. (1976). Idiosyncratic cardiovascular response of human neonates to acoustic stimuli. *Journal of the American Audiology Society, 1,* 185–192.

Greenberg, D. B., Wilson, W. R., Moore, J. M., & Thompson, G. (1978). Visual reinforcement audiometry (VRA) with young Down's syndrome children. *Journal of Speech and Hearing Disorders, 43,* 448–458.

Hardy, W. G., & Pauls, M. D. (1952). The test situation of PGSR audiometry. *Journal of Speech and Hearing Disorders, 17,* 13–24.

Haskins, H. L. (1949). A phonetically-balanced test of speech discrimination for children. Unpublished master's thesis, Northwestern University, Evanston, IL.

Hayes, D., & Jerger, J. (1978). Response detection in respiration audiometry. *Archives of Otolaryngology, 104,* 183–185.

Hoversten, G., & Moncur, J. (1969). Stimulus and intensity factors in testing infants. *Journal of Speech and Hearing Research, 12,* 687–702.

Hyde, S., & Engle, D. (1977). *The Potomac program: A curriculum for the severely handicapped deaf-hearing impaired-non-verbal.* Beaverton, OR: Dormac.

Jerger, J., Burney, P., Mauldin, L., & Crump, B. (1974). Predicting hearing loss from the acoustic reflex. *Journal of Speech and Hearing Disorders, 39,* 11–22.

Jerger, J., Hayes, D., & Jordan, C. (1980). Clinical experience with auditory brainstem response audiometry in pediatric assessment. *Ear and Hearing, 1,* 19–25.

Keith, R. W., Murphy, K. P., & Martin, F. (1976). Acoustic impedance measurement in the otological assessment of multiply handicapped children. *Clinical Otolaryngology, 1,* 221–224.

Kenworthy, O. T. (1982). Integration of assessment and management processes: Audiology as an educational program. In B. Campbell & V. Baldwin (Eds.), *Severely handicapped/hearing impaired students.* Baltimore: Paul H. Brookes.

Lamb, L. E. (1975). Acoustic impedance measurement. In R. T. Fulton & L. L. Lloyd (Eds.), *Auditory assessment of the difficult to test.* Baltimore: Williams and Wilkins.

Lamb, L. E., & Dunckel, D. C. (1976). Acoustic impedance measurement with children. In A. S. Feldman & L. A. Wilber (Eds.), *Acoustic impedance and admittance: The measurement of middle ear function.* Baltimore: Williams and Wilkins.

Lamb, L. E., & Norris, T. (1969). Acoustic impedance measurement. In R. T. Fulton & L. L. Lloyd (Eds.), *Audiometry for the retarded.* Baltimore: Williams and Wilkins.

Lamb. L. E., & Norris, T. (1970). Relative acoustic impedance measurements with mentally retarded children. *American Journal of Mental Deficiency, 75,* 51–56.

Langford, C. L., Bench, J., & Wilson, I. (1975). Some effects of prestimulus activity and length of prestimulus observations on judgments of newborns' responses to sounds. *Audiology, 14,* 44–52.

Ling, D., Ling, A. H., & Doehring, D. G. (1970). Stimulus, response, and observer variables in the auditory screening of newborn infants. *Journal of Speech and Hearing Research, 13,* 9–18.

Lloyd, L. L. (1966). Behavioral audiometry viewed as an operant procedure. *Journal of Speech and Hearing Disorders, 31,* 128–136.

Lloyd, L. L. (1977). The assessment of auditory abilities. In P. Mittler (Ed.), *Research to practice in mental retardation* (Vol. II). Baltimore: University Park Press.

Lloyd, L. L., Spradlin, J. E., & Reid, M. J. (1968). An operant audiometric procedure for difficult-to-test patients. *Journal of Speech and Hearing Disorders, 33,* 236–245.

Martin, F. N., & Coombes, S. (1976). A tangibly reinforced speech reception threshold procedure for use with small children. *Journal of Speech and Hearing Disorders, 41,* 333–338.

Matkin, N. D. (1977). Assessment of hearing sensitivity during the pre-school years. In F. H. Bess (Ed.), *Childhood deafness: Causation, assessment and management.* New York: Grune and Stratton.

Matkin, N. D. (1981). Hearing aids for children. In W. R. Hodgson & P. H. Skinner (Eds.), *Hearing aid assessment and use in audiologic habilitation.* Baltimore: Williams and Wilkins.

McCoy, D. F., & Lloyd, L. L. (1967). A hearing aid orientation program for mentally retarded children. *Training School Bulletin, 64,* 21–30.

Moncur, J. P. (1968). Judge reliability in infant testing. *Journal of Speech and Hearing Research, 11,* 348–357.

Moore, E. J., Miltenberger, G. E., & Barber, P. S. (1969). Hearing aid orientation in a state school for the mentally retarded. *Journal of Speech and Hearing Disorders, 34,* 142–145.

Morgan, D., Dirks, D., & Bower, D. (1979). Suggested threshold sound pressure levels for frequency modulated (warble) tones in the sound field. *Journal of Speech and Hearing Disorders, 44,* 37–54.

Niemeyer, W., & Sesterhenn, C. (1974). Calculating the hearing threshold from the stapedius reflex for different sound stimuli. *Audiology, 13,* 421–427.

Northern, J. L., & Downs, M. P. (1978). *Hearing in children* (2nd ed.). Baltimore: Williams and Wilkins.

Pascoe, D. P. (1975). Frequency responses of hearing aids and their effects on the speech perception of hearing-impaired subjects. *Annals of Otology, Rhinology and Laryngology, 84* (Suppl. 23), (5, Pt. 2).

Poole, R., Goetzinger, C., & Rousey, C. (1966). A study of the effects of auditory stimuli on respiration. *Acta Otolaryngologica, 16,* 143–152.

Potocki, P. A., & Miller, B. (1980). *Hands on: A manipulative curriculum for teaching multiply-handicapped hearing impaired students.* Tucson: Communication Skill Builders.

Reiter, L. I., Goetzinger, C. P., & Press, S. E. (1981). Reflex modulation: A hearing test for the difficult-to-test. *Journal of Speech and Hearing Disorders, 46,* 262–266.

Resnick, S. B. (1982). Speech recognition testing: Non-conventional testing techniques and their application to children. Invited paper presented at the NINCDS Workshop on Speech Recognition by the Hearing Impaired, Bethesda, MD.

Resnick, S. B., Friedrich, B. W., Heinz, J. M., & Talkin, D. (1981). Techniques for quantification of ABR waveforms in multi-handicapped children. Paper presented at the Convention of the American Speech-Language-Hearing Association, Los Angeles, CA.

Resnick, S. B., Friedrich, B. W., Smyke, A. T., & Heinz, J. M. (1980). Application and interpretation of ABR measures in multiply handicapped children. Paper presented at the Convention of the American Speech-Language-Hearing Association, Detroit, MI.

Ross, M., & Lerman, J. (1970). A picture identification test for hearing-impaired children. *Journal of Speech and Hearing Research, 13,* 44–53.

Ross, M., & Tomassetti, C. (1980). Hearing aid selection for preverbal hearing-impaired children. In M. C. Pollack (Ed.), *Amplification for the hearing impaired* (2nd ed.). New York: Grune and Stratton.

Ruth, R. A., & Niswander, P. S. (1976). Application of the differential loudness summation test for estimating hearing thresholds in mentally retarded subjects. Paper presented at the Convention of the American Speech-Language-Hearing Association, Houston, TX.

Salamy, A., Mendelson, T., Tooley, W., & Chaplin, E. (1980). Differential development of brainstem potentials in healthy and high risk infants. *Science, 210,* 553–555.

Sanders, J. W., & Josey, A. F. (1970). Narrow-band noise audiometry for hard-to-test patients. *Journal of Speech and Hearing Research, 13,* 74–81.

Sanderson-Leepa, M. D., & Rintelmann, W. F. (1976). Articulation functions and test-retest performance of normal-hearing children on three speech discrimination tests: WIPI, PBK-50, and N. U. Auditory Test, No. 6. *Journal of Speech and Hearing Disorders, 41,* 503–519.

Schulman, C. A., Smith, C. R., Weisinger, M., & Fay, T. H. (1970). The use of heart rate in the audiological evaluation of non-verbal children: 1. Evaluation of children at risk for hearing impairment. *Neuropaediatrie, 2,* 187–196.

Schwartz, A. H., & Goldman, R. (1974). Variables influencing performance on speech-sound discrimination tests. *Journal of Speech and Hearing Research, 17,* 25–32.

Shimizu, H. (1981). Editorial: Clinical use of auditory brainstem response: Issues and answers. *Ear and Hearing, 2,* 3–4.

Skinner, P., & Glattke, T. J. (1977). Electrophysiologic response audiometry: State of the art. *Journal of Speech and Hearing Disorders, 42,* 179–198.

Spradlin, J. E., Locke, B., & Fulton, R. T. (1969). Conditioning and audiological assessment. In R. T. Fulton & L. L. Lloyd (Eds.), *Audiometry for the retarded.* Baltimore: Williams and Wilkins.

Stream, R., & Dirks, D. (1974). Effect of loudspeaker position on differences between earphones and free-field thresholds (MAP and MAF). *Journal of Speech and Hearing Research, 17,* 549–568.

Thompson, G., & Folsom, R. (1981). Hearing assessment of at-risk infants. *Clinical Pediatrics, 20*, 257–261.

Thompson, G., & Weber, B. A. (1974). Responses of infants and young children to behavioral observation audiometry (BOA). *Journal of Speech and Hearing Disorders, 39*, 140–147.

Thompson, G., Wilson, W. R., & Moore, J. M. (1979). Application of visual reinforcement audiometry (VRA) to low-functioning children. *Journal of Speech and Hearing Disorders, 44*, 80–90.

Tillman, T. W., Johnson, R. M., & Olsen, W. O. (1966). Earphone versus sound-field threshold sound-pressure levels for spondee words. *Journal of the Acoustical Society of America, 39*, 125–133.

Tucker, D. J., & Berry, G. W. (1980). Teaching severely multihandicapped students to put on their own hearing aids. *Journal of Applied Behavior Analysis, 13*, 65–75.

Weaver, N. J., Wardell, F. N., & Martin, F. N. (1979). Comparison of tangibly reinforced speech-reception and pure-tone thresholds of mentally retarded children. *American Journal of Mental Deficiency, 83*, 512–517.

Weber, B. A. (1969). Validation of observer judgments in behavioral observation audiometry. *Journal of Speech and Hearing Disorders, 34*, 350–355.

Wilson, W. R., & Moore, J. M. (1978). Pure-tone earphone thresholds of infants utilizing visual reinforcement audiometry (VRA). Paper presented at the Convention of the American Speech-Language-Hearing Association, San Francisco, CA.

Wilson, W. R., Moore, J. M., & Thompson, G. (1976). Sound-field auditory thresholds of infants utilizing visual reinforcement audiometry (VRA). Paper presented at the Convention of the American Speech-Language-Hearing Association, Houston, TX.

Worthington, D., & Peters, J. (1980). Quantifiable hearing and no ABR: Paradox or error? *Ear and Hearing, 1*, 281–285.

Chapter 9

Improving Evaluation of Vision

Pamela J. Cress, Charles R. Spellman, and
Holly A. Benson

There are a number of individuals with hearing impairments and developmental disabilities who experience the additional handicapping condition of undetected or untreated visual impairments. In consultation with various state officials and during visits throughout the United States to programs serving individuals with multiple handicaps, the authors have found that there are many with impaired hearing and developmental disabilities who have never received any type of vision services. Historically, such infants, preschoolers, and school-age individuals have been excluded from existing vision services. When otherwise conscientious service providers neglect to address an area so critical to the learning process, one can assume that one or more of the following factors are operating.

- A general lack of awareness regarding the importance of good vision care. For hearing-impaired developmentally disabled people, an additional and uncorrected impairment in the visual modality can have detrimental and pervasive effects upon their ability to function at a maximum level of independence. Vision plays an especially critical role in communication for these individuals; their ability to learn and use such alternative communication modes as speechreading and signed or printed symbols is dependent upon vision.
- A lack of information regarding the specialized assessment techniques currently available for testing individuals who have hearing impairment and developmental disabilities.
- Lack of interdisciplinary cooperation among such professionals as teachers, early education specialists, social workers, school nurses, pediatricians, and professional eye examiners (optometrists and ophthalmologists). Such cooperation is essential to the provision of adequate services to hearing-impaired developmentally disabled people.

The purpose of this chapter is to provide information regarding vision and the importance of conscientious vision care. Available objective and subjective methods for

The activities described in this chapter were partially supported by the U.S. Department of Education, USOSE Grant No. G008102115, Bureau of Education for the Handicapped. The views expressed herein do not necessarily represent the official position of that agency.

assessing vision, and procedures for selecting appropriate screening tools, are described. The authors further propose a process for the design and implementation of a vision care system that decreases the probability that vision problems remain undetected and ensures that appropriate treatment and follow-up services are provided.

Background Information

The incidence of vision problems in the hearing-impaired developmentally disabled population is not well documented. Some data are available regarding the incidence of visual impairment within the separate populations of those with hearing impairment and those with developmental disabilities, but, to date, no such data have been collected for the population with both hearing impairment and other developmental disabilities. This lack of information probably reflects the difficulties of testing that population for possible visual impairment and also may be due to corresponding difficulties in assessing hearing within the population with developmental disabilities; thus, the hearing-impaired developmentally disabled population has not been clearly distinguished from the general developmentally disabled population for research purposes. Many of the prenatal, postnatal, and environmental factors that place a person at risk for other handicapping conditions are essentially the same as those which place one at risk for visual impairments (Woodruff, 1972); thus, one would speculate that the probability of a hearing-impaired developmentally disabled person having a vision problem would be significantly higher than for the nonhandicapped population.

For example, individuals with Down's syndrome are known to have a much higher evidence of vision problems than do nonhandicapped populations (Smith & Wilson, 1973). Donlon (1966) reported that 75 percent of all children with cerebral palsy may have a significant visual impairment. These data, coupled with the known risk of common medications (muscle relaxants, tranquilizers, and many anticonvulsant drugs) which have potential visual side effects, suggest that people with hearing impairment and developmental disabilities who have a history of using medications with transient or permanent vision side effects are at even greater risk of having vision problems. Barker and Barmatz (1975) found that myopia and prenatal cataracts occur more frequently in premature children. They also found that blindness and visual impairments in children from poverty level families were double those of middle-income families. Even without specific studies of people with impaired hearing and developmental disabilities, one may assume that the incidence of visual impairment is much higher than in the general population; for the group, the incidence probably falls within the 65 percent to 85 percent range reported by Fletcher and Thompson (1961), Woodruff (1977), and Ellis (1979) for the developmentally disabled population.

The most common types of visual impairments are those caused by refractive errors and muscle imbalance (strabismus). Those caused by refractive errors generally can be corrected with prescriptive lenses. Unfortunately, many hearing-impaired developmentally disabled individuals do not currently receive this relatively common treatment. Refractive errors include myopia, hyperopia, and astigmatism. Myopia (near-sightedness) affects how well one sees at a distance as compared to hyperopia (far-sightedness) which affects near vision. In myopia the distance between the eye's lens and the retina is too long, causing the light rays to focus in front of the retina rather than on the retina. Conversely, with hyperopia the distance between the eye's lens and the retina is too short to allow the light rays to focus on the retina. Astigmatism is caused by an uneven curvature of the cornea and generally affects near vision more than distance vision. The uneven curvature results in light rays being distorted so thay they do not focus directly on the retina. With astigmatism one has difficulty in focusing on both horizontal and vertical rays at the same time. People with astigmatism will fatigue quickly when doing close work and often experience burning and squinting when engaged in prolonged near-focusing as required in many school activities. When refractive errors go undetected or untreated for long periods of time they can lead to permanent reduction in vision (Stangler, Huber, & Routh, 1980; Woodruff, 1977).

Muscle imbalance, or strabismus, refers to a variety of conditions which result in misalignment of the eyes in a manner that causes them to deviate from the midline in any direction. These deviations make it impossible for the person to fixate both eyes in a coordinated manner and to produce a single image. Strabismic conditions are classified as either tropias or phorias. Tropias are obvious deviations in the alignment of the eye(s) that are consistently present. According to a number of authors (e.g., Harley, 1975; McGuire, 1966), tropias must always be considered abnormal, and, without appropriate treatment, vision will be compromised. Phorias refer to those muscle imbalances that are not apparent to the observer and are only present when binocular vision is interrupted, as seen during administration of the Cover-Uncover Test (briefly described later). Generally, phorias are not considered significant unless the child complains of headaches or has symptoms of eye strain; nonetheless, children with suspected phorias should be referred for professional eye care to monitor the condition.

Prefixes used to describe the direction of deviation of both tropias and phorias include *eso* (inward), *exo* (outward), *hetero* (upward), and *hypo* (downward). Therefore, a child diagnosed as having exotropia would have consistently obvious out-turned eye alignment. Eye patching, surgery, and glasses are the most typical treatments for muscle imbalances. The importance of early identification and treatment of strabismus is magnified by the fact that this condition can be effectively treated in the young child, but, if left untreated up to age 6 or after, the chance for obtaining normal binocular vision is significantly reduced.

Another vision problem with a critical period for treatment is amblyopia. Amblyopia refers to a condition wherein the child's two eyes do not see equally well, either because of unequal refractive errors, strabismus, or other causes. This condition, if left untreated, can result in reduced functioning of one eye leading to possible blindness. Thus, as with strabismus, amblyopia must be identified and treated in the preschool years to avoid needless loss of sight.

Visual Assessment

The types of visual assessment and other specialized vision services that are appropriate for hearing-impaired developmentally disabled individuals vary greatly. Ideally, the individual's chronological age and level of handicapping condition should determine which assessments and services are most appropriate. For instance, individuals who are relatively proficient in using traditional communication modes will probably not require special services to benefit from existing vision care systems. Others who have significant communication deficits or use atypical communication modes will need varying degrees of assistance to obtain appropriate vision care. The following section provides an overview of alternative assessment tools that may be appropriate.

Visual Acuity Tests

There are a number of recently developed products and procedures that provide the medical community with faster, more sophisticated, and more precise ways of objectively measuring a number of different parameters of the vision system (i.e., retinoscopy, ophthalmoscopy, visually evoked response). Unfortunately, the educational implications that can be gleaned from these objective procedures are quite limited. Answers to the most critical educational questions cannot be obtained through the use of objective procedures; rather, a subjective measurable response is required to indicate whether or not a specific visual signal has been detected. Without these subjective data, educators must speculate about the level of useful vision.

Likewise, professional eye examiners (optometrists and ophthalmologists) cannot determine whether many of their interventions, such as glasses, eye patching, or surgery, improved, worsened, or had no effect upon the person's vision. There are many hearing-impaired developmentally disabled individuals from whom the professional eye examiner cannot obtain this important assessment information. Most teachers, psychologists, speech/language pathologists, and others who frequently interact with hearing-impaired developmentally disabled people can obtain this critical subjective data relatively easily with little or no additional training. By selecting and administering one of the subjective visual acuity tests described in this section, one can obtain this information for use by medical and educational specialists.

Subjective tests for visual acuity require the individual being assessed to answer questions regarding the test stimuli, for example, "What letter is this?" There are some individuals who cannot verbally label letters on a wall chart at a distance of 20 feet. By modifying the response from verbal labeling to manual signing, some of those individuals can complete the testing. For those who cannot sign letters, other procedures described later are available that will allow most hearing-impaired developmentally disabled people to indicate how well they see the stimuli presented at several standard sizes. If test results indicate that an individual can discriminate one size but not the next smallest test target, accurate visual acuity data can be obtained.

One of the most important tasks of the vision screener when assessing difficult-to-test individuals is the selection of the appropriate screening tool. The Snellen E is the most commonly used test for people who don't read. However, it is not appropriate for many people with handicaps, due to the difficult responses and the discriminations (directionality) that are required. Most other visual acuity tests were designed to meet the needs of verbal young children and have not taken into consideration the language limitations of the target population. Only in the past few years have visual acuity test procedures that use nonverbal responses been readily available (Cress, Spellman, DeBriere, Sizemore, Northam, & Johnson, 1981; Faye, 1968; Lippmann, 1971; Sheridan, 1960). These tests yield visual acuity scores while requiring a less difficult response from the person being tested. Table 1 (next page) describes several visual acuity tests that may be appropriate for people with impaired hearing and developmental disabilities who are unable to perform on standard tests. Visual acuity can be measured at near-point, generally 13 to 16 inches, and at far-point, 10 to 20 feet. The exact viewing distance varies between tests and is specified in each test's instructions. Ideally, individuals should be tested for both near and far visual acuity. Regardless of what test and test distance are used, it is important that each eye be tested separately. Only by testing each eye separately can certain types of amblyopia (a significant difference between the two eyes) be detected.

Most of the acuity tests listed in Table 1 are simple to administer and can be completed within 10 minutes. Several of these tests for distance acuity, including the HOTV, Lighthouse, and others, require the person to label or match pictures or letters at a distance of 10 to 20 feet. While some individuals with handicaps can perform these tests successfully, many of them have difficulty attending and responding to stimuli at a distance.

Many people who are unable to perform the preceding tests reliably can perform the Parsons Visual Acuity Test (PVAT; Cress, Johnson, Sizemore, Spellman, & Shores, 1982). However, the PVAT requires a significantly longer period of testing time than do the other tests and requires additional skill on the part of the screener. Most screeners who are familiar with principles of operant conditioning and individualized training techniques can teach themselves to administer the PVAT; others require more extensive training in the techniques for administering the test. In addressing the problem of distance testing, this test uses a 13-inch test distance and optically simulates a 20-foot distance by using a +3 diopter lens. The person being tested is required to touch or place a match card on a picture of a hand or make some other available operant response when presented with a card showing a hand, a cake, and a bird. [A sample of this card is shown in Figure 1. These test targets were originally developed for use with verbal preschool children by Allen (1957).]

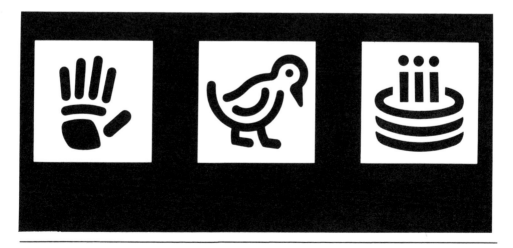

Figure 1. Sample pretest card (card number 10 in Figure 2). Developed by Allen (1957) and incorporated into the Allen Preschool Vision Test (American Optical).

Table 1. Visual Acuity Tests (Arranged in order of difficulty of required response)

Test	Appropriate for Ages[a]	Near or Far Test	Information Yielded	Commercial Availability
1. Snellen E	4 years-Adult	Screening—available for both near- and far-point testing	Directional response of labeling, pointing (can be modified to include matching)	American Optical Buffalo, NY 14215 Western Optical 1200 Mercer Street Seattle, WA 98109 Bernell Corp. 422 East Monroe Street South Bend, IN 46601
2. Sjogen Hand	4 years-Adult	Screening—available for both near- and far-point testing	Directional response of labeling, pointing (can be modified to include matching)	American Optical Western Optical Bernell Corp.
3. HOTV	3 years-Adult	Screening—available for far-point testing only	Labeling or matching letters	Good-Lite Company 1540 Hannah Avenue Forest Park, IL 60130
4. Blackhurst Test	3 years-Adult	Screening—available for both near- and far-point testing	Labeling pictures (can be modified to include matching)	Spectrum Products, Inc. 17451 Mt. Elliott Detroit, MI 48212
5. Allen Preschool Vision Test	3 years-Adult	Screening—available for far-point testing only	Labeling pictures (can be modified to include matching)	American Optical Western Optical
6. Lighthouse Flashcard	2 years-Adult	Screening—available for both near- and far-point testing	Labeling pictures (can be modified to include matching)	New York Association for the Blind 111 East 59th Street New York, NY 10022 Good-Lite Company

Test		Near or Far Test	Information Yielded	Commercial Availability
7	Parsons Visual Acuity	18 months-Adult	Screening—available for both near- and far-point testing	Pointing, labeling, or operant yes-no response (training program included)	Bernell Corp.
8	Stycar	6 months-Adult	Screening—includes battery of tests at various distances	Mixed: responses differ with portion used	NFER Publishing Company 2 Jennings Building Thames Avenue Windsor, Berks, SL4 1QS England

aLower age limit dependent on performance

Table 2. Vision Assessments

Test	Appropriate for Ages	Near or Far Test	Information Yielded	Commercial Availability
1. Bayley Scales of Infant Development (portions of)	0-6 months	Mixed: including fixation, tracking, head turning, reaching	Child's visual development compared to norms	Psychological Corp. 304 East 45th Street New York, NY 10017
2. Denver Developmental	0-6 years	Mixed: including fixation, tracking, head turning, reaching	Child's visual development compared to norms	LADOCA Project & Publisher East 51st Avenue & Lincoln Denver, CO 80216
3. Low-Functioning Vision Assessment Kit	0-Adult	Assessment	Performance data for most visual skills	NW Illinois Assessment for Hearing, Vision, and Physically Handicapped Children 145 Fisk Avenue DeKalb, IL 60115
4. Functional Vision	0-Adult	Mixed: including fixation, tracking, head turning, reaching, labeling, or matching testing	Performance data for most visual skills with suggested interventions	Stoelting Company 1305 South Kostner Avenue Detroit, MI 48212

Two discrimination training programs have been developed for people who are initially unable to perform on the PVAT. These discrimination training procedures were based upon previous research in errorless learning such as reported by Terrace (1963), Sidman and Stoddard (1966), and Dorry and Zeaman (1975). Figure 2 provides selected examples of the stimulus-shaping discrimination training program. The program consists of 30 cards (3 stimulus cards at each of 10 stages of completion). The figure being trained (hand) is always complete, and segments of the other two figures are gradually introduced until all three figures are complete.

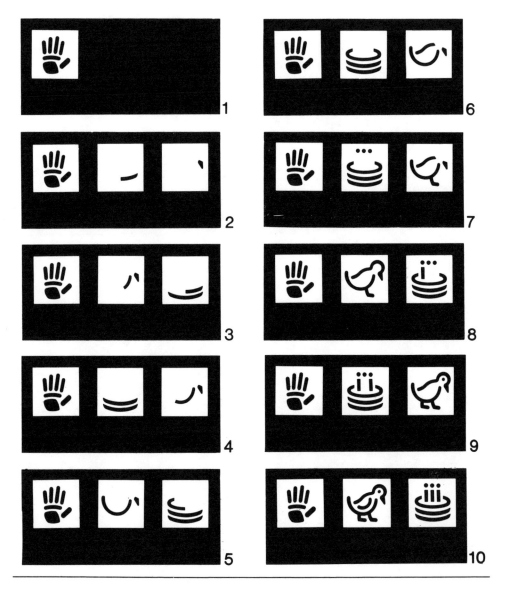

Figure 2. Selected trials from the stimulus shaping program. Developed by Allen (1957) and incorporated into the Allen Preschool Vision Test (American Optical).

A second discrimination training program uses an intensity fading approach in which the figure being trained is always at full intensity (black), and the other two figures gradually become darker, beginning with a very light gray and ending in black. Initial data indicate that some people with handicaps are more successful when trained with this program than with the stimulus shaping approach and vice versa. All errorless learning discrimination procedures initially allow the learner to base the discriminative response upon an irrelevant dimension of the stimuli; eventually these additional cues are faded until the learner is required to respond only to the relevant dimension of the discrimination. In the programs being discussed, the stimulus-shaping procedure requires a transfer of discriminative control from the size or completeness of the stimuli to their shapes. In the intensity-fading approach, the transfer is from the dimension of blackness to that of shape (Spellman, Cress, & Sizemore, 1983).

People who can reliably discriminate among the three figures, or can do so after training, are presented a series of cards that systematically reduce the size of the test targets, with the target sizes corresponding to equivalent Snellen visual acuity ratings. Results from field-testing of the PVAT with handicapped preschoolers showed that 90 percent of a group of 447 children served in preschool special education programs were able to perform on this test. Another finding was that approximately 40 percent of these children could also perform on the Lighthouse Flashcard Test (Spellman et al., 1983). This suggests that a fairly large number of preschoolers and older people will not require the use of the PVAT and can be tested for acuity with one of the tests previously mentioned.

When attempting to determine which visual acuity test to use, the screener should begin by selecting one of the acuity tests described in Table 1, where they are arranged according to the difficulty of the required response. A pretest of the required responses should be administered to determine whether or not to use a particular test. For example, to pretest the HOTV the child should demonstrate labeling or matching of the four letters before the actual test is given. If an individual fails to respond correctly to a given test format and set of targets, a test requiring an easier response should be pretested.

Some hearing-impaired developmentally disabled people, either because of their age or because of the severity of their handicapping conditions, are unable to perform on any of these acuity tests. They should still be assessed for visual impairment as thoroughly as possible by using a functional vision assessment and tests for muscle balance, procedures described in the following sections.

Functional Vision Assessment

Unlike the acuity tests previously described that measure a specific visual skill (visual acuity), a variety of functional vision assessments have been developed to determine an individual's ability to perform several other vision functions. Because this type of assessment involves observation of an individual who is performing various visual tasks, the findings may more closely reflect the person's use of vision in everyday activities. Test items on functional vision assessments generally cover at least the following:

1. Reflexive visual responses. Examples include pupillary reflex to light and blink reflex to the tester's hand as it is moved toward the eyes.

2. Earliest developing visual skills. Sample test items would include momentary and prolonged fixation on an object or light and turning toward a light or object entering the periphery of the visual field.

3. Visual pursuit (tracking). Eye mobility and the coordination of the two eyes are typically assessed by eliciting tracking responses to lights and objects which are moved vertically, horizontally, diagnoally, and circularly; ability to track different-sized objects at various distances may also be assessed.

In addition to these assessment areas, most of the available functional vision assessments include a modified test for visual field (the area that can be seen when the eyes are centrally fixated) and an acuity test for those people who can make a reliable response on such tests. While the administration of a functional vision assessment is most critical for those whose age or severity of disability prevents them from performing on an acuity test, these procedures can also be used with people who complete acuity testing. This may be done to detect other problems in visual functioning. For example, an individual may have good central visual acuity and still experience difficulty in visual pursuit tasks. The authors recommend that anyone who is unable to perform acuity tests should be assessed for functional vision and referred for professional eye care. Moreover, people who pass acuity tests but are still suspected of having difficulty with visual tasks should receive a functional assessment. On a functional assessment, failure on one or more items appropriate for a person's age would warrant a referral.

The functional vision assessments included in Table 2 (page 159) have each been developed for a different population of difficult-to-test people. Portions of the Bayley Scaler of Infant Development (Bayley, 1969) and the Denver Developmental Screening Test (Frankenburg & Dodds, 1975) were designed to assess visual skills of the young child. Children who fail to develop visual skills at the normal ages can be detected and referred for the earliest possible treatment of their visual impairments. The Low-Functioning Vision Assessment Kit (Northwestern Illinois Association, 1982) was developed for use with the severely multihandicapped, particularly those with cerebral palsy. The Functional Vision Inventory for the Multiple and Severely Handicapped (Langley, 1980) includes an assessment procedure and a section with detailed information on activities designed to teach deficit visual skills.

Muscle Balance Tests

As previously mentioned, eye muscle imbalance is one of the most common types of vision problems. Muscle imbalance, often called strabismus, can take a number of forms depending on the direction and angle of deviation and whether the imbalance is latent (phorias) or manifest (tropias). The probability of effectively correcting muscle imbalance decreases with the age of the person. Individuals whose eyes are obviously out of alignment should always be referred for professional eye care at least once every two years. Those who show no obvious eye muscle imbalance should be assessed by using two procedures, the Corneal Light Reflex Test and the Cover-Uncover Test (Frankenburg &

Camp, 1975), Fortunately, both of these procedures are quick, easy to administer, and do not require complex responses from the person being assessed.

The Corneal Light Reflex Test involves shining a penlight into the eyes of the person being tested from about 13 inches away. The tester observes the reflections of the light in both eyes simultaneously with the normal result being reflections in the center of both pupils. Any difference between the locations of the reflections in the two eyes is cause for referral. This test is effective in identifying individuals with possible tropias (manifest deviations). Testers should be aware of the discomfort caused by this procedures in persons who are photosensitive. Individuals who exhibit discomfort due to light should be referred with a description of their behavior when exposed to the light.

Another procedure for detecting muscle imbalance is the Cover-Uncover Test. This test is useful in detecting phorias (latent muscle imbalance) in individuals older than 6 months. The Cover-Uncover Test is preferably done at both near distance (13 to 16 inches) and at far distance (20 feet or more). The person being assessed must maintain fixation on a target object while the tester covers and uncovers each eye separately, each time covering the eye for a sufficient time to disrupt fusion of the two eyes (at least 3 seconds). The tester observes for any monocular movement (one eye only) when the cover is removed. To pass the Cover-Uncover Test the person must exhibit no monocular movement in either eye.

An Interdisciplinary Process

For the past seven years the authors have been involved in (1) research and development of a visual acuity test for the difficult-to-test, (2) nationwide field-testing activities, (3) inservice training of vision testers, and (4) designing systems of service delivery in a variety of community-based and institutional settings. As such, the authors have had unique opportunities to observe various existing vision service delivery systems. After synthesizing the information gained by these experiences, the authors wish to make recommendations about how best to provide vision services to people who are considered difficult to test.

The Need for Individualization

Systems for providing vision services to hearing-impaired developmentally disabled persons must, of necessity, be individualized to meet each person's needs. Not all individuals will require the full range of services to be described. For example, a teenager with hearing impairment and a mild developmental disability may be able to access existing vision service systems without special assistance. However, by understanding the possible range of service needs, the vision care advocate will be better able to identify those specialized services which are appropriate for each individual. To assist the vision care advocate in this regard, a process will be described which indicates components that may need to be modified for individuals with specialized vision care needs. Figure 3 on the next page illustrates this process.

First, an initial vision screening or assessment should be conducted on any student or young child who is suspected of having hearing impairment, developmental disability, or both. The rationale for completing an assessment prior to referring the person

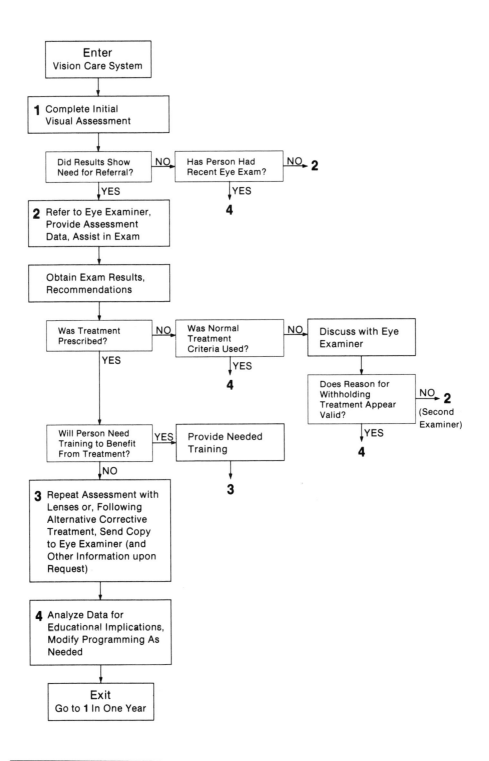

Figure 3. Vision care process.

for a professional eye examination is that it provides information about the person's vision that may not be obtainable in the examination setting or within the time constraints of the examination. In addition, the completion of an initial assessment helps prepare the individual for the professional eye examination by providing a number of experiences, such as making responses to visual targets and tolerating the shining of light into the eyes.

Next, all individuals who have completed the initial assessment should be referred for a professional eye examination regardless of test results if they have not been examined within the past two years. The results of assessment should be provided to the eye examiner prior to the examination. Following the examination, most professional eye examiners will recommend a time interval for a return visit. A return visit should be scheduled sooner in cases in which the annual assessment results show an unexpected worsening in visual acuity, eye muscle balance, or vision related skills.

The eye examiner may be unfamiliar with the unique communication modes of an individual with moderate and severe disabilities. Therefore someone familiar with the individual's responses and communication modes, such as the vision tester, teacher, or parent, should accompany the individual to the professional eye examination. The person accompanying the hearing-impaired developmentally disabled individual can provide assistance by modeling, physically assisting, reinforcing the desired responses, or suggesting or interpreting alternative response and communication modes for the examiner. Some individuals will require systematic pretraining in such examination related behaviors as holding their heads still, sitting in a hydraulic chair, or fixating on a distant target. Thus, communication and cooperation between the professional eye examiner and other service providers is necessary to ensure that the hearing-impaired developmentally disabled person will receive adequate vision care.

Once the examination is completed, the results and recommendations of the eye examiner should be sent to the professionals responsible for developing intervention programs for the client. If treatment has been prescribed (i.e., glasses, eye patching, surgery, orthoptic exercises), it is recommended that a follow-up assessment be conducted. A follow-up assessment serves to provide educators and significant others with information regarding changes in the person's visual capabilities following treatment. This information may be valuable as well to the eye examiner in determining the effectiveness of prescribed treatment(s). The authors have found that professional eye examiners frequently wish to receive the results of visual acuity testing following surgical procedures, eye patching, or the use of various prescriptive lenses. Examples of additional information which could be provided to the professional eye examiner upon request include observation of the effects of vision treatment on daily activities or school performance, and the provision of specific assessment data in cases where vision is expected to deteriorate or when a change in visual capabilities has diagnostic significance to the eye examiner.

Educational Implications

The educational implications of the eye examination and other assessment data should be carefully considered as they relate to possible modifications in the services or programs being provided. Such modifications might include the design and implementation of a program to teach the wearing of glasses, changes in seating or lighting, or the use of larger or higher contrast visual stimuli for those whose visual impairment is not totally correctable. Those with impaired hearing and developmental disabilities who are found to have a severe visual impairment should probably be considered deaf-blind, a population whose needs cannot be addressed fully here. Readers who wish to provide service to individuals who are deaf-blind should seek further information from their regional deaf-blind center or their state department of education.

The interpretation of eye examination reports by other professionals is sometimes difficult due to a lack of knowledge of vision terminology. Some explanation of common vision terms has already been provided here; if the reader wishes more information on how to interpret eye examination reports, he or she should consult with the eye examiner or other available resources such as special educators of the visually impaired.* At least two authors have developed lists of questions to ask the eye examiner in order to obtain more relevant information for educating an individual with handicaps (Efron & Duboff, 1980; Mt. Plains, 1980). Examples of such questions (from Efron, 1977, p. 25) are

1. What is the cause of the visual impairment?
2. Is any special treatment required? If so, what is the general nature of the treatment?
3. Is the visual impairment likely to get worse, better, or stay the same?
4. Should the teacher be alert to any particular symptoms (such as eye rubbing and so forth) that would signal the need for professional attention?
5. What restrictions should be placed on the child's activities?
6. Should the child wear glasses or contact lenses? If so, under what circumstances?
7. Were you able to make an accurate measurement of visual acuity? If so, what was the child's visual acuity?
8. If a visual acuity measurement was not possible, what is your opinion regarding the child's visual functioning?
9. Are the child's focusing ability and eye muscle balance adequate? If no, please describe.
10. Were you able to determine the field of vision? If so, were there areas of no vision in the field? Where?
11. Was the child able to follow visually a moving object? Were there any directions in which he or she could not track moving objects?
12. Will the child work better with large or small objects and pictures? At what distance?
13. What lighting would be optimal for his or her visual functioning?

---

*The National Society to Prevent Blindness sells many inexpensive educational materials on vision, including a dictionary of vision terms. A catalog can be obtained by writing to National Society to Prevent Blindness, Inc., 79 Madison Avenue, New York, NY 10016.

14. What are your specific recommendations concerning this child's use of vision in learning situations?

15. When should this child be examined again?

While interpreting the educational implications of the examination results, one should be aware that some eye examiners will not use the same criteria for prescribing treatment for patients with handicaps as they do for their nonhandicapped patients. If the vision care advocate believes that different criteria for treatment are being used for the hearing-impaired developmentally disabled person, or has other questions about some aspect of the report, the eye examiner should be consulted. If, after consultation with the eye examiner, the vision care advocate decides that appropriate treatment is being withheld due to the person's disabilities, a second opinion should be obtained from a different eye examiner. In this event, more attention should be given to selecting an examiner who fully understands the importance of good vision to individuals with disabilities.

Summary and Discussion

In summary, the authors would like to stress the importance of comprehensive vision care for people with hearing impairment and developmental disabilities. There are many individuals in our schools and communities who continue to experience visual impairments that have not been detected. Many of these impairments could be significantly reduced, or eliminated altogether, with appropriate prescriptive lenses. Some of the more serious impairments, no longer correctable, might have been arrested if identification and treatment had occurred prior to the age of six. The technology to identify and treat most vision problems is available, yet good comprehensive vision services remain the exception rather than the rule.

In some cases, dramatic changes in the availability and quality of vision care services have been affected by the availability of information regarding good vision care. It is not uncommon for some administrators, parents, teachers, and professional eye examiners to become determined to alter the existing system once they realize that the hearing-impaired developmentally disabled person is not receiving adequate services. Others will be inspired and motivated when they realize that the population can benefit significantly from the treatment afforded nonhandicapped people. It is not uncommon to find professional eye examiners who do not realize that people with developmental delays, and particularly those with concomitant hearing impairments, can benefit from corrective treatments; this is evidenced by the diagnosis "vision is adequate for needs" still found in many developmentally disabled individuals' medical files today.

In recent years, several states have begun to plan and implement statewide systems for provision of vision services to people with handicaps, including those with hearing impairment and developmental disabilities. Naturally, these systems were designed to utilize the state's existing resources and services whenever possible. Vermont, for example, has a state interdisciplinary assessment team for the severely handicapped. By training the team's educational specialist and nurse to conduct specialized vision assessment and by increasing communication with the team's ophthalmologist, Vermont has developed a system that can meet the vision care needs of all school-age youth with severe handicaps. In a similar vein, Ohio chose to train members of the 18 regional low-incidence assessment teams to conduct alternative vision assessments. In Iowa, most area education agencies that provide special education services employ special education nurses who are trained to conduct specialized vision assessment of those with handicaps. Other states, including Indiana and Missouri, are using school nurses to provide vision care services. In Kansas, one or more individuals from each of the eight special education regions were selected to serve as backup vision testers; students who cannot be tested by the regular vision screening methods can be referred to the regional specialist for visual assessment.

Unfortunately, the provision of information regarding the whys and hows of comprehensive vision care does not alter the availability or quality of vision services in all cases. Some agencies and individuals choose not to provide this needed service unless it is mandated. In these cases, publishing rules, regulations, or guidelines can often affect the availability of services. To ensure the improvement of the quality of services, it is frequently necessary to take measures to identify individuals who can provide quality vision services or to provide comprehensive skill training to those who are responsible for providing the service. Identifying eye examiners who are interested in and experienced with testing people with handicaps is often difficult, especially in agencies that have stated policies against referring clients to specific professional service providers. For example, many public schools have policies that do not allow the school nurse to suggest that a parent take his or her child to a specific eye examiner.

Likewise, the notion of improving quality of vision services through training appears reasonable until one attempts to locate programs, agencies, or indivuals who can provide training for those who wish to learn to provide screening and assessment for the difficult to test. People who are knowledgeable about vision assessment often do not have experience with those who are hearing impaired and developmentally disabled. Professionals working with hearing-impaired developmentally disabled individuals generally do not have experience or training with the various technologies available for vision testing. In the area of hearing, there is a long history of professionals in speech/language pathology and audiology interacting with developmentally disabled populations; there is no parallel in the area of vision. It is not surprising that the availability and quality of vision services are substandard when there is no single professional responsible for providing vision related services within most education programs.

Another factor that appears to contribute to substandard vision services for those with impaired hearing and developmental disabilities is that those responsible for monitoring compliance to rules and regulations often do not have the skills to judge the quality of vision care. This problem is frequently exemplified in institutional settings. For example, many institutions serving hearing-impaired developmentally disabled individuals are not cited for deficiencies in their vision care services despite data showing that very few of the residents wear corrective lenses. It is not uncommon to find that residents referred for comprehensive eye examinations are referred by consensus of staff members rather than through a systematic vision screening and identification process.

Over the past few years, some local and state agencies have made substantial improvements in providing quality vision care services for hearing-impaired developmentally disabled people. There are many more agencies that still need to evaluate the current status of their systems and to establish realistic goals for improvement.

References

Allen, H. F. (1957). Testing of visual acuity in preschool children: Norms, variables and a new picture test. *Pediatrics, 19,* 1093–1100.

Barker, J., & Barmatz, H. (1975). Eye function. In W. Frankenburg & B. Camp (Eds.), *Pediatric screening tests.* Springfield, IL: Charles C. Thomas.

Bayley, N. (1969). *Bayley scales of infant development: Manual.* New York: The Psychological Corporation.

Cress, P. J., Johnson, J. L., Sizemore, A. C., Spellman, C. R., & Shores, R. E. (1982). The development of a visual acuity test for persons with severe handicaps. *Journal of Special Education Technology, 5*(3), 11–19.

Cress, P., Spellman, C., DeBriere, T., Sizemore, A., Northam, J., & Johnson, J. (1981). Vision screening for persons with severe handicaps. *Journal of the Association for Severely Handicapped, 6,* 41–50.

Donlon, E. T. (1966). Implications of visual disorders. In W. M. Cruickshank (Ed.), *Cerebral palsy: Its individual and community problems* (2nd ed.). Syracuse, NY: Syracuse University Press.

Dorry, G. W., & Zeaman, D. (1975). Teaching a simple reading vocabulary to retarded children: Effectiveness of fading and non-fading procedures. *American Journal of Mental Deficiency, 6,* 711–716.

Efron, M. (1977). Hints for examining and reporting the vision of deaf-blind children. In *Proceedings of the Workshop for Ophthalmologists, Optometrists, and Educators.* Sacramento, CA: Southwestern Regional Deaf-Blind Center.

Efron, M., & Duboff, E. (1980). *A vision guide for deaf-blind children.* Raleigh: North Carolina Department of Public Instruction.

Ellis, D. (1979). Visual handicaps of mentally handicapped people. *American Journal of Mental Deficiency, 5,* 497–511.

Faye, E. E. (1968). A new visual acuity test for partially-sighted non-readers. *Journal of Pediatric Ophthalmology, 5,* 210–212.

Fletcher, M. C., & Thompson, M. M. (1961). Eye abnormalities in the mentally defective. *American Journal of Mental Deficiency, 66,* 242–244.

Frankenburg, W. K., & Camp, B. W. (Eds.). (1975). *Pediatric screening tests.* Springfield, IL: Charles C. Thomas.

Frankenburg, W. K., & Dodds, J. B. (1975). *Denver developmental screening test: Reference manual* (rev. ed.). Denver: LADOCA Project and Publishing Foundation.

Harley, R. D. (1975). *Pediatric ophthalmology.* Philadelphia: W. B. Saunders.

Langley, M. B. (1980). *Functional vision inventory for the multiple and severely handicapped.* Chicago: Stoelting.

Lippmann, O. (1971). Vision screening of young children. *American Journal of Public Health, 61*(8), 1586–1601.

McGuire, J. (1966). Refraction. In S. Leibman & S. Gellis (Eds.), *The pediatrician's ophthalmology* (pp. 57–72). St. Louis: Mosby.

Mt. Plains Regional Center for Services to Handicapped Children. (1980). *Visual assessment of deaf-blind children*. Denver: Author.

Northwestern Illinois Association for Hearing, Vision, and Physically Handicapped Children. (1982). *Low-functioning vision assessment kit: Procedural manual*. DeKalb, IL: Author.

Sheridan, M. D. (1960). Vision screening of very young or handicapped children. *British Medical Journal, 5196,* 453–456.

Sidman, M., & Stoddard, L. T. (1966). Programming perception and learning for retarded children. In N. R. Ellis (Ed.), *International review of research in mental retardation* (Vol. 2). New York: Academic Press.

Smith, D. W., & Wilson, A. A. (1973). *The child with Down's syndrome (mongolism): Causes, characteristics, and acceptance.* Philadelphia: W. B. Saunders.

Spellman, C. R., Cress, P. J., & Sizemore, A. C. (1983). *Final report from the project for research and development of subjective visual acuity procedures for handicapped preschool children* (Grant No. G007901961). Washington, DC: U.S. Office of Education.

Stangler, S. R., Huber, C. J., & Routh, D. K. (1980). *Screening growth and development of preschool children: A guide for test selection.* New York: McGraw-Hill.

Terrace, H. S. (1963). Discrimination learning with and without errors. *Journal of the Experimental Analysis of Behavior, 6,* 1–27.

Woodruff, M. E. (1972). *A list of children termed "visually at risk" in terms of possible vision defects.* Waterloo, Ontario: University of Waterloo.

Woodruff, M. E. (1977). Prevalence of visual and ocular anomalies in 1968 noninstitutionalized mentally retarded children. *Canadian Journal of Public Health, 68,* 225–232.

Chapter 10

Developmental Approaches to Communication Assessment and Enhancement

Mary Pat Moeller

Obtaining a reliable and valid comprehensive evaluation of the communicative skills of hearing-impaired children is problematic. The assessment process is complicated by lack of standardized instruments designed for this population and the unknown effects of the sensory deficit on test performance. A test battery approach, combining both formal and informal measurements, has been suggested in view of these problems (Miller, 1981; Moeller, McConkey, & Osberger, 1983). When a hearing-impaired child has additional handicapping conditions, the problem of assessing and interpreting language performance is intensified. Adequate assessment of the hearing-impaired developmentally disabled child requires teamwork, flexible adaption of procedures, and application of a developmental perspective. This chapter discusses an adaptive approach to assessment, special considerations in test use and interpretation, and the importance of an approach that integrates evaluation and treatment.

Adaptive Evaluation Procedures

Hearing-impaired developmentally disabled children often present a highly individual profile of needs and behaviors. The clinician must use traditional procedures adaptively to obtain a description of the child's developmental status in comprehension, production, and communication (Miller, 1981). When possible, performance is measured in the areas of the form (syntax, phonology), content (vocabulary, semantics), and function of language (Bloom & Lahey, 1978; Kretschmer & Kretschmer, 1978; Miller, 1981). Perhaps the most complex aspect of evaluating the language skills of the hearing-impaired developmentally disabled child is that the effects of combined disorders on behavioral responses are not known. Most clinical tools have been developed for children with normal hearing. When sensory deficits co-occur, or occur in combination with motor or cognitive impairments, the synergistic consequences may have dramatic and complex effects on language learning. An adaptive approach implies flexible modification of procedures to fit the unique needs of the child and interpretation of test findings in light of the child's unique problems. The role of the clinician includes determination of strengths and current limitations in the child's approach to language learning and in the child's use of language. This goal requires attention to variables involving both the child and the diagnostic procedures.

Issues of Sensory Organization

Children with multiple disabilities vary in their capabilities for selective attention and in their state of arousal at any particular time. The clinician should make systematic observations of factors that appear to influence attention and arousal; this information affects interpretation as well as program planning. For example, some children "overload" to extraneous visual or auditory stimuli in the environment. Others may demonstrate lethargy due to seizures or medication problems. Adaptations might include reduction of stimuli (reducing talking when the child is concentrating on a motor task) or changing the child's position to heighten arousal (rocking from supine to sitting position; Fieber, 1975).

A child who is functioning at a low sensorimotor stage of development may require consideration of prerequisite attending behaviors. For example, what is the status of the child's visual fixation abilities (Robinson & Robinson, 1978)? Is looking self-regulated? Will selective positioning of the child enhance attention?

Another concern in the area of sensory organization is response time. The hearing-impaired developmentally disabled child may require more than the usual amount of response time. For example, if the child appears to be nonresponsive when performing an object selection task, the clinician may need to wait for a short period before providing repetition of the item or placing new demands on the child. Short-term memory constraints may also interfere with task completion, especially if a motor response is involved. The clinician should keep detailed records of observational data and behavioral impressions to examine the effects of response latency or potential short-term memory constraints on language performance.

Self-stimulatory behaviors may also interfere with the child's responses. Fieber (1975) suggested that adaptive observations of such behavior may lend further insight into the child's sensory organization. For example, a visually impaired child who moves fingers or a shiny object close to his or her eyes may be demonstrating perception of light, shadow, or movement capabilities. Fieber suggests that the clinician make note of what happens when a self-stimulating behavior is interrupted. Can the child stop the behavior when presented with an interesting alternative?

Response Modes Available to the Child

Careful observation of the motor repertoire of the child may guide the clinician in selecting an appropriate response task. Even mild visual-motor coordination deficits can adversely affect performance on object manipulation tasks, distracting the child from linguistic performance and yielding questionable results. Response tasks also must be modified to accommodate for the child's motor problems. For example, the cerebral palsied hearing-impaired child may be capable of giving an eye-gaze response as a substitute for object selection. Teamwork in such a case is essential; the accommodative task chosen should be in synchrony with other developmental goals. That is, if the occupational therapist is working toward reduction of spastic extension of the arm, language response tasks should reinforce this goal.

Cognitive Status. Integral to the interpretation of rate of progress, or degree of delay, is a comprehensive understanding of the child's cognitive skills (see Chapter 12).

For further information, Robinson and Robinson (1978) presented a detailed description of adaptive methods for evaluation of cognitive skills which they consider to be prerequisites to formal language use. Miller (1978) also discussed this issue.

Modality Concerns. Little is known about the comprehension of language through the visual modality. In particular, the developmental aspects of auditory-visual processing are not well understood. F. C. Caccamise (personal communication, November 1981) has stressed the importance of considering the visual modality when presenting tests through sign language. His findings suggest that the clinician must pace the rate of signing and clearly distinguish signs that are minimally contrastive (e.g., *big* may look like *open* if signed rapidly). Sign precision or clarity and rate of signing are particularly important issues to be monitored when evaluating the hearing-impaired developmentally delayed population.

Meaningfulness of the Stimuli. Clinicians dealing with this population are frequently confronted with the problem of lack of skill generalization. The child may recognize or use a linguistic meaning in a single restricted context but not in other contexts. Language progress may be reflected only with familiar tasks; less familiar materials may distract the student from the task at hand. Two procedures are suggested when this problem occurs. First, observation of the behavior in varied contexts is recommended to determine generalizability and "representativeness" of the skill. Second, incorporation of teacher suggestions in planning task and object selection is helpful. Teacher input also should be solicited to determine the optimal type of reinforcement for the student.

Variables Related to Formal Tests

Moeller et al. (1983) described a number of concerns when formal tests are used with hearing-impaired children. Among these concerns were item length, number of practice items, number of test items at each developmental level, and effects of presentation mode. These concerns are intensified with hearing-impaired children who have additional handicaps. Our experience indicates that adaptations to enhance the evaluation include the following:

- The child's performance should be analyzed beyond the test scores to identify characteristics or skills that are important educationally.
- Age scores should be interpreted with extreme caution, particularly if the test procedures are modified (for example, by changes in presentation of test instructions and test items in sign language, repetition of test items, and reinstruction of the task). Although these modifications are critical to obtaining an accurate impression of the child's abilities, they nevertheless invalidate test norms.

  When repetition of items or addition of extra practice items is necessary to ensure focus and attention, a double scoring procedure is suggested. This procedure yields two age scores: The standard or first administration of the item is indicated as one score, and the results of the repeated administration are reported as a second score.

- The length and syntactic structure of test items may need to be adjusted because undesirable linguistic effects, such as complex syntactic structures, may prevent the child from demonstrating semantic or conceptual knowledge.
- If testing is performed in a quiet and controlled environment, the clinician must consider what impact a more distracting environment, both acoustically and visually, may have on performance. Ideally, the evaluation should include classroom observation.

Few formal tests of language are appropriate for use with this population. The clinician must augment or, in some cases, replace norm-referenced tests with criterion-referenced procedures, informal probes, and behavioral charting. In the following sections, formal and informal tasks that have been found to have clinical applicability are described. The discussion focuses on four distinct periods or language levels: (1) the prelinguistic child, (2) the child using one- and two-word utterances, (3) the child using simple utterances, and (4) the school-age child using simple and complex utterances.

Evaluation Considerations at the Prelinguistic Level

The multihandicapped child may give the appearance of having no language or of being noncommunicative. Teamwork, attention to prerequisite cognitive and social behaviors, and observation of the caregiver and child in natural contexts are critical for assessing communicative needs. Recent developments in the areas of pragmatics and caregiver-child interaction have led to a greater understanding of the earliest communicative behaviors that may be observed clinically (Bates, 1976; Dore, 1974; Greenfield & Smith, 1976; Snow, 1977). Preverbal communication is recognized as providing a basis for later linguistic communication, as do the child's sensorimotor explorations and social accomplishments. McLean and Snyder-McLean (1978) noted that the child learns to convey linguistically those functions that already have been accomplished nonlinguistically. This notion has important implications for evaluation and intervention.

Robbins and Steinquist (1967) described a hierarchy of spontaneous interpersonal communications that assist a clinician in determining a child's level of preverbal communication. They divided these early communicative behaviors into classes of *signals* and *protosymbolic behaviors*. Signals refer to a low level of communication which indicates wants and involves physical immediateness (Fieber, 1975). Symbols, on the other hand, involve mental representations and the ability to think about objects without manipulating them. The term protosymbolic behavior describes prerequisite nonverbal behaviors that are representational in nature and follow a sequence of development (Fieber, 1975).

Robbins and Steinquist (1967) described a sequence of signals that may be helpful to guide the clinician in observations of nonverbal prerequisite language benchmarks. These are summarized in Table 1.

Fieber (1975) noted that a child does not develop signal behaviors until he or she is able to anticipate and has the beginnings of mental representations of events. Intervention programs should work to design events that will lead to this anticipation,

Table 1. Preverbal Signaling Behaviors Observed in Young Children

Signals	Examples
1. Cries, smiles	Smile reflects or signals feeling or state—"I enjoy this"
2. Anticipates daily routine (time sense based on physical needs)	Child gets excited at usual feeding time
3. Tugging, pulling at, pushing vaguely about	Tugs and fusses at mother (wants out of highchair)
4. Leads people; places adult hand on objects	Puts mother's hand on jack-in-the-box to get it to work again
5. Anticipates based on physical situation; definite participation	Gets excited; tugs on own pants when sees bath preparation

Note. From *The Deaf-Blind "Rubella" Child* (Pub. No. 25) by N. Robbins and G. Steinquist, 1967, Watertown, MA: Perkins School for the Blind. Adapted by permission.

deliberately planning signifiers (events or prompts that signal the child to act) for the child. The diagnostician should include teacher and parent interviews in the test battery to determine cues and events that elicit signaling behaviors from the child. Situations may also be contrived to determine the child's responsiveness to attempts to elicit signaling behavior. Fieber (1975) offered some examples of these, which appear in Table 2.

Initial signals may be person-directed or object-directed (swats at the toy for more action; smiles at Mother when asked, "Want more?"). Later, signals become more complex as the child combines simple signal schemes (e.g., looks at Mother and touches her hand). Person-oriented and object-oriented schemes also combine later (e.g., signals

Table 2. Examples of Signaling Behaviors Elicited by Familiar Social Routines

Event	Signifier	Child's Response	Assumed Meaning to Child
Game Ritual	Mom asks, "Pat-a-cake?", moving child's hands a little	Looks expectant and smiles	"Going to play pat-a-cake or something
Daily Sequence	On mat, sight of baby food jar	General excitement, eye contact, movements	"I'm going to eat"
Feeding	Child holds mother's little finger during feeding	Learns to pull hand toward mouth to signal "more"	"I want more"

Note. From *Movement in Communication and Language Development of Deaf-Blind Children* by N. Fieber, 1975, paper presented at National Deaf-Blind Workshop, Dallas, TX. Adapted by permission.

first to person, then to object; Fieber, 1975). Observations of typical social routines between caregiver and child may reveal the extent to which the child is engaging in signaling and the caregiver's sophistication in responding to these early responses. The clinician or teacher should retain cumulative records of signals by sampling varied situations and specific signifiers (Fieber, 1975).

Protosymbolic Behaviors

As the child's interactions become more intentional, early communicative behaviors become more complex and varied (cf. Chapman, 1981, for a comprehensive review). Bates (1976) discussed early gestures and vocal behaviors as protosymbolic behaviors. *Protodeclaratives* refer to the child's preverbal effort to direct the adult's attention to some event or object in the world. "This includes exhibiting the self, showing objects and pointing or giving sequences which attract an adult's attention" (Chapman, 1981, p. 114). *Protoimperatives* are defined as the child's use of means to cause the adult to do something. Chapman (1981) noted that such behaviors grow out of more instrumental skills in which the child attempts to get the object for him- or herself—reaching, opening and closing the hand, etc. These behaviors also become gradually more complex, so that a protoimperative might include glancing from object to parent, reaching, and vocalizing. *Protosymbols* are more advanced than signaling behaviors in that they are representational in nature. For example, pointing indicates some separation or distancing of the child from concrete (grasping or taking the object) behavior. Smiling is no longer a reflection of state, but a pleasurable, shared activity or form of greeting (Fieber, 1975).

Vocalizations also serve as protosymbols in early communicative attempts. Ricks (1975) described request (call) noises, frustrated noises, and greeting and surprise noises in 8- to 11-month-old babies.

The clinician evaluating the hearing-impaired developmentally disabled child should observe the child in ritualized situations with the caregiver to observe instances of signaling and protosymbolic behaviors. An effort should be made to determine (1) how well the child makes use of the situational context to aid comprehension (e.g., sees coat and then anticipates going bye-bye); (2) the level of generalization of signals or protosymbols; (3) the complexity of behaviors (pointing vs. looking, vocalizing, and pointing); and (4) the pragmatic functions of the communication.

A useful system for accomplishing such a description has been developed by Coggins and Carpenter (1981) in the Communicative Intention Inventory. The inventory is an observational system for describing children's early gestural, vocal, and verbal communicative behaviors. The inventory comprises eight intentional behaviors based on the writings about pragmatic language development by Bates (1976), Dore (1974), Greenfield and Smith (1976), and Halliday (1975). Coggins and Carpenter have selected definable categories so that clinicians may distinguish intentional behaviors from unintentional sensorimotor sequences. Two other features of the inventory make it appealing for use with the hearing-impaired developmentally disabled child. Because the inventory is designed to classify uses of language in developmentally young children, behavioral descriptions are given for gestural, gestural/vocal, and verbally encoded intentions. Also, it is intended to be used as a criterion-referenced measure, which provides information on behaviors felt to be necessary for acquisition of subsequent conversational skills. The latter point supports a primary evaluation goal—the determination of emergent skills on which to base intervention.

McLean and Snyder-McLean (1978) described useful guidelines for the assessment and integration of findings in the cognitive, social, and linguistic domains. Information on the child's cognitive basis for language (such as development of means-ends and causality and knowledge of functional attributes) and social bases for language (maintaining interaction, joint referencing, etc.) is considered essential to understanding receptive and expressive language performance.

In summary, children at prelinguistic levels present varied cognitive, social, and vocal or gestural behaviors that constitute targets of evaluation. Too often, such children are described as untestable because they are unable to perform on conventional tests or tasks. Informal evaluation of prerequisite, nonlinguistic behaviors is essential.

An example of this point is 2½-year-old E. M., a severely cerebral palsied hearing-impaired child, who was referred for evaluation due to "noncommunication." His language age was estimated by his teacher at a two- to four-month development level. Observation of this child in varied contexts revealed that although he had limited motor skills, he was highly communicative and demonstrated intentional eye-gaze sequences to obtain desired objects (look at Mom; look at toy; fuss; look at Mom). E. M. demonstrated intentional avoidance of foods he disliked and engaged in limited reciprocal vocal play. He used a generalized "want" gesture to request; used an eat sign (gross approximation) and lip smacking to express hunger (even when food was not present). E. M. also rocked his torso to indicate a desire to ride his rocking horse. The many instances of this child's intentional communication were encouraging. Because of his severe motor impairment, he was unable to respond conventionally to receptive language tasks. Yet, the examiner found that E. M. had a wide range of potential receptive responses (e.g., eye gaze, gesture in response to "What do you want?"). Observation of parent-child interaction revealed that the parents rarely gave the child opportunities to respond receptively to their comments. They were instructed in adapting the environment and their strategies to facilitate E. M.'s active participation (e.g., making sure his coat was within visual range so that he could search for it visually and point in answer to "Wanna go bye-bye?"). At this stage, the diagnostician should consider what responses are available to the child and how such responses may have maximum utility for the child.

Early Language Development: Evaluation Considerations

Several formal and informal procedures may be adapted for use with hearing-impaired developmentally disabled children who are functioning at early symbolic language stages (one- and two-word simple utterances). The discussion here will center on four areas: (1) prerequisite behaviors for language learning, (2) early content comprehension/lexical use, (3) caregiver skills, and (4) phonological concerns.

Before discussing these areas, it should be mentioned that the Minnesota Child Development Inventory (Ireton & Thwing, 1972) is a useful measure. This comprehensive parent questionnaire surveys developmental skills in the areas of gross and fine motor, self-help, personal-social, conceptual and situation comprehension, and expressive language. Most of the items are applicable to the target population, with the exception of the child with severe motor impairments. Information from the Minnesota should be viewed in combination with that obtained from the parent interview and a comprehensive case history.

In addition, before undertaking formal assessment, the clinician may also want to use the Oliver: Parent-Administered Communication Inventory (Environmental Prelanguage Battery, Horstmeier & MacDonald, 1978). This inventory assesses the child's communication skills in his or her natural environment through caregiver and teacher reports. The clinician gains information on the child's usual means of communicating, typical utterance content, length, attention, imitation abilities, and knowledge of object function. This inventory has been particularly useful with parents who accept rudimentary signals from their hearing-impaired developmentally disabled child and are unaware of the potentially more complex language interaction that could develop.

Prerequisites for Language Learning

Bricker and Dennison (1978) discussed the importance of developing behaviors in developmentally disabled children that are necessary prerequisites to formal, symbolic language development. They viewed four steps as being initial targets in the gradual development of a generative language system: (1) on-task behavior (consistent focus of attention on selective tasks for a reasonable, predetermined time period); (2) imitation; (3) discriminative use of objects (e.g., pound with a hammer, eat with a spoon); and (4) word recognition (association of meaningful verbal stimuli with appropriate events). The authors suggested behavioral charting procedures as a means of evaluating the child's readiness for language learning tasks. They also discussed a comprehensive approach to training these skills if weaknesses in these prerequisite areas are identified.

The Environmental Prelanguage Battery (EPB; Horstmeier & MacDonald, 1978) is a semantically based instrument useful for the child functioning at or below a single-word level. Readiness or "entry" skills surveyed include attention, response to simple commands, imitation, and interaction with adults and objects in the environment.

A relatively new instrument, the GAEL-P (Grammatical Analysis of Elicited Language—Pre-sentence Level) includes a language "readiness" section. This test has been standardized with severely and profoundly hearing-impaired young students by Moog, Kozak, and Geers (1983). Motivating diagnostic teaching tasks are used to probe (1) general response to speech (or manual sign), (2) differentiation of words in a small set, and (3) imitation of motor actions and speech sounds. The large-scale, realistic toys used in this task make it particularly useful for the developmentally young hearing-impaired child.

A useful aspect of both the GAEL-P and the EPB is the potential for diagnostic teaching. The clinician may ascertain by probing which activities elicit responses (and, potentially, learning) from the child.

Early Content Comprehension and Lexical Development

Miller (1978) stressed the need for careful consideration of developmental data to make "informed clinical decisions." Chapman (1978a) presented a compilation of receptive and expressive language achievements in normally developing children from Sensorimotor Stage 5 (12–18 months) to Stage 6 (18–22 months). Miller added that the diagnostician's focus throughout this stage should be on semantic functions, the child's dependence on nonlinguistic context in early comprehension of language, and the rapid growth in language after the child's cognitive development advances to Sensorimotor Stage 6 (Miller, 1978).

Developmental charts, such as that designed by Chapman, are extremely useful for the qualitative analysis of the child's communicative interactions and free speech. Early syntactic accomplishments may be coded following the Assigning Structural Stage procedure, described by Miller (1981). The reader is referred to these developmental schedules, which are extremely useful for interpretation of the child's performance. Because a complete review of the issues at this stage of development is beyond the scope of this chapter, the remaining comments will focus on practical issues and concerns particularly germane to the hearing-impaired developmentally disabled population.

First, as Chapman (1978b) has so aptly described, children rely on a variety of comprehension strategies while learning language. The young child's "knowledge of the world" predisposes him or her to certain responses (e.g., putting things *in* containers, but *on* flat surfaces). At times the child appears to understand complex language messages when his or her responses are actually based on situational context or a strategy. Some hearing-impaired developmentally disabled children fail to make the best use of their "worldly knowledge" or cues from the environment which support comprehension. The diagnostician should observe if the child is making appropriate use of nonlinguistic information to support language learning.

Second, the diagnostician should be attuned to problems of generalization in the hearing-impaired developmentally disabled child. It is important to probe whether object selection is restricted to a particular set of toys, or whether the targeted object can be retrieved from another room. Similarly, comprehension of directions may be tied to specific eliciting situations. Our clinical experience has shown two tests to be particularly useful in probing receptive and expressive language developments in varied contexts. One is the Sequenced Inventory of Communication Development (SICD; Hendrick, Prather, & Tobin, 1975). If the test is employed with a child who has minimal residual hearing, however, it is recommended that the auditory items be deleted. A second test that has been useful is the Ski-Hi Language Development Scale (Watkins, 1979). This criterion-referenced scale of receptive and expressive development is completed through caregiver interview and direct observation. It is based on modification of other early language scales (e.g., the Receptive/Expressive Emergent Language Scale, Bzoch & League, 1970) to meet the unique needs of the hearing-impaired child. Certain auditory items are deleted, and credit is given for a signed or verbal response.

Third, the examiner may need to determine the effects of the materials on the child's responses because this may provide useful teaching information. For example, reducing a set size from six to four objects may increase successful responding. Large-scale realistic toys may be preferable to small-scale representational ones, depending on the child's cognitive skills. Pictured materials should be used with caution until the examiner is certain the child recognizes such representations of objects.

Fourth, a number of issues should be considered in assessing vocabulary. Distribution of lexical learning is a critical issue with this population. Too often, hearing-impaired developmentally disabled children learn an abundance of noun labels (due to their concrete referents), but they learn few semantic notions that have more communicative relevance (e.g., rejection terms, possessives, action terms). The diagnostician should attempt to survey the distribution of semantic meanings in the child's lexicon. This may be accomplished through diaries kept by the caregiver or teacher or through free-speech analysis. In our clinic, an informal vocabulary survey was developed to address this issue. Lexical items commonly used in the first words of children and representing eight semantic classes are incorporated in an object selection and manipulation task. The results provide useful information for planning lexical expansion.

The GAEL-P, described earlier, has a simple vocabulary recognition and production task that uses large-scale realistic toys. This may be useful for children with limited vocabularies. A limitation of the test, however, is that only nouns are surveyed.

Fifth, the Environmental Language Inventory (ELI; MacDonald, 1978) and the GAEL-P and GAEL-S (simple sentence level) tests utilize a method of analogous prompting to determine whether spontaneous one- and two-word utterances may be expanded through directed modeling procedures. Each of these tests has application for determining useful therapy techniques.

Caregiver Skills. A great deal of interest in recent years has been centered on caregiver-child interaction and the potentially nurturing effects of this interaction on language development. Concern has been expressed, on the other hand, for differences in the communicative style of caregivers of handicapped children (Collins, 1969; Gross, 1970). The informal parent-child interaction survey, shown in Appendix A, has been developed by the author to assess the effectiveness of the caregiver in providing a nurturing linguistic environment. This informal assessment is particularly relevant when a parent is attempting to use sign language with the child and is not yet proficient in its use. In this instance, professional efforts need to be directed toward the language used in interaction with the child.

Phonologic Skills. Evaluation of the oral mechanism should be completed as part of the communication assessment. Articulatory and nonarticulatory speech skills can be assessed using procedures described by Ling (1976), procedures developed for normally hearing children, or both. For a discussion of considerations for testing and test selection in this area, the reader is referred to Moeller et al. (1983).

Simple Utterances Level: Test Considerations

Once a student's comprehension and attending behaviors advance, a number of standardized tests, designed for use with younger hearing children, may be modified to determine a child's progress and assist in design of therapy goals. Some measures that have been useful with this population are described in Appendix B. The limitations of standardized instruments should be considered when analyzing results. Because of the limitations, formal test results should never be viewed in isolation from other developmental observations. The test battery should also include a free-speech analysis. An excellent resource for such procedures appeared in Miller (1981). Informal procedures, which augment a comprehensive battery, are described by Moeller et al. (1983). In the remaining section, key issues relevant to this stage of analysis are highlighted.

The first issue, raised in the previous section, concerns comprehension strategies. This issue also needs to be considered when testing older hearing-impaired developmentally disabled students. Older students may bring to the closed-set testing task more sophisticated strategies than the young child for whom the test was designed. This may inflate test results. On the other hand, some hearing-impaired students rely on developmental comprehension strategies and situational context well beyond the point where these are productive. Some students, for example, attend to key words in a message to the exclusion of more important semantic or syntactic features. Reliance on particular comprehension strategies may be counterproductive to comprehension. The diagnostician should watch for such problems.

Second, some children present significant memory constraints. If this occurs, the examiner should seek to determine the effect of stimulus length on information processing. Does chunking of the information assist the student? Does reduction of signing or speaking rate help? Is repetition useful?

Third, a number of researchers suggest the need to assess the communicative functions used by the student. Chapman (1981) presented a comprehensive review of taxonomies for describing communicative functions and speech acts. In summarizing this body of literature, Chapman urged diagnosticians to take communicative contexts into account, to use discourse levels of analysis, and to note the child's observance of the rules governing speech acts (Chapman, 1981, p. 134). Thus, the clinician must be attuned to whether the student's comments are appropriate to the context and to the conversational content. The student's ability to seek clarification or repair broken communication should also be explored (Moeller et al., 1983). Prutting and Kirchner (1983) presented a charting procedure for analyzing speech acts. Moeller et al. (1983) described a discourse charting procedure that concentrates on a frequent discourse problem of the hearing-impaired population: question comprehension. Using this procedure, the clinician tabulates the percentage of correct and incorrect responses to a variety of conversational questions. When transcribing free-speech samples, the clinician is instructed to include both examiner and student comments, unintelligible segments, and the student's attempts at clarifying the message.

Fourth, a critical point with the hearing-impaired developmentally disabled student is one of relevance. The diagnostician must develop an evaluation plan that is sensitive to the priority needs of the older student. This requires careful integration of effort with the classroom teachers and careful study of the student's needs in various environments.

A brief case illustration supports this point. Three hearing-impaired developmentally disabled adolescents were enrolled in a residential school for the deaf. The students were profoundly hearing impaired, below average intellectually, and had varying degrees of visual impairment. Formal structured evaluation revealed language levels ranging from three to five years developmentally. The students could follow directions and understand simple questions; they also had a large core of sign vocabulary and could express simple ideas. The most valuable portion of the evaluation was the charting of their pragmatic behaviors and functional uses of language. A major deficit was noted in their initiation of communicative exchange with each other. They rarely commented or questioned. Language functioned primarily for satisfaction of needs and answering direct requests, but it was used for no apparent social purposes. Diagnostic teaching tasks were devised by reviewing the students' theoretical pragmatic needs and considering their life-skill needs. Several tasks evolved as useful in expanding their communicative performance; they are described in Table 3. For children like this, qualitative improvement of communication directed toward improved life-skills may be far more important than quantitative growth of syntactic skills or vocabulary.

Table 3. Tasks Contrived to Target Social Language Use

Task	Target Language Use
Role-play going to the doctor to explain an illness	Description, specific explanation, comprehension of interpreter's instructions
Barrier game where specific instructions result in communication partner completing a task appropriately (after Simon, 1979)	Following and giving instructions, repairing communication, questioning
Role-play selling at concession at the school basketball game; deliberately give customer the wrong item	Polite requests, questioning repair strategies
Role-play store; describe item desired on the shelf (group of items presented)	Provide salient description

The importance of setting priorities was also apparent in the case of a 6-year-old hearing-impaired developmentally disabled youngster who was referred for evaluation because of limited language growth and a tendency to "ignore" the teacher. Neurological examination revealed that the student was experiencing frequent psychomotor seizures. Once the seizures were controlled, J. M. was a "teachable" youngster. He had a relatively large core of sign vocabulary which he used in single-word productions for varied purposes (labeling, commenting, requesting). A semantic and pragmatic analysis revealed gaps in his communicative content, however. For example, he had no mechanism for rejecting, except situation avoidance. Focus was placed on his communicative needs, and situations were contrived in which his communication attempts were rewarded by obvious results, as suggested by McLean and Snyder-McLean (1978). With this help J. M. quickly learned to incorporate negation in his language. He learned that expressing "put away" would bring an end to a boring activity, and this was so powerful and rewarding that he readily generalized it to several contexts. Use of "no white" earned a drink of chocolate milk.

Too often hearing-impaired developmentally disabled children learn highly ritualized or stereotypic programmed responses. If the goal is generative language use and flexible communication, then an evaluation goal is determination of functional gaps and strategies that will help fill the gaps.

Fifth, if it is possible for the diagnostician to be in close contact with the teacher, rates of learning should be monitored. The teacher might be assisted in setting up feasible charting procedures to note how long the student typically takes to achieve and generalize a goal. These data may be critical for determining if the communication modality being used is appropriate for the student. (See Chapter 14 for a discussion of augmentative communication techniques and their evaluation.)

In summary, although a number of formal procedures may be administered and may be useful with the older student, descriptive procedures and informal analysis continue to be essential. A high priority is determination of how language is used by the student in varied contexts and how identified weaknesses translate into therapy goals. Goal determination should be based on an understanding of each student's present and future communicative needs. The clinician should determine how useful the potential language goal will be to the student's overall functioning.

Beyond Simple Utterances: Evaluation Considerations

A primary focus of this chapter has been evaluation of the developmentally young and/or low functioning hearing-impaired child. Hearing-impaired students with milder degrees of secondary impairment also require an adaptive and integrated approach to evaluation.

One group of hearing-impaired developmentally disabled students has received considerable professional attention in recent years. The hearing-impaired child with specific learning problems has presented new challenges to diagnosticians and educators. Space in this chapter does not permit a comprehensive discussion of the hearing-impaired learning disabled population (a topic that merits a separate volume). However, several key issues germane to these and other school-age students will be highlighted. Differential diagnostic procedures take on increased importance in an age when educational labels and consequent services are "restrictive." For example, many states will not certify a student (for placement purposes) as hearing impaired *and* learning disabled. This places an increased burden on the educator of hearing-impaired children to seek information on the effect of a child's learning problem on his or her language and academic progress.

Integration of evaluation findings is essential to effective management of this group of children. The teacher must have opportunities to view the child's language and learning profile in light of performance data in the areas of memory, processing, and academics. A visual memory problem, for example, may contribute to excessive delays in lexical, semantic, and syntactic acquisition. Full understanding of the interrelated problems is necessary for the development of compensatory, remedial strategies.*

A second consideration is the need to structure the evaluation with sensitivity to the discourse demands of a classroom situation. Simon (1979) offered many practical guidelines in this area. Principally, the clinician must consider the impact of the language and learning problems on academic development. Pursuant to this goal, the language evaluation should be multifaceted and should include emphasis on the following areas.

---

*A complete description of learning skills evaluations used with hearing-impaired students will be included in a special monograph to be published in the near future by the Boys Town National Institute for Communication Disorders research department.

Classroom "Survival Skills." Is the student able to answer both convergent and divergent questions posed by the teacher in classroom discussions? The Preschool Language Assessment Instrument (PLAI), described in Appendix B, is often useful to address this concern. Charting of question and answer routines may also be useful for describing this important discourse skill. Is the student able to follow directions? Teacher-made tasks or subtests from the Detroit Tests of Learning Aptitude are useful in answering this question. The clinician should attend closely to the student's level of organization and strategy in attempting to follow directions. The clinician should also note if the student adopts an impulsive or reflective approach to school-like tasks.

Lexical Skills. Many hearing-impaired learning disabled students exhibit problems retaining or recalling information; evaluation therefore should include a focus on lexical skills. Assessment of single, literal meanings for isolated vocabulary terms is incomplete. The clinician should determine if the student has developed any independence in the lexical learning process. (For example, does he or she derive information from context to figure out less familiar terms?) Organization of the lexicon should be investigated by probing classification skills: ability to group, regroup, define, and exclude members from a group. Specific procedures are described by Moeller et al. (1983) and Simon (1979). Ability to retrieve familiar lexical terms is assessed using word latency measures (rapid naming upon confrontation).

Skill Application. Another area of concern is whether learned language skills can be applied to novel situations and daily living or classroom problems. Thus, mathematics concepts are evaluated singly as well as in the context of applied math problems (see Woodcock-Johnson Quantitative Concepts, Appendix B). Conjunctions are surveyed in the context of cause-effect solutions (Kellman, Flood, & Yoder, 1977). Are time concepts useful for helping the students plan ahead and evaluate past experiences?

Thought-Related Language Skills. In the later primary grades, academic content requirements increase in their cognitive abstraction and demands for thought-related reasoning. Evaluation should include tests that probe the student's ability to discern and describe relationships, make predictions, and reason with language. The PLAI and TCU tasks described in Appendix B and the Inventory of Language Assessment Tasks (Kellman, Flood, & Yoder, 1977) have provided insights in this area.

Formulation Skills. Expressive language analysis with this population should focus on the student's overall organization of information relay. Word retrieval problems, for example, may lead to false starts, verbal mazes, semantic errors, or unorganized, unintelligible explanations. Incoherence may result from inability to recall semantic concepts or syntactic rules. The clinician should attend to the effect of the retrieval problems on automatic rule use and organization of discourse.

The advocated approach, then, is to coordinate findings from various perspectives or disciplines and to view language skills in light of the discourse demands of the learning environment. By integrating test findings and relating them to classroom needs, the clinician may more easily define therapy priorities.

The hearing-impaired learning disabled child often presents a complex profile of strengths and weaknesses. Comprehensive evaluation and diagnostic teaching may be necessary to "tease" out factors important to an integrated therapy effort. As the following case example illustrates, the problems are rarely straightforward or singular in their effect.

B. H., age 12 years, was seen for an interdisciplinary evaluation due to concerns for delayed academic progress. B. H. had a moderate-to-severe sensorineural hearing loss in both ears. He was placed in a fourth grade self-contained class for hearing-impaired children. Psychological test results indicated a performance IQ of 126 with a verbal IQ of 62. The psychologist expressed significant concern about B. H.'s memory and thought-related language skills. The learning disabilities specialist documented severe memory and retrieval problems. Results of language evaluation revealed receptive and expressive language delays in excess of what would be anticipated for B. H.'s age and degree of hearing loss. He was functioning at approximately a 4- to 4½-year-old level in language skills. Qualitative analysis of the language supported the findings of the psychologist and the learning disabilities specialist. Expressive language sampling revealed extensive retrieval and formulation problems causing superficial descriptions, poorly organized simple utterances, and frequent semantic errors.

For example, the following scenario resulted when B. H. was asked about his Halloween costume.

	Discourse	Concern
Clinician:	What are you going to dress up like for Halloween?	Question
B. H.:	Candy—bunch one.	Comprehension
Clinician:	Listen to my question. What will you wear?	
B. H.:	Um, the red one all over.	Retrieval
Clinician:	What is that, B.?	
B. H.:	I forgot it.	
Clinician:	What has red all over?	
B. H.:	Like this one (gesture) have a tail and this thing . . . a. . . a. . . /dir/?	Retrieval
Clinician:	A devil?	
B. H.:	Yeah.	

B. H. was given the PLAI. On this measure he evidenced significantly reduced thought-related language skills. Due to his formulation problems, he had difficulty conceptualizing relationships, retrieving category examples, and providing explanations and descriptions. His memory and retrieval problems also affected his concept application. He exhibited extreme confusion of basic time concepts (yesterday, now, next, tomorrow), creating conversational problems. He demonstrated limited classification skills, difficulties solving story problems, and frustration with verbal tasks. (While looking at a picture of a Christmas tree, he excitedly labeled it "trick or treat," then reported sadly, "No, that's not it.")

Recommendations for this seriously learning disabled hearing-impaired boy resulted from a team effort. Isolated work on weak areas was not likely to influence language organization or classroom learning. Diagnostic teaching revealed certain compensatory strategies (visualizing, using recognition to recall, or multiple choice prompts) to be helpful. These were illustrated to B. H.'s teacher. Importantly, language remediation suggestions were incorporated into the content of the academic program. For example, time concept development was to be stressed during daily planning and scheduled review times; vocabulary development was related to word associations and application of concepts to solving simple word problems. Although individual therapy time with this youngster was useful, the most effective strategy was the therapist illustrating to the teacher how the language problems could be addressed in the daily academic curriculum. The teacher gained a better understanding of how the related language/learning problems were at the base of B. H.'s academic difficulties.

Much further research is needed to determine optimal procedures for differential diagnosis of hearing-impaired students with learning disabilities. Until such information is available, clinicians must rely on a cautiously interpreted test battery, integrated professional efforts, and a knowledge of the child's most important classroom communication needs.

Summary

This chapter has described a number of issues and considerations that apply when evaluating hearing-impaired developmentally disabled children. Little is known about the effects of combined impairments on language development. Even less is known about the most appropriate procedures for assessing language needs and progress in these children. The clinician must flexibly adapt and apply existing clinical procedures to evaluate the hearing-impaired developmentally disabled child. Key considerations include (1) the need to expand the contexts in which communicative behaviors are observed (either directly or indirectly); (2) the need to integrate data from social, cognitive, and linguistic domains; and (3) the need to consider the relevance of the language skill when planning therapy goals.

References

Bangs, T. E. (1975). *Vocabulary comprehension scale*. Boston: Teaching Resources.

Bates, E. (1976). *Language and context: The acquisition of pragmatics*. New York: Academic Press.

Blank, M., Rose, S., & Berlin, L. (1978). *Preschool language assessment instrument*. New York: Grune and Stratton.

Bloom, L., & Lahey, M. (1978). *Language development and language disorders*. New York: John Wiley.

Boehm, A. (1971). *Boehm test of basic concepts.* New York: Psychological Corporation.

Bornstein, H., Saulnier, K., & Hamilton, L. (1980). Signed English: A first evaluation. *Americans Annals of the Deaf, 125,* 467–481.

Brenza, B., Kricos, P. B., & Lasky, E. (1981). Comprehension and production of basic semantic concepts by older hearing-impaired children. *Journal of Speech and Hearing Research, 24,* 414–420.

Bricker, D., & Dennison, L. (1978). Training prerequisites to verbal behavior. In M. E. Snell (Ed.), *Systematic instruction of the moderately and severely handicapped.* Columbus, OH: Charles E. Merrill.

Bzoch, K., & League, R. (1970). *Receptive/expressive emergent language scale (REEL).* Gainesville, FL: Anhinga Press.

Carrow, M. A. (1973). *Test for auditory comprehension of language.* Austin, TX: Urban Research Group.

Chapman, R. (1978a). Chart in J. Miller, Assessing children's language behavior. In. R. L. Schiefelbusch (Ed.), *Bases of language intervention.* Baltimore: University Park Press.

Chapman, R. (1978b). Comprehension strategies in children. In J. F. Kavanaugh (Ed.), *Speech and language in the laboratory, school and clinic.* Cambridge, MA: MIT Press.

Chapman, R. (1981). Exploring children's communicative intents. In J. Miller (Ed.), *Assessing language production in children.* Baltimore: University Park Press.

Coggins, T., & Carpenter, R. (1981). The communicative intention inventory. *Applied Psycholinguistics, 2,* 235–251.

Collins, J. (1969). *Communication between deaf children of preschool age and their mothers.* Unpublished doctoral dissertation, University of Pittsburgh.

Crager, R., & Spriggs, A. (1972). *The development of concepts: The test of concept utilization.* Los Angeles: Western Psychological Services.

Crystal, D., Fletcher, P., & Garman, M. (1976). *The grammatical analysis of language disability: A procedure for assessment and remediation.* New York: Elsevier-North Holland.

Davis, J. (1974). Performance of young hearing-impaired children on a test of basic concepts. *Journal of Speech and Hearing Research, 17,* 342–351.

Davis, J. (1977). Reliability of hearing-impaired children's responses to oral and total presentations of the test of auditory comprehension of language. *Journal of Speech and Hearing Disorders, 4,* 520–527.

Dore, J. (1974). A pragmatic description of early language development. *Journal of Psycholinguistic Research, 4,* 343–350.

Dunn, L. (1959). *Peabody picture vocabulary test.* Circle Pines, MN: American Guidance Services.

Fieber, N. (1975). *Movement in communication and language development of deaf-blind children.* Paper presented at National Deaf-Blind Workshop, Dallas, TX.

Foster, R., Gidden, K., & Stark, J. (1973). *Assessment of children's language comprehension.* Palo Alto: Consulting Psychologists Press.

Gardner, M. (1979). *Expressive one word picture vocabulary test.* Novato, CA: Academic Therapy Publications.

Geers, A. E., & Moog, J. S. (1979). *CID grammatical analysis of elicited language* (CID Pub. No. 104). St. Louis: Central Institute for the Deaf.

Geffner, D., & Freeman, L. (1980). Assessment of language comprehension of six-year-old deaf children. *Journal of Communication Disorders, 13*(6), 445–470.

Greenfield, P., & Smith, J. (1976). *The structure of communication in early language development.* New York: Academic Press.

Gross, R. (1970). Language used by mothers of deaf children and mothers of hearing children. *American Annals of the Deaf, 115,* 93–95.

Halliday, M. A. K. (1975). *Learning how to mean.* New York: Elsevier-North Holland.

Hedrick, D. L., Prather, E. M., & Tobin, A. R. (1975). *The sequenced inventory of communication development.* Seattle: University of Washington Press.

Horstmeier, D., & MacDonald, J. (1978). *Environmental prelanguage battery.* Columbus, OH: Charles E. Merrill.

Ireton, H., & Thwing, E. (1972). *Minnesota child development inventory.* Minneapolis: Behavior Science Systems.

Kellman, M., Flood, C., & Yoder, D. (1977). *Inventory of language assessment tasks.* Madison, WI: Waisman Center, University of Wisconsin.

Kirk, S., McCarthy, J., & Kirk, W. (1968). *Illinois test of psycholinguistic abilities.* Urbana, IL: University of Illinois Press.

Kretschmer, R., & Kretschmer, L. (1978). *Language development and intervention with the hearing impaired.* Baltimore: University Park Press.

Lee, L. (1974). *Developmental sentence analysis.* Evanston, IL: Northwestern University Press.

Lillie, S. M. (1976). *Rules of talking.* Nashville: Bill Wilkerson Hearing and Speech Center, Intersect.

Ling, D. (1976). *Speech for the hearing-impaired child: Theory and practice.* Washington, DC: A. G. Bell Association.

MacDonald, J. (1978). *Environmental language inventory.* Columbus, OH: Charles E. Merrill.

McLean, J., & Snyder-McLean, L. (1978). *A transactional approach to early language training.* Columbus, OH: Charles E. Merrill.

Mehrabian, A., & Moynihan, C. (1979). *Child language ability measures.* Los Angeles: University of California Press.

Miller, J. (1978). Assessing children's language behavior. In R. L. Schiefelbusch (Ed.), *Bases of language intervention.* Baltimore: University Park Press.

Miller, J. (1981). *Assessing language production in children.* Baltimore: University Park Press.

Miller, J., & Yoder, D. (1975). *Miller-Yoder test of grammatical comprehension.* Unpublished experimental edition, University of Wisconsin, Madison.

Moeller, M., McConkey, A., & Osberger, M. (1983). Evaluation of the communicative skills of hearing impaired children. *Audiology, VIII*(8), 113–127.

Moog, J., Kozak, V., & Geers, A. (1983). *The grammatical analysis of elicited language—Presentence level.* St. Louis: Central Institute for the Deaf Press.

Newcomer, P., & Hammill, D. (1977). *Test of language development.* Los Angeles: Western Psychological Services.

Peddicord, R. S. (1977). *Evaluation of the effectiveness of a multi-media parental education course.* Unpublished doctoral dissertation, University of Nebraska.

Prutting, C., & Kirchner, D. M. (1983). In T. Gallagher & C. Prutting (Eds.), *Pragmatic assessment and intervention strategies.* San Diego: College-Hill Press.

Quigley, S., Steinkamp, M., Power, D., & Jones, B. (1978). *Test of syntactic abilities.* Beaverton, OR: Dormac.

Raffin, M., Davis, J., & Gilman, L. (1978). Comprehension of inflection morphemes by deaf children exposed to a visual English sign system. *Journal of Speech and Hearing Research, 21,* 387–400.

Reynell, J. K. (1977). *Reynell developmental language scale.* Windsor, England: NFER Publishing.

Ricks, D. (1975). Vocal communication in pre-verbal normal and autistic children. In N. O'Conner (Ed.), *Language, cognitive deficits and retardation.* London: Butterworths.

Robbins, N., & Steinquist, G. (1967). *The deaf-blind "rubella" child* (Pub. No. 25). Watertown, MA: Perkins School for the Blind.

Robinson, C., & Robinson, J. (1978). Sensorimotor functions and cognitive development. In M. Snell (Ed.), *Systematic instruction of the moderately and severely handicapped.* Columbus, OH: Charles E. Merrill.

Saulnier, K., & Heidinger, V. (1980). Signed English morphology test. *American Annals of the Deaf, 125*(4), 480–481.

Scherer, P. (1981). *Sign vocabulary test.* Chicago: Center on Deafness.

Simon, C. (1979). *Communicative competence: A functional-pragmatic approach to language therapy.* Tucson: Communication Skill Builders.

Snow, C. (1977). The development of conversation between mothers and babies. *Journal of Child Language, 4,* 1–22.

Thoms, C., & Moeller, M. P. (1978). *Parent-child interaction checklist.* Unpublished.

Trammell, J. L., Farrar, C., Francis, J., Owens, S. L., Shepard, D. E., Thiers, T. L., Wilten, R. P., & Faist, L. H. (1976). *Test of auditory comprehension.* N. Hollywood: Foreworks.

Watkins, S. (1979). *The Ski-Hi language development scale.* Logan, UT: Ski-Hi Outreach, Utah State University.

Woodcock, R., & Johnson, M. B. (1977). *Woodcock-Johnson psychoeducational battery.* Boston: Teaching Resources.

Appendix A
Informal Evaluation of Parent/Child Interaction

Name: Date:

Date of Birth: Clinician:

Activity Description:

Key: "Frequent"—Observed 10 + times in 30-minute interaction

"Occasional"—Observed 5–8 times

"Infrequent"—Less than 3 observations

"Not Observed" (N.O. for no opportunity)

Structured Segment (from Peddicord, R., 1977):

Free Play

Game Interaction

Parent "Occupied"

Direct Clean Up

Child's Social/Interactional Skills (after McLean & Snyder-McLean, 1978)

1. Child attends visually to adult for sustained period

2. Child attends selectively to an object the parent is regarding

3. Child shifts attention to alternate speakers/signers

4. Child seeks communicative interaction

5. Child initiates interaction:

   a) verbally (signed or spoken)

   b) gesturally

   c) combined

6. Complies with parent request given

   a) verbally (signed or spoken)

   b) gesturally

   c) combined

7. Imitates when prompted

8. Requests assistance

9. Requests information

10. Requests repetition or clarification

Parent/Caregiver Strategies (after Lillie, 1976; McLean & Snyder-McLean, 1978; Thoms & Moeller, 1978)

Parent/Listener Role:

1. Comprehends _____% of child's spoken utterances (quantify from tape)

2. Comprehends _____% of child's signed utterances

3. Describe how parent handles utterances that are not intelligible (e.g., requests clarification, ignores, queries with key word)

4. Does parent provide or maximize opportunities for child to assume spoken role? Describe.

Parent Communication Strategies:

  A. Interaction (social/emotional aspects)

    1. Able to elicit compliant behavior

    2. Able to maintain child's interest in activity

    3. Able to follow child's lead/shift activities to maintain child's interest

    4. Provides opportunity for creative representational play

    5. Facial expression and vocal tone is natural and conveys interest

    6. Uses natural gestures in communication

    7. Lets child actively participate

    8. Pauses for child's action and/or verbal response; gives child a chance to show he/she understands

    9. Talks about child's and own feelings

    10. Maintains behavior control; deals effectively with inappropriate behavior

  B. Verbal Stimulation

    1. Uses vocabulary, phrases, and sentences appropriate to the child's language level

    2. Provides natural language appropriate to the activity; focuses on the "here and now"

    3. Announces or cues topic and topic shifts

    4. Communicates about and directs child's attention to demonstrable referents (if appropriate level)

    5. Provides expansion of child's utterances

    6. Provides expatiation of child's utterances

    7. Is able to modify level of linguistic input to match child's needs. Comments:

    8. Provides repetition of key language concepts

    9. Repair strategies

      a) paraphrases

      b) repeats

      c) increases visual support

      d) gives examples

      e) "gives up" (does not pursue)

      f) other

Appendix B

Formal Tests: A Review of Considerations in Adapting for Use with Hearing-Impaired Children

To Assess Receptive Lexical/Semantic Skills

Instrument	Findings	Test Considerations
Peabody Picture Vocabulary Test (Dunn, 1959)	(1) Data suggest this measure is sensitive to developmental change with age (see Moeller et al., 1983), although gains are not linear. (2) Clinical experience suggests alternate forms of this test may not be of equal difficulty in hearing-impaired population. (3) Clinical experience suggests experimental/informational gaps are reflected in scattered profiles of abilities.	(1) May allow comparing child against him- or herself and evaluating mainstreamed students who are competing with hearing peers. (2) Results may reflect specific lexical knowledge. Signed administration needs to be interpreted with caution.
Test of Language Development (TOLD) Picture Vocabulary subtest (Newcomer & Hammill, 1977).	(1) Not sensitive enough to developmental change beyond nine years of age on deaf students, due to low ceiling and too few items (Moeller et al., 1983).	(1) Was designed as a screening instrument and is not meant to be used as a diagnostic or prescriptive measure.
Receptive Sign Vocabulary Test (Scherer, 1981).	(1) Has normative information on hearing-impaired children but standardization sample is small. (2) Clinical experience suggests that the results are often inconsistent with age scores on other measures.	(1) Cautious interpretation is required since the standardization sample is small.
Boehm Test of Basic Concepts (Boehm, 1971)	(1) Data on school-age profoundly hearing-impaired students revealed best scores on spatial concepts, followed by miscellaneous and quality concepts. Time concepts were the most difficult (Moeller et al., 1983). (2) Beyond 10 years of age, this test was insensitive to developmental change in most residential hearing-impaired	(1) Useful for testing a range of concepts in two-dimensional space. (2) Useful within a restricted age range; less sensitive to change when given to hearing-impaired children age 10 or older.

students tested (Moeller et al., 1983).

(3) Studies of hard-of-hearing 6–8-year-olds revealed the same order of difficulty as reported above. In comparison to hearing students, the subjects were delayed in their development (Davis, 1974).

(4) A study of 15 orally trained deaf 13–14-year-old students revealed that four-fifths of the group scored lower than the 10th percentile for second-grade hearing children. Comprehension exceeded production. Of the concepts surveyed on the Boehm, 80% appeared in the student's textbooks (Brenza, Kricos, & Lasky, 1981).

Vocabulary Comprehension Scale (Bangs, 1975)	(1) No obvious relationships between age level expectancies and profoundly hearing-impaired subjects' performance (Moeller et al., 1983). (2) Clinical experience suggests that differences may be due to the instructional priorities for preschool hearing-impaired children and to gaps in development.	(1) Useful for surveying a range of concepts in three-dimensional space. (2) Motivating test format.

To Assess Receptive Syntactic Skills

Instrument	Findings	Test Considerations
Test of Language Development— Grammatic Understanding subtest	(1) For individual subjects, results of this measure may be higher than those obtained on other syntax measures. It has been noted that students older than the standardization sample are able to use key words and the pictured choices available to "guess" at meaning. It is uncertain if syntactic comprehension is always reflected in the results. Collectively, hearing-impaired	(1) Response strategies should be critically analyzed.

students performed similarly to findings on the CLAM (Moeller et al., 1983).

Test of Syntactic Abilities (TSA; Quigley et al., 1978)

(1) Normed on hearing-impaired students, the authors' findings are in agreement with the order of acquisition of forms reported by Quigley et al. (Moeller et al., 1983).

(1) The screening test is presented in orthography; conclusions about oral language performance cannot be drawn directly from such data.

Child Language Ability Measures (Mehrabian & Moynihan, 1979)—Grammatic Comprehension subtest

(1) Hearing-impaired students from a residential program demonstrated limited growth in syntactic skill with age. An average developmental age score of 6.8 years was obtained on students 12 to 19 years of age (Moeller et al., 1983).

(1) Few items sampling each structure are presented.

(2) Several test items have only one foil, increasing the child's chances of guessing the correct answer.

Test of Auditory Comprehension of Language (TACL; Carrow, 1973)

(1) Data on 18 hearing-impaired students (10 educated orally, 8 educated in total communication) revealed similar, developmentally expected performance for both oral and TC groups. The author concludes that this is an appropriate, reliable instrument for use with hearing-impaired children (Davis, 1977).

(1) Item length on this test is fairly well controlled and a multiple choice is provided. This level of redundancy may not represent typical language demands facing older hearing-impaired students.

Assessment of Children's Language Comprehension (ACLC; Foster, Giddan, & Stark, 1973)

(1) A group of 6-year-old hearing-impaired children show a delayed but developmental pattern, with reception of four critical elements being the most difficult task (Geffner & Freeman, 1980).

(2) Six-year-old hearing-impaired children's performance was closest to hearing 3- to 4-year-olds (Geffner & Freeman, 1980).

(3) Little information is available on presentation of this test in sign language.

(1) Useful test for determining how increased length or syntactic complexity influences understanding.

(2) May assist in screening for evidence of memory deficits.

(3) May be useful for comparing performance in separate modes (e.g., oral/TC).

Signed English Morphology Test (Saulnier & Heidinger, 1980)

(1) Was developed to assess understanding and production of certain signed inflections by deaf children.

(1) A methodological problem with this measure is that it samples only the marked feature, which may lead

(2) Authors of the test evaluated 20 hearing-impaired students over a 4-year period. Receptive syntactic knowledge improved and accelerated over the four years, as reflected by the *Signed English Morphology Test* and other measures. Students continued to have difficulty comprehending regular past, participle, irregular plural, and irregular past (Bornstein, Saulnier, & Hamilton, 1980).

(3) Raffin, Davis, and Gilman (1978) developed another test of morpheme-based concepts to evaluate 67 deaf children using Seeing Essential English (SEE-1). They found the following order of acquisition: plural -*s*, past -*ed*, present progressive -*ing*, possessive -'*s*, third person -*s*, comparative -*er*, superlative -*est*, and present perfect -*en*.

students to develop a response bias.

(2) Test may be useful to survey student's competence in this area; may not reflect typical "performance" in running conversation, however.

Instrument	Findings	Test Considerations
Miller-Yoder Test of Grammatical Comprehension (Miller & Yoder, 1975)	(1) Data suggest this measure is sensitive to developmental change in syntactic growth with age (Moeller et al., 1983). (2) This nonstandardized, experimental procedure was developed to assess structures emerging at ages 4, 5, 6, and 6+ years.	(1) Test administration guidelines require that both the marked and unmarked features of a stimulus pair be identified for the syntactic structure to be credited as correct. Each structure is sampled several times. Both of these features reduce the effects of guessing on the child's score. (2) Clinical experiences suggest this is a useful measure with hearing-impaired children.

To Assess Receptive Functional Communication Skills

Instrument	Findings	Test Considerations
Reynell Developmental Language Scale—Verbal Comprehension Scale (Reynell, 1977)	(1) A group of profoundly hearing-impaired children did not show expected relationship between performance and item difficulty due in part to the students' semantic knowledge	(1) Very useful in assessing the level of abstraction and length/complexity the child is able to handle. (2) Motivating test for children (object manipulation).

exceeding their ability to process lengthy syntactic messages (Moeller et al., 1983).

(2) Clinical experience suggests the test is less sensitive to developmental change in children having difficulty processing lengthy syntax.

(3) Informal probing with the items gives insight to the child's comprehension strategies.

To Assess *Functional Auditory Skills*

Instrument	Findings	Test Considerations
Test of Auditory Comprehension (Trammell et al., 1976)	(1) Investigates processing of speech at a linguistic rather than a phonetic level. (2) This test was designed for and normed on hearing-impaired children ages 4 years to 12 years, 11 months.	(1) A very useful test for obtaining prescriptive information for planning auditory management programs. (2) An instructional program, *Auditory Skills Instructional Planning System,* is available to be used in conjunction with the TAC.

To Assess *Expressive Lexical/Semantic Skills*

Instrument	Findings	Test Considerations
Woodcock-Johnson Psychoeducational Battery—Picture Vocabulary subtest (Woodcock & Johnson, 1977)	(1) Clinical experience suggests that hearing-impaired children may perform better on the expressive than receptive vocabulary measure because the expressive measure allows for varied responses (*ship* or *oceanliner*), making the task more child-controlled.	(1) Because few items are sampled at each level, the results may be affected by gaps in specific lexical knowledge.
Expressive One Word Picture Vocabulary Test (Gardner, 1979)	(1) The authors have consistently noted somewhat inflated performance on this measure by hearing-impaired students. This may relate to scatter within the lexicon.	(1) Caution must be exercised in interpreting signed responses to ensure that the child is using a formal sign rather than pantomime.
Test of Language Development (TOLD)—Oral Vocabulary subtest	(1) On a group of deaf residential students, similar performances were found on the TOLD and Woodcock-Johnson subtests measuring expressive vocabulary (Moeller et al., 1983).	(1) This test is useful for evaluating the child's ability to isolate specific attributes to define words. Information on formulation may also be obtained.

| Woodcock-Johnson Quantitative Concepts and Antonyms/ Synonyms | (1) These measures assess specific vocabulary skills relative to academic grade and age.

(2) The math concepts test surveys math vocabulary, which appears to correlate with applied math skills. | (1) These measures provide additional insight on vocabulary skills needed in academic settings. |

To Assess Expressive Syntactic/Morphological Skills

Instrument	Findings	Test Considerations
Grammatical Analysis of Elicited Language— Simple and Complex levels (Geers & Moog, 1979)	(1) Geers and Moog comprehensively discuss hearing-impaired children's performance on these measures relative to hearing children.	(1) Analogous prompt and controlled context methods used on these tests address the problems inherent in spontaneous language sampling. (2) A child's performance may be compared to norms for hearing-impaired children. (3) Uses referential communication tasks to elicit questions which at times are hard to elicit from hearing-impaired children. (4) The authors recommend using this measure in conjunction with a spontaneous language sample.
TOLD Grammar Completion subtest; ITPA Grammatic Closure subtest (Kirk et al., 1968); Signed English Morphology Test	(1) Measures appear to identify strengths and weaknesses in the student's use of morphological rules. The authors advocate viewing the results in conjunction with a spontaneous language sample.	(1) The authors have found that many hearing-impaired students have difficulty with oral administration of the TOLD subtest (due to length and topic shifting). The same students are often successful in taking the test in print (written/read). (2) The ITPA subtest format is useful with this population, since the pictured referents reduce the demands for processing lengthy directions.
Structural Analysis Methods; e.g., DSS (Lee, 1974) and LARSP (Crystal et al., 1976)	(1) Geers and Moog (1979) found some deviation from expected performance by hearing-impaired children when	(1) For any of these structural analysis measures, one should consider problems in obtaining a representative sample (e.g., Is

the Developmental Sentence Scoring was used to analyze their language.

this sample representative of the child's typical performance?).

(2) Low intelligibility of speech or sign may impede interpretation, particularly if context is not available to support the child's message.

(3) Structural methods based on English grammar are inappropriate for describing American Sign Language.

Test of Concept Utilization (TCU; Crager & Spriggs, 1972)

(1) Hearing-impaired students are challenged to identify a variety of relationships between pictured object pairs. The authors have observed that hearing-impaired students often identify the relationship but have difficulty explaining it.

(1) A useful measure for investigating how well older hearing-impaired students solve and discuss abstract verbal problems.

(2) Pictures available often aid the hearing-impaired student in focusing on the relationship. That is, understanding of the task is not wholly dependent on language.

(3) Information can be gained as to the student's ability to shift flexibly his or her perspective.

Preschool Language Assessment Instrument (PLAI; Blank, Rose, & Berlin, 1978)

(1) Assesses the young (late preschool to early primary grades) hearing-impaired child's ability to respond to questions on a variety of levels of abstraction.

(1) This test provides a significant amount of information regarding the child's discourse skills and task approach to solving verbal problems. It is especially recommended for mainstreamed children. Again, the pictured referents cue the relationship being discussed, reducing the pure linguistic demands of the task and allowing the child to focus on the semantic content.

Woodcock-Johnson Analogies subtest

(1) Hearing-impaired students are often able to demonstrate conceptual relationships among meanings on this task, particularly since the vocabulary is somewhat controlled.

(1) Examiner descriptions are supported visually (in print: mother, father, sister, _____), which assists the student in solving the verbal analogy.

(2) Vocabulary deficits may affect performance as the test proceeds to higher levels.

Chapter 11

Physical and Occupational Therapy Models for Motor Evaluation

Susan Harryman and Lana Warren

Motor assessment of a hearing-impaired child with a developmental disability may contribute significant information in the development of an individualized treatment program. Physical therapists are concerned with overall posture and movement abilities while occupational therapists focus more on upper extremity skills and activities of daily living. Information related to development of the sensorimotor system, as well as assessment and intervention strategies used in physical and occupational therapy, will be reviewed in this chapter. Special focus will be placed upon the implications of motor impairments upon the development of manual and oral communication skills.

Motor Development

The development of the motor system is the most easily observed and recorded aspect of human growth and development. Motor maturation proceeds in a predictable and sequential manner with minimal environmental influence compared with other aspects of development. Although the appearance of motor milestones is dependent to some degree on an intact musculoskeletal system, the development of the motor system primarily reflects maturation of the central nervous system.

The cephalocaudal progression of motor development results in the child initially gaining control of the head and eyes, with development then proceeding to the upper trunk and arms, then to the lower trunk, and finally to the lower extremities by the end of the first year. In addition, motor development proceeds in a proximodistal fashion with the child first gaining control of the musculature closest to the trunk. Therefore, control of the shoulder region is gained before hand control, and control is gained of the hip region prior to control of the foot.

Although information regarding motor development is remembered by parents more frequently than information about other areas of development, it is not sufficient merely to collect documented case history information relative to milestones when assessing a hearing-impaired child exhibiting developmental delay. For example, to know only that a child is not walking does not provide enough information to plan an individual intervention program. Analysis of the specific motor problem, in this situation walking, is necessary to determine why the skill has not developed. Muscle weakness, aberrations in muscle tone, joint contractures, or immaturity of equilibrium reactions could each prevent the development of independent walking and would each require a different type of intervention. It is therefore necessary that the examiner have an understanding of, and explore the underlying prerequisites for, development of perceptual motor function. This complex process reflects neurological maturation of both the sensory and motor systems. It is necessary to be familiar with early reflex behavior in infants as well as the later-developing automatic movement reactions that serve as a basis for postural stability and coordinated movement.

The infant is under control of the lower brain centers at birth. Thus the newborn exhibits relatively little voluntary movement and is primarily controlled by reflexive behavior. These reflexes of the motor system in the newborn are frequently referred to as primitive reflexes. The primitive reflexes as a group generally involve changes in distribution of muscle tone which result in a postural change or stereotypic movement. These early reflexes are significant to the infant; they provide initial movement experiences in a predictable and organized manner. During the first few months of life, as the central nervous system matures, these primitive reflexes are gradually integrated and the intact infant develops voluntary motor control. The primitive reflexes that are of primary concern in the newborn period (Capute et al., 1978) include:

Asymmetrical tonic neck reflex. The proprioceptive stimulus for this reflex is rotation of the head. The response is an increase of extensor tone/posture in the extremities on the face side and an increase in flexor tone/posture in the extremities on the skull side (see Figure 1). Asymmetries in trunk tone/posture related to the asymmetrical tonic neck reflex may also be observed.

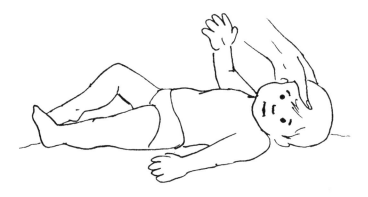

Figure 1. The asymmetrical tonic neck reflex.

Symmetrical tonic neck reflex. The stimulus for this reflex is flexing/extensions of the head. With head flexion the response is an increase of flexor tone/posture of the arms and extensor tone/posture of the legs. With head extension the response is an increase of extensor tone/posture of the arms and flexor tone/posture of the legs.

Tonic labyrinthine reflex. The stimulus for this reflex is the position of the labyrinth in the inner ear. When the head is in extension or the child is on his or her back, extensor tone/posture predominates throughout the body. When the head is flexed or the child is on his or her stomach, flexor tone/posture predominates.

Grasp reflex. The stimulus for this reflex is touching the palmar surface of the hand, which results in automatic closing of the fingers.

The automatic movement reactions that support the development of normal postural control and movement are developing during the first year of life as higher brain centers, including the cortex, mature. These righting, equilibrium, and protective reactions primarily serve three functions: to keep the body in alignment in space, to allow transitions from one position to another, and to support coordinated movement. The automatic movement reactions (Bobath, 1971) include:

Head righting. The person maintains the head in a vertical position in space.

Derotative righting reactions. The person maintains the head in line with the body and parts of the body in line with each other.

Equilibrium reactions. The body as a whole responds to maintain position in space when the center of gravity is shifted. These reactions develop in a sequential fashion beginning in prone (see Figure 2) and supine, progressing through sitting and hands and knees, and finally appearing in standing positions.

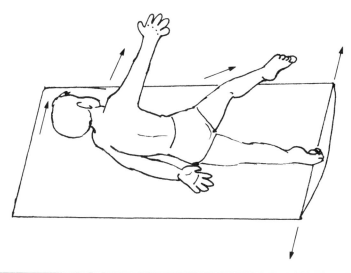

Figure 2. Equilibrium reactions in prone.

Protective reactions. When the center of gravity is suddenly disturbed, the arms protectively extend to prevent a fall. These reactions also develop in a sequential manner, beginning in the anterior direction, then lateral, and finally the posterior direction.

Developmental disabilities affecting the sensorimotor system are initially reflected in a delayed rate of development of perceptual motor skills. In many cases, this delay is further complicated by abnormalities in muscle tone affecting the quality of posture and movement. Two common developmental disabilities resulting in deviant motor performance are mental retardation and cerebral palsy.

Hearing-impaired children with mental retardation often exhibit a delay in the development of perceptual motor skills concomitant with their overall delay in development, although the normal sequence of attainment of motor milestones should not be affected nor should there be major defects in the quality of performance. However, it is not unusual for children with significant cognitive delay to exhibit little or no delay in attainment of early gross motor milestones (Hreidarsson, Shapiro, & Capute, 1983; Shapiro, Accardo, & Capute, 1979). When assessing fine motor development, such as the ability to build a block tower, it is necessary to remember the close relationship of fine motor coordination to problem-solving abilities. Delayed attainment of fine motor skills in a child with mental retardation may actually reflect delayed development of cognitive or visual abilities rather than the presence of motor disability. If fine motor problems are present, this may have a significant impact on a child's ability to use an expressive sign language system. This is an issue in the development of manual communication skills to be discussed later in this section.

Delayed achievement of gross motor milestones due to vestibular dysfunction in infancy has been reported in the literature. Vestibular impairment has also been reported to be more prevalent in children with severe hearing loss, especially those with a history of meningitis, although the correlation is not precise (Rabin, 1974). Vestibular dysfunction may be assessed by electronystagmography, caloric response, and close clinical attention to development of righting and equilibrium reactions. In a hearing-impaired child presenting with delayed sitting or walking, these measures may assist in differentiating vestibular dysfunction from associated handicaps of mental retardation and cerebral palsy.

Cerebral palsy is defined as a disorder of posture and movement due to a nonprogressive lesion of the brain which occurs in the developing central nervous system. Readily recognizable deviations from normal motor development, related to quality of posture and movement as well as acquisition of motor milestones, are present. Cerebral palsy is characterized primarily by abnormalities in quality and distribution of muscle tone, persistence of primitive reflexes, and impaired maturation of automatic movement reactions. These deviations from normal development lead to restrictions in voluntary movement and a paucity of movement patterns.

The spectrum of motor disability related to cerebral palsy is broad. At one end of the spectrum are children who continue to be dominated by reflexive behavior and who develop minimal voluntary control of movement resulting in few, if any, functional skills, relegating them to a life of total physical dependency. At the opposite end of this spectrum are children with minimal cerebral dysfunction who may be described as uncoordinated or clumsy. Although these latter children will have no major long-term motor disability problems, they may develop a poor self-concept due to their motor incoordination, especially in group physical activities with peers.

Assessment

As with any evaluation, accurate findings are crucial to effective program planning and to establishing a baseline for the measurement of subsequent progress. Occupational and physical therapists obtain critical assessment data through observation of structured play activities. Unlike other areas of developmental evaluation, motor assessment does not rely heavily upon the use of language. Use of gestures and imitation often is adequate to elicit the desired motor performance of the hearing-impaired or otherwise language-delayed child. The following areas should be considered during motor assessment.

Reflex and Postural Mechanisms

This portion of the motor assessment provides a basis for understanding the neuro-developmental level of the child. Such information aids in distinguishing the delayed child from the child with abnormal neurological development. In the presence of abnormal reflex activity, appropriate postural management is critical to maximize performance during all aspects of assessment.

Selected evaluation tools include:

- The Milani-Comparetti Motor Development Screening Test (Kliewer et al., 1977)
- Primitive Reflex Profile (Capute et al., 1978)
- Reflex Testing Methods for Evaluating CNS Development (Fiorentino, 1972)
- Movement Assessment of Infants (Chandler et al., 1980)

Musculoskeletal System

Hearing-impaired children with central nervous system disorders frequently have abnormal muscle tone and structural deformities; the tone may be increased, decreased, or of a variable nature. Increased muscle tone may lead to limitations in movement resulting in musculoskeletal deformity. A child with low tone or weakness may have difficulty with endurance and fatigue. Maintenance of posture and modulation of movement may be compromised in the presence of low or variable tone. Muscle tone, range of motion, and strength must all be considered in developing overall positioning and in determining realistic expectations with respect to posture and movement. Checklists are usually available for documentation of range of motion and strength. If desired, standardized information can be found in Daniels and Worthingham (1972) and American Academy of Orthopedic Surgeons (1972).

Developmental Milestones

This portion of the assessment focuses on attainment of specific motor abilities, such as sitting unsupported, walking, eating with a spoon, picking up a pellet. In the motor-impaired child, it is critical to assess developmental milestones in relationship to neurodevelopmental maturation. To know that a child cannot feed him- or herself is not sufficient. The neurological readiness for self-feeding must also be analyzed as a basis for appropriate program planning. Utilizing information from the neurodevelopmental assessment will provide insight to determine specific areas for intervention; e.g., a child with immature equilibrium reactions in sitting is going to have difficulty self-feeding if he or she is working on both keeping upright and managing a spoon.

Selected evaluation tools include:

- Bayley Scales of Infant Development (Bayley, 1969)
- Brigance Diagnostic Inventory of Early Development (Brigance, 1978)
- DeGangi-Berk Test of Sensory Integration (Berk & DeGangi, 1983)
- Denver Developmental Screening Test (Frankenburg, 1975)
- Manual of Developmental Diagnosis (Knoblock et al., 1980)
- Vulpe Assessment Battery (Vulpe, 1969)

Upper Extremity Skills

Although upper extremity abilities are included in the assessment areas already mentioned, specific focus may be indicated for the child for whom the use of manual communication is being considered. Shane and Wilbur (1980) review a procedure for determining signing potential based on motor function (see Shane, Chapter 15 in this text.) They consider the factors of sign location, hand shape, and movement. The possibility of sensory deficits, including the inability to accurately perceive touch and movement, may also need to be considered in addition to data on fine motor development.

Selected evaluation tools include:

- Erhardt Developmental Prehension Assessment (Erhardt, 1982)
- Jebson-Taylor Hand Function Test (Jebson & Taylor, 1969)

Perceptual Motor/Sensorimotor Integration

Perceptual motor and sensorimotor integration evaluation tools are more commonly used with the child having minimal cerebral dysfunction or the child described as being clumsy. These assessments focus on the child's ability to use his or her body in an efficient and well-coordinated manner. Many factors are involved when determining which sensorimotor test should be used for a given child. These include the child's age and major problem(s), the purpose of the evaluation, and the specific skill/background of the evaluator.

Selected evaluation tools include:

- Bruininks-Oseretsky Test of Motor Proficiency (Bruininks, 1978)
- Hughes Basic Gross Motor Assessment (Hughes, 1975)
- Miller Assessment for Preschoolers (Miller, 1982)
- Purdue Perceptual Motor Survey (Roach & Kephart, 1966)
- Southern California Sensory Integration Test (Ayres, 1972)

Intervention

Treatment of the hearing-impaired developmentally disabled child with motor impairment can be examined from a variety of perspectives. The initial step in planning intervention is to distinguish between the two major groups of children exhibiting motor delay. The children in the first of these two groups are delayed across all spheres of development, including the attainment of motor skills. These children often appear relatively normal as they exhibit no deviant motor behaviors; that is, motor skills develop in a normal sequence, and motor patterns are of essentially normal quality. The second group of children, more obviously handicapped, exhibit delay in development of motor skills due to impaired motor systems. These children also demonstrate disordered sequence of development and abnormal quality of movement. The differences in planning intervention for these two groups of motor-delayed children are discussed in the following section.

Motor Delay with Normal Quality of Movement

The developmentally disabled child who is motor delayed but who has normal quality of movement is frequently functioning at his or her potential and may not need an active intervention program. However, the child who has a neurodevelopmental level that exceeds the present level of function may indeed benefit from specific stimulation activities to enhance emergence of skills for which the underlying components are already present. For example, if a child exhibits equilibrium reactions at the level of maturity which should allow unsupported sitting, and he or she is not yet sitting, a motor stimulation program is highly recommended. Children in this category often have decreased muscle tone and tend to be less active than the typical child; yet they often quickly gain new skills when provided a stimulation program offering the opportunity to experience motor activities compatible with their neurodevelopmental level. Children in this category may also have inefficiencies in sensorimotor processing that may adversely affect efficiency and coordination of motor skills. Intervention strategies with this type of child focus on provision of controlled sensory input to elicit a specific adaptive response.

The majority of intervention strategies for the motor-delayed child with normal quality of movement are not significantly different for the hearing-impaired and the normal-hearing child, with the exception that movement in the hearing impaired is primarily stimulated through visual tracking and tactile stimulation rather than orientation to amplified sound. For example, when teaching a severely hearing-impaired child to roll over, it is essential to gain his or her visual attention with a desired object; the object is then moved through the visual field to encourage head rotation in the specific direction which initiates rolling. This is in contrast to a child with normal hearing, who may be stimulated to initiate movement by shaking a rattle toward the side to which he or she is to roll. Obviously, for those children whose residual hearing with amplification permits cuing with auditory signals, stimulation of movement via the auditory modality will be employed.

Delayed motor development frequently results in children who are delayed in attaining independent sitting. A severely hearing-impaired child who is limited to prone and supine positions will have a restricted environment, because his or her visual field may be limited to people and objects placed in the line of vision. It is therefore important that hearing-impaired babies who are not stimulated to turn to sound, and so inspect their surroundings, are provided with a supported seating arrangement which can greatly expand their visual interaction with the environment.

Motor Disorder with Abnormal Quality of Movement

Treatment planning and intervention for the developmentally disabled child with abnormal quality of movement and delayed development of righting/equilibrium presents a much more complex problem. Information gained from the neurodevelopmental assessment will assist in defining underlying components of posture and movement, not yet spontaneously utilized, which may be facilitated through treatment. Various neuromuscular techniques (Trombly & Scott, 1977) are used as intervention strategies for managing abnormal postural tone and movement. These techniques promote the maintenance and development of muscle tone approximating normal developmental sequence as much as possible to enhance the development of postural control and the expression of voluntary coordinated movement.

Concepts of normal development, including cephalocaudal and proximodistal progression, must also be considered when planning a treatment program. Articulation and fine hand skills are frequently of paramount importance in the hearing-impaired child, but it must be remembered that these are the most refined aspects of movement and require that more proximal structures are functioning adequately. Controlled hand movement is based on a stable wrist and shoulder. Shoulder stability is achieved through a posturally stable trunk. Head control, providing a basis for both visual function and articulation, is also of key importance in the linkup of eye-hand coordination. It becomes obvious that hearing-impaired children with proximal postural problems may have significant difficulties using their hands and mouth. The extent of these problems must be carefully evaluated when considering the use of a manual or oral expressive language system. The child with inability to control his or her trunk will therefore not only experience difficulty maintaining a sitting position but will also lack a point of stability for developing upper extremity skills and may have poor respiratory support for spoken language.

In the presence of abnormal muscle tone, the primary concerns are positioning and handling to allow the child to function at his or her maximum potential. Provision of adaptive seating is extremely important; sitting is our most functional position. Proper support and alignment of our head and trunk in sitting are critical to allow maximal use of our visual abilities as well as to maximize respiratory functions, which are so important for any type of oral program. Adaptive seating also provides the necessary proximal stability for arm/hand control. From another perspective, this support is critical in reducing energy expenditure and improving efficiency of motor output. A child who is working to maintain his or her head upright while attempting to talk is being asked to work considerably harder and less efficiently than a child with normal postural abilities. In the presence of primitive reflexes, the influence of the head position on function of the upper extremities must be considered as well as the boundaries of the visual field. Rotation of the head in the presence of an asymmetrical tonic neck reflex or tonic labyrinthine reflex may result in tone and/or postural changes throughout the body. A child who turns his or her head to the side to look at a switch he or she is attempting to activate, or to look at a specific place on a communication board, may elicit an asymmetrical tonic neck reflex and be unable to activate the switch or to point due to arm stiffness. Children who frequently go into abnormal posturing when engaged in such functional activities as activating a switch are at high risk for developing deformities which may require orthopedic surgery.

If muscle tone is variable or head-righting reactions not fully developed, the ability to maintain a steady position of the head will be hindered. In this situation, children will spontaneously attempt to find a head position that offers increased stability. The habitual position is frequently hyperextension of the neck, which limits the visual field to the ceiling, or flexion of the neck, which allows only inspection of the floor. In the hearing-impaired child for whom visual information is critical, it is essential that adequate head support be provided. This support must not only ensure an adequate resting position but must also allow controlled movement for optimum visual access of the environment.

Arm and hand skills of the physically handicapped hearing-impaired child are often of particular concern to those children needing an augmentative communication system—particularly those who will be signing, activating a switch, or pointing. The evaluation of hand skills, which is often an ongoing process, must be done in the context of the child's overall postural abilities, including influence of primitive reflexes and abnormal muscle tone. Only after a child is well positioned, with tone as normal as possible, can potential for arm and hand use begin to be assessed accurately. Factors that need to be considered include range of movement, ability to reach with control and accuracy, bilateral arm use, ability to sustain grasp or a position, isolated finger movement, manipulation abilities, and ability to release objects. For example, a child with increased tone may have a limited range of pointing, which may restrict the size of a communication board. That same child may have difficulty with isolated finger movements, which may compromise signing abilities. However, as the occupational therapist is working to improve arm/hand function, new skills may emerge that necessitate ongoing team interaction and problem solving around the choice of a communication modality. Some children with severe motor involvement will never have enough dexterity for a manual system and may only be able to activate a single switch. Hand splinting or use of a head-pointer may also be considerations to optimize function for these children.

Cooperation and Continuity

Planning a communication program for the developmentally disabled hearing-impaired child should be a team process to ensure that all aspects of potential function are addressed. Representatives from the disciplines of audiology, education, occupational therapy, pediatrics, physical therapy, psychology, and speech/language pathology may all have unique contributions to the individualized treatment program of which effective communication is such an important aspect. In severely physically handicapped hearing-impaired children who are dominated by reflexive behavior, and who exhibit limited voluntary movement, physical and occupational therapists may be an essential resource to the audiology and speech/language professionals as well as teachers concerned with developing an augmentative means of communication. Representatives from occupational and physical therapy also may play a key role in interpreting specific body movements currently used for communication purposes as well as evaluating and establishing those voluntary movements which could be used for efficient communication.

It is also necessary to understand that neither assessment nor planning for intervention can be completed at one point in time. To ensure that optimal functioning —including seating, visual interaction, and communication—continues in all environments, it is essential that a method for ongoing assessment be addressed as part of the initial intervention plan. It is only through this ongoing interactive interdisciplinary process that the unique needs of this significantly disabled population may be met.

References

American Academy of Orthopedic Surgeons. (1972). *Joint motion.* Chicago: Author.

Ayres, J. (1972). *Southern California sensory integration test.* Los Angeles: Western Psychological Services.

Bayley, N. (1969). *Bayley scales of infant development.* New York: Psychological Corporation.

Berk, R., & DeGangi, G. (1983). *DeGangi-Berk test of sensory integration.* Los Angeles: Western Psychological Services.

Bobath, B. (1971). *Abnormal postural reflex activity caused by brain lesions.* London: William Heinemann.

Brigance, A. (1978). *Brigance diagnostic inventory of early development.* Newton, MA: Curriculum Associates.

Bruininks, R. (1978). *Bruininks-Oseretsky test of motor proficiency.* Circle Pines, MN: American Guidance Service.

Capute, A., Accardo, P., Vining, E., Rubenstein, J., & Harryman, S. (1978). *Primitive reflex profile.* Baltimore: University Park Press.

Chandler, L., Andrews, M., & Swanson, M. (1980). *Movement assessment of infants.* Rolling Bay, WA: Authors.

Daniels, L., & Worthingham, C. (1972). *Muscle testing.* Philadelphia: W. B. Saunders.

Erhardt, R. (1982). *Erhardt developmental prehension assessment.* Laurel, MD: RAMSCO.

Fiorentino, M. (1972). *Reflex testing methods for evaluating CNS development.* Springfield, IL: Charles C. Thomas.

Frankenburg, W. (1975). *Denver developmental screening test.* Springfield, IL: Charles C. Thomas.

Hreidarsson, S., Shapiro, B., & Capute, A. (1983). Age of walking in the cognitively impaired. *Clinical Pediatrics, 22,* 248–250.

Hughes, J. E. (1975). *Hughes basic gross motor assessment.* Golden, CO: Author.

Jebson, R., & Taylor, N. (1969). Jebson-Taylor hand function test. *Archives of Physical Medicine and Rehabilitation, 50,* 311–319.

Kliewer, D., Bruce, W., & Trembath, J. (1977). *The Milani-Comparetti motor development screening test.* Omaha: Meyer Children's Rehabilitation Institute.

Knoblock, H., Stevens, F., & Malone, A. (1980). *Manual of developmental diagnosis.* New York: Harper and Row.

Miller, L. (1982). *Miller assessment for preschoolers.* Littleton, CO: Foundation for Knowledge in Development.

Rabin, I. (1974). Hypoactive labyrinth and motor development. *Clinical Pediatrics, 13*(11), 922–937.

Roach, E., & Kephart, N. (1966). *Purdue perceptual motor survey.* Columbus, OH: Charles E. Merrill.

Shane, H., & Wilbur, R. (1980). Potential for expressive signing based on motor control. *Sign Language Studies, 29,* 331–348.

Shapiro, B., Accardo, P., & Capute, A. (1979). Factors affecting walking in a profoundly retarded population. *Developmental Medicine and Child Neurology, 21,* 369–373.

Trombly, C., & Scott, A. (1977). *Occupational therapy for physical dysfunction* (pp. 70–105). Baltimore: Williams and Wilkins.

Vulpe, S. (1969). *Vulpe assessment battery.* Toronto: National Institute on Mental Retardation.

Chapter 12

Creative Assessment in the Psychological and Educational Domains

Lynne Blennerhassett

This chapter focuses on cognitive, psychoeducational, social-emotional, and adaptive behavior assessment. The discussion will be guided by three objectives: to present criteria for selection of appropriate assessment instruments, to discuss adapting techniques for more effective evaluation outcomes, and to provide guidelines for interpreting assessment results so that they will be useful to those responsible for educational program implementation.

Any discussion of assessing handicapped children must be prefaced with an understanding that there are both legislative and pragmatic considerations guiding the assessment process. The legislative concerns are those addressed in the Education for All Handicapped Children Act of 1975 (Public Law 94-142). In contrast, the pragmatic concerns center on providing assessment results that meet the needs of both administrators and teachers, who must act upon the assessment findings in different ways.

The impact of PL 94-142 on testing and evaluation procedures has been the subject of discussion and training for school psychologists and other professionals who evaluate cognitive, psychoeducational, social-emotional, and adaptive functioning (Barnett, 1983; Bersoff, 1982; Sattler, 1982). Specifically with regard to evaluation procedures, the regulations require that

1. Tests and other evaluation material
   a. Are provided and administered in the child's native language or typical mode of communication, unless it is clearly not feasible to do so;
   b. Have been validated for the specific purpose for which they are used; and
   c. Are administered by trained personnel in conformance with instructions provided by their producer.
2. Tests and other evaluation materials include those tailored to assess specific areas of educational need and not merely those which are designed to provide a single general intelligence quotient.
3. Tests are selected and administered so as best to ensure that when a test is administered to a child with impaired sensory, manual, or speaking skills, the test results accurately reflect the child's aptitude or achievement level or

whatever other factors the test purports to measure, rather than reflect the
child's impaired sensory, manual, or speaking skills (except where those
skills are the factors which the test purports to measure . . .). (Office of
Education, 1977, pp. 42,496–42,497)

These legal regulations provide a special challenge when applied to hearing-impaired
developmentally disabled children. In other words, the clinician must not only take into
account the child's language level and mode of communication during test selection, but
must also attempt to bypass other known (or suspected) impairments when trying to
evaluate underlying aptitude or abilities.

This challenge is illustrated when attempting to measure cognitive skills of a
hearing-impaired developmentally disabled child with known visual perceptual processing and/or motoric expression problems. It has been recommended practice to omit
verbal scales and subtests from cognitive and intellectual tests when working with
hearing-impaired children. In other words, cognitive measurements are based only on
the performance-based sections of these tests (Levine, 1981; Sullivan & Vernon, 1979).
However, since such performance-based tools rely heavily on visually presented stimulus
items and on motoric responses, attempting to assess cognitive abilities through these
channels may merely result in measuring the impaired channel rather than in establishing a valid estimation of the child's cognitive and/or intellectual abilities. As has been
argued elsewhere (Forcade, Matey, & Barnett, 1979), the assessment of low-incidence
populations, including hearing-impaired developmentally disabled children, requires
creative use of standardized instruments. Creative assessment procedures, for example,
might involve modifying test administration strategies so as to assess the dynamic
problem-solving skills of the child rather than merely stating the product of the child's
performance (Feuerstein, 1979).

In addition to adhering to legislative guidelines, the clinician must select assessment procedures while considering such pragmatic ends as meeting the needs of both
administrators and teachers. Salvia and Ysseldyke (1981) stated that "assessment information is communicated to different audiences, and those audiences have different,
although not mutually exclusive, needs" (p. 516). Teachers and administrators are
among the most frequent consumers of assessment information.

Because administrators are faced with placement decisions, they "need scores and
interpretations of pupil performance on norm-referenced tests to document placement
decisions" (p. 516). Teachers, however, are more interested in assessment information
that offers guidance for classroom management. Salvia and Ysseldyke (1981) explained:

Teachers typically want and need to know specifically what to do instructionally for
students. They usually do not receive that information. Teachers have long expressed
concern that mere knowledge of the extent to which a student deviates from normal is of
little help in their efforts to devise an appropriate educational program for that student.
They repeatedly ask for effective strategies to move students from where they are to
where teachers want them to be. (p. 517)

Most tests of cognitive, psychoeducational, social-emotional, and adaptive functioning are designed to yield norm-referenced interpretations, which may serve the needs

primarily of administrators. As will be discussed later, the challenge with norm-referenced tests is to employ tests that have appropriate norms for hearing-impaired children as well as for hearing children. In addition, the use of norm-referenced tests implies that appropriate norms exist for the full range of children served under PL 94-142 across a variety of functioning domains—an assumption that is not necessarily supported by the current state of test development. With regard to meeting the needs of teachers, it will be argued that use of criterion-referenced instruments and creative modifications in administration of standardized tests provides more useful information for teachers. Before discussing alternate assessment techniques, criteria for selecting appropriate assessment instruments will be presented.

Criteria for Selecting Appropriate Assessment Instruments

A number of researchers have offered guides for the selection of appropriate assessment instruments. Levine (1981) recommended that during test selection, examiners carefully evaluate the nature and quality of the standardization followed during test construction.

> There are well-standardized tests, poorly standardized ones, and some for which the term "standardization" is simply window dressing. Whatever modifications need to be made to adapt a test to a deaf subject, the least that can be asked is that the test be well constructed. A good indication of a test's soundness can be found in its standardization details, which are described in the manuals of all responsible tests. (p. 265)

Standardization details that warrant attention include test validity and reliability and reference to special populations for whom normative data are provided. It is of specific concern when working with hearing-impaired school children to note which tests offer norms for the hearing-impaired or low-incidence populations, as well as for the population of children with normal hearing.

Finding appropriately standardized tests for use with hearing-impaired children may not be an easy task. The problem is illustrated with reference to the area of cognitive/intellectual assessment. For example, a test such as the Leiter International Performance Scale (Leiter, 1980) appears to be appropriate for use with hearing-impaired children in that the items are administered and responded to nonverbally by means of block manipulations, pointing, and demonstrations. However, the final performance score can only be compared to the performance of populations with normal hearing, and no norms for those with impaired hearing have been developed. Another example is the Hiskey-Nebraska Test of Learning Aptitude (Hiskey, 1966). This test was specially designed for use with hearing-impaired individuals and, as such, has specialized standard administration procedures and norms for those with impaired hearing. In addition, standard administration procedures and norms are presented for use with hearing children. The standardization procedures for both populations are not the same: The hearing normative sample received verbal instructions that resulted in more information being communicated than is possible in the standardization procedures with hearing-impaired people (procedures which included use of pantomime and gesture). Also, the final score for the hearing-impaired group is interpreted in terms of a learning quotient (LQ) that is derived from a ratio of attainment to chronological age; with the procedures for hearing individuals, one derives a deviation IQ. Deviation IQs have an advantage over ratio IQs (or similarly derived quotients) in that they more accurately reflect the real "amount by which a subject deviates above or below the average performance of individuals of his own age group" (Wechsler, 1974).

Another example is the Wechsler Intelligence Scale for Children–Revised (Wechsler, 1974), one of the most popular tests of intelligence used with school-age children. The Performance Scale of this test has been used successfully with the hearing impaired, and norms for that population have been available since 1977 (Anderson & Sisco, 1977). Although those norms provide useful guides for comparing the performance of individual children to that of hearing-impaired peers, the norms were collected without making certain that comparable administration procedures were followed during the data collection. That is, uniformity in administration was not controlled with regard to the kinds of alterations used in administration, the number and types of demonstrations and practice items used, and the degree to which examiners altered verbal directions to guarantee that the hearing-impaired children understood the task instructions. More recently, Ray (1979) developed standard procedures for administering the Performance Scale of the Wechsler Intelligence Scale for Children–Revised to hearing-impaired children. His standard instructions may be especially useful when working with hearing-impaired developmentally disabled children in safeguarding (through additional practice items) that the instructions are understood. Thus, it is often necessary to piece together the efforts of various researchers in an attempt to select instruments that satisfy standardization criteria for use with hearing-impaired children.

When working with hearing-impaired developmentally disabled children, the goal of finding appropriately normed test instruments may not, in reality, be easily satisfied. As was mentioned earlier, the use of norm-referenced tests carries the assumption that norms exist for the full range of children addressed in PL 94-142—an assumption that exceeds the current state of norm-referenced test development. For example, although it may be possible to assess the nonverbal cognitive abilities of a hearing-impaired child through a performance-based test with norms for that population, such norms would not be appropriately applied to a hearing-impaired child with cerebral palsy and/or additional impairments of a perceptual/motor nature. Such a child would be at risk of performing less efficiently than his or her hearing-impaired peers due to the perceptual demands of the test rather than to cognitive capabilities. However, special norms for hearing-impaired children with additional perceptual/motor impairments are not available for the major nonverbal, performance-based intelligence tests used with children having a significant hearing loss.

In addition to standardization concerns, Levine (1981) recommended that communication requirements of the tests be scrutinized when selecting instruments for use with hearing-impaired individuals. This is necessary to ensure that the child understands the test instructions. Without such safeguarding, "poor test performance may be due as much to a misunderstanding of directions as to mental inability" (p. 273). Toward this end, evaluators may seek instruments with standardized instructions that account for the child's language level and mode of communication (Ray, 1979), or that permit the examiner to communicate task requirements through the use of pointing, gestures, demonstrations, pantomime, or practice items (Hiskey, 1966; Leiter, 1980; Smith & Johnson, 1977).

Another guideline for selecting appropriate assessment instruments relates to the goal of achieving balance in the nature of the total battery of instruments used with any particular child. With regard to objective tests, this would mean selecting both norm-referenced and criterion-referenced instruments. In addition to using objective measures, such techniques as observation and interview are important data-collecting strategies from which valuable information can be obtained relative to educational goals and objectives (Barnett, 1983; Diebold, Curtis, & DuBose, 1978; Forcade, Matey, & Barnett, 1979; Levine, 1981).

Researchers have provided summary listings of a variety of evaluation techniques used with hearing-impaired children to assess cognitive, psychoeducational, social-emotional, and adaptive behavior (Hasenstab & Horner, 1982; Levine, 1981; Ray, O'Neill, & Morris, 1983; Spragins, Spencer Day, & Blennerhassett, 1982; Sullivan & Vernon, 1979; Zieziula, 1982). The assessment instruments surveyed include standardized tests that yield norm-referenced or criterion-referenced interpretations, observational techniques, and interview sources of information collection.

What follows are brief descriptions of selected assessment techniques that are typically used with hearing-impaired school children and, with adaptations, may be of value with hearing-impaired developmentally disabled children. This list is abbreviated from a review of individually administered assessment instruments originally presented by Spragins et al. (1982). The review collectively covered a variety of functional areas, not all of which are presented here.*

Developmental Scales

1. Adaptive Performance Inventory (Gentry et al., 1980). This inventory is a 650-item, criterion-referenced scale that measures skills and provides goals for areas of physical intactness and reflexes and reactions and gross motor, fine motor, self-care, sensorimotor, social, and communication skills. The authors recommend its use for children up to the chronological age of nine years; it is designed for use with children functioning developmentally under two years of age. Data are collected through observations of the child in routine situations.

Although this inventory is a somewhat lengthy measurement technique, the authors report that an abbreviated version is currently under development which, in its shorter form, may be preferable to evaluators. Regardless of its length, this inventory offers the following advantages: small skill increments are measured so that even very slow

---

*This review of assessment instruments is limited to those intended for individual administration. Group administered tests for hearing-impaired students, such as the Stanford Achievement Test, Special Edition for Hearing Impaired Students (Madden, Gardner, Rudman, Karlsen, & Merwin, 1972), the Metropolitan Achievement Test (Durost, Bixler, Wrightstone, Prescott, & Balow, 1971), and the Brill Educational Achievement Test for Secondary Age Deaf Students (Brill, 1977), are not reviewed. Discussion of group administered tests can be found in Levine (1981), Sullivan and Vernon (1979), and Zieziula (1982).

progress is recognized; and special adaptations of item administration are provided for use with children who are motor impaired, hearing impaired, and/or visually impaired.

2. Callier-Azusa Scale (Stillman, 1978). This developmental scale was specifically designed for assessing deaf-blind and profoundly handicapped children. It is an observational measurement composed of 18 subscales in five areas: motor development; perceptual development; daily living skills; cognition, communication, and language; and social development.

Although this scale is not normed, it offers the following advantages: measurement of small skill increments that recognizes even very slow progress; and behavior examples that were taken from those actually observed in deaf-blind and multihandicapped hearing-impaired children.

3. Developmental Activities Screening Inventory (DuBose & Langley, 1977). This inventory contains 55 items grouped into nine developmental levels. The developmental levels range from 6 to 60 months of age, grouped in 6-month intervals. Areas assessed include fine motor coordination, cause-effect and means-end relationships, association, number concepts, size discrimination, and seriation. The authors state that the inventory has been used with more than 200 multihandicapped children.

An advantage of this scale is that adaptations are provided for administering the items to visually impaired children.

4. Developmental Profile II (Alpern & Shearer, 1980). This scale includes 217 items grouped in five subscales: physical skill, self-help ability, social competence, academic skills, and communication ability. Items are developmentally ordered, ranging from birth to the nine-year level. Information may be gathered through observation, testing, and parent interview. Children with handicaps were specifically excluded from the standardization so that items would represent normal developmental expectations. The standardization group included more than 3,000 children. The standardization sample was most heavily represented by children from urban areas in Indiana and Washington state.

Although some items (e.g., telephone use, rhyming words, listening skills) may not be appropriate for use with hearing-impaired children, attempts were made to eliminate items believed to discriminate due to race, social class, and sex. In addition, this profile provides a useful table for determining significance of observed delays for each age interval and each subscale.

5. Ordinal Scales of Psychological Development (Uzgiris & Hunt, 1975). This instrument assesses a wide range of behaviors based on Piagetian sensorimotor levels of cognitive development, including play, gestural and vocal imitation, causality, spatial relationships, object permanence, and purposeful problem solving.

Although the developmental range is limited on this instrument (0–2 years), it offers an advantage in that no verbal instructions are necessary. Object manipulations and interactive play situations elicit responses. No norms are provided, but Dunst (1980) provided "developmental stages" and "estimated developmental ages" for each item.

*6. **Uniform Performance Assessment System*** (Haring et al., 1981). This is a "curriculum-referenced" instrument, from which it is possible to establish educational goals, rather than a norm-referenced test. Observable behaviors under investigation include preacademic, fine motor, communication, social/self-help, and gross motor skills.

A possible disadvantage of this instrument is that the skill increments may not be detailed enough for some low-functioning children. However, given that the skill range is at an appropriate level for the child being evaluated, guidelines and scoring procedures allow for such adaptations as providing support and demonstrations.

*7. **Southern California Ordinal Scales of Development*** (Ashurst et al., 1977). This instrument assesses behaviors across the areas of cognition, communication, fine motor, gross motor, social-affective, and life skills. It relates each area to Piagetian developmental stages. The scales are not normed, but general developmental ages or stages are provided from normal child development. Instructions vary from scale to scale and item to item, but flexibility in administration is allowed in order to elicit the appropriate responses.

Disadvantages of this system include that it is lengthy to administer and that some higher level items on the cognitive scale are difficult to administer when the child's language level is far below his or her nonverbal abilities. Nevertheless, this instrument has been used successfully with hearing-impaired and developmentally disabled children because of the flexibility in administration procedures.

Standardized Tests of Intelligence/Mental Abilities

*1. **Hiskey-Nebraska Test of Learning Aptitude*** (Hiskey, 1966). This nonverbal test is designed for use with both hearing and hearing-impaired children ages 3 to 18½ years old. Norms for both hearing and hearing-impaired children are available. A median learning age and learning quotient (LQ) are reported for those with impaired hearing; learning ages and a deviation IQ are reported for children with normal hearing. Various cognitive areas are tested, including memory, spatial reasoning, picture matching, classification, visual analysis and synthesis of parts into wholes, and form completion. Instructions for hearing-impaired children are entirely nonverbal, involving pointing, gesturing, pantomime, and occasional demonstrations.

Although administration of this test can be time-consuming, the variety of subtests tends to hold the child's interest. Few of the subtests are timed, and those that are allow generous time limits.

*2. **Kaufman Assessment Battery for Children*** (Kaufman & Kaufman, 1983). This is an individually administered test of both intelligence and achievement for children 2½ to 12½ years old. It consists of 16 subtests, 10 of which yield a global Mental Processing Score; 6 subtests yield a global Achievement Score. The Mental Processing Scale is divided into two subscales: Simultaneous Processing and Sequential Processing, representing holistic and temporal mental abilities, respectively. This instrument offers advantages in that language plays a minimal role in the mental processing assessments, and standardization allows for teaching some failed items so as to facilitate the child's performance. Although hearing-impaired children were not included in the original standardization sample, the authors provided a technique for summing 6 of the 10 mental processing subtests to yield a Nonverbal Score; this is recommended for use with hearing-impaired children. The feasibility and appropriateness of using all 10 mental processing subtests with hearing-impaired children is currently under investigation at Gallaudet College in Washington, D.C. (S. Gibbins, personal communication, January 31, 1984).

3. Leiter International Performance Scale (Leiter, 1980). This is an untimed, nonverbal measure of intelligence designed for use with children ages 2 through 18 years. Most of the task requirements are self-evident, but some items are demonstrated. All items are administered nonverbally. Cognitive skills being assessed at the very early age levels include basic matching of form, number, color, and pictures; visual discrimination; seriation; and classification. Apparently no hearing-impaired children were included in the various standardization samples, and, to date, no norms exist for such children.

4. Merrill-Palmer Scale of Mental Tests (Stutsman, 1948). This is a general intelligence test for preschool children from ages 19 months to 6 years. More than 30 different subtest items are included. They cover such areas as fine motor skills, language, puzzles, block building, form boards, peg boards, color matching, and picture matching. Scoring standards allow for the omission of items that the child refuses or that cannot be administered due to handicapping conditions, while a final score can still be calculated through prorating procedures. Performance items can be administered nonverbally by gesture and demonstration. The task requirements for many of the nonverbal items are self-evident. No hearing-impaired children were included in the normal standardization sample, and there are no separate norms for that population. Score interpretations are mental age comparisons to a standardized group of 631 preschoolers between the ages of 18 and 77 months and of unreported ethnicity and socioeconomic levels. The Extended Merrill-Palmer Scale (Stutsman Ball, Merrifield, & Stott, 1978) assesses four dimensions of cognitive processes across the 3- to 5-year-old levels. The cognitive dimensions tested include semantic production, semantic evaluation, figural production, and figural evaluation.

5. Raven's Progressive Matrices (Raven, 1956; Raven, Court, & Raven, 1976, 1977). The Raven's matrices provide a nonverbal measure of thinking skills for ages five through adulthood. The Coloured Progressive Matrices (1956) are recommended for younger children. Test booklets present visual displays in which a part is missing; the child points to his or her answer from among multiple choices. Task requirements are usually self-evident, and, because only pointing responses are required, motor requirements are at a minimum. The thinking skills tapped include simple pattern completion; pattern completion with closure; concrete reasoning by analogy; and, at the upper levels, abstract reasoning by analogy. The norms for young children include only a sampling of hearing populations.

The Raven's offers advantages in that only a short administration time is required and the multiple choice format may allow for informative observations regarding the child's problem-solving abilities on recognition versus recall tasks. However, the tests may not be valid for use with impulsive children, as they may respond randomly.

6. Smith-Johnson Nonverbal Performance Scale (Smith & Johnson, 1977). This is a nonverbal developmental measurement for preschool children ages 24–48 months. The scale includes 65 items gathered from a number of standardized tests and grouped into 14 categories. Performance is recorded in terms of percentage of items passed at each month level from 24 to 48 months. Separate norms are provided for girls with normal hearing, girls with impaired hearing, boys with normal hearing, and boys with impaired hearing.

Although only a two-year developmental period is covered, this scale offers advantages in that administration is brief enough to stay within the fatigue limit of most preschoolers, and it yields comparative performance descriptions without relying on an overall intelligence quotient.

7. Wechsler Intelligence Scale for Children—Revised (WISC-R; Wechsler, 1974). The Performance Scale of the WISC-R provides a measurement of nonverbal intelligence for children ages 6 to 16½ years. Nonverbal subtests include picture completion, picture arrangement, block design, object assembly, coding, and mazes. Hearing-impaired children were not included in the original norms, but separate norms for that group are available (Anderson & Sisco, 1977). The standardized administration procedure for the Performance Scale involves verbal instructions; however, separate administration procedures for hearing-impaired persons are available, and they take into account the child's language level and mode of communication (Ray, 1979).

A downward extension of the WISC-R, the Wechsler Preschool and Primary Scale of Intelligence (WPPSI), that covers ages 4 to 6½ is available (Wechsler, 1967). Like the WISC-R, the WPPSI has a Performance Scale that includes tasks considered appropriate for those with impaired hearing. Also like the WISC-R, the WPPSI Performance Scale did not include hearing-impaired children in the original standardization, however, and verbal administration procedures were used. Separate standardized administration procedures for hearing-impaired individuals, which take into account the child's language level and mode of communication, are currently available (Ray & Ulissi, 1982). For both the WISC-R and WPPSI, performance results are interpreted in terms of deviation IQs and standard deviations which allow for norm-referenced comparisons of standards for both normal-hearing and hearing-impaired children.

Although the Wechsler tests do not attempt to measure cognitive skills below the age four level, the Performance Scales are among the most frequently used instruments for assessing cognitive/intellectual skills of hearing-impaired children.

Tests of Social-Emotional and Adaptive Behavior Functioning

1. AAMD Adaptive Behavior Scale, Public School Version (American Association on Mental Deficiency, 1974). This scale is both a norm- and criterion-referenced measurement of adaptive behavior for children ages 7 years, 3 months to 13 years, 2 months. The scale contains two parts: Part I includes 54 items that measure self-reliance and social development; Part II includes 39 items that give an assessment of social adaptation, relying on the nature of the child's affective characteristics. Parent and teacher interviews are used for data collection. The original standardization sample included 2,800 public school children with normal hearing representing regular, educable mentally retarded, and trainable mentally retarded children. Norms for those with impaired hearing are currently unavailable. The basic AAMD Adaptive Behavior Scale (American Association on Mental Deficiency, 1975) is appropriate for ages 3 to 21 and includes 66 items in Part I and 44 items in Part II.

2. Joseph Preschool and Primary Self-Concept Screening Test (Joseph, 1979). This test provides a general measure of self-concept for children 3½ to 12 years old. It includes 15 items, each providing a choice between two pictures representing children doing something. The question posed to the child is, "Which is most like you?" The instructions can be pantomimed, although such administration was not in the original standardization process. Norms are based on a standardization group of 1,200 mid-western children receiving special education. No norms for hearing-impaired children are available.

3. Meadow/Kendall Social-Emotional Assessment Inventory for Deaf Students (Meadow, 1980). This inventory is a 59-item behavior checklist for children 7 to 21 years old. Teachers and other school personnel are raters of the behaviors. Raw scores convert to percentiles on three scales: social adjustment, self-image, and emotional adjustment. Norms available for those with impaired hearing are based on a standardization sample of more than 2,000 hearing-impaired students in residential and day schools in the U.S.

4. Vineland Social Maturity Scale (Doll, 1965). This scale is a norm-referenced measure of functioning from birth to 30 years. It is designed to assess six major areas: self-help, locomotion, communication, self-direction, occupation, and socialization. Information is obtained through interviews with people who are very familiar with the child. Scores are expressed as social age equivalents (SAs), and the age scores are converted to an overall social quotient (SQ). No norms for those with impaired hearing were included in the original scale; however, Altepeter and Moscato (1982) reported that inquiry into use of the Vineland Adaptive Behavior Scale has been initiated with hearing-impaired children in residential settings.

Individually Administered Tests of Basic Educational Skills

1. Behavior Characteristics Progression (Santa Cruz Special Education Management System, 1973). This inventory is a criterion-referenced assessment and instructional reference. It includes assessment of 59 areas or "behavioral strands." Each strand contains approximately 25 to 50 "characteristics" or subskills against which the child's performance is rated. Data are collected through child observations and interactional situations by school personnel. The behavioral strands assess functioning across the following areas: perceptual/motor, language, self-help, recreational, vocational, social, and academic. Academic strands cover such areas as reading, math, practical math, writing, and spelling. The specific "characteristics" or objectives within each of these strands identify behaviors that might be displayed by children with various mental, physical, sensory, and behavioral handicaps. Thirteen of the 59 behavioral strands focus specifically on assessing areas educationally relevant to children with special needs (wheelchair use, speech/reading, articulation, fingerspelling, sign language, etc.).

2. Brigance Diagnostic Inventory of Basic Skills (Brigance, 1977). This criterion-referenced inventory covers a total of 140 items of school-related skills from kindergarten to sixth grade levels. It provides a systematic structure for informal assessments and can be used to generate educational goals. The inventory contains four scales: readiness (color recognition, body identification, etc.); reading (sight vocabulary, comprehension, etc.); language arts (handwriting, grammar, spelling, etc.); and mathematics (counting, writing numbers, operations, etc.). Single tests and items may be used separately. Many items, such as phonetic decoding measures and oral reading, may not be appropriate for use with hearing-impaired children. Performances for each skill are rated as either mastered or unmastered. Examiners are allowed to adapt administration procedures to ensure that they get a valid assessment of mastery.

3. Criterion Test of Basic Skills (Lundell, Brown, & Evans, 1976). This criterion-referenced instrument assesses basic reading and arithmetic skills and suggests teaching strategies for each educational objective resulting from the assessment. In assessing basic reading skills, this profile places a strong emphasis on phonic word attack skills. It breaks the reading process down into a unit analysis that may not prove beneficial with hearing-impaired children. In assessing basic arithmetic skills, it focuses on such abilities as identifying and sequencing numbers, printing numbers, telling time, handling money measurements, and doing basic arithmetic operations. Performance interpretations are expressed on three levels: Mastery Level, where the child succeeds on 90–100 percent of the items; Instructional Level, where 50–89 percent mastery is demonstrated; and Frustration Level, where the child succeeds on less than 50 percent of the items in the skill category under consideration.

4. Keymath Diagnostic Arithmetic Test (Connolly, Nachtman, & Pritchett, 1976). This is a norm-referenced instrument of 14 subtests that profile a student's math skills in three areas: content, operations, and applications. Instructions for some items (e.g., word problems) require that the child process syntactically complex verbal language even though test materials are presented in a picture-book easel. No norms for hearing-impaired students are available. The standardization sample was 1,222 school children with normal hearing in kindergarten through Grade 7 in eight states. Raw scores are converted into grade levels for each of the 14 arithmetic subtests; an overall math grade level is computed from the child's summative performance profile.

5. Peabody Individual Achievement Test (Dunn & Markwardt, 1970). This is a norm-referenced screening test of achievement across five areas: mathematics, reading recognition, reading comprehension, spelling, and general information. Although some subtests require only pointing responses, many parts of the test require complex syntactic abilities. No standardization for hearing-impaired children is available. The standardization sample for this test was 2,889 children in regular public school programs from kindergarten through high school. Raw scores are converted into grade equivalents, age equivalents, percentile ranks, and standard scores.

6. Reading Miscue Inventory (Goodman & Burke, 1972). In this approach to the assessment of reading skills, the child is given story passages to read aloud. Following the reading, comprehension is evaluated by having the child retell the story. During the child's reading, the evaluator notes the occurrence of substitutions, omissions, etc., made by the child; these miscues are then analyzed according to whether semantic and syntactic meaning was either preserved or altered in significant ways that might affect comprehension of the story. This system is preferable to other reading assessment approaches in that the preservation of meaning and the goal of comprehension of the passage take precedence over a unitary analysis and frequency count of "errors" in reading which characterize so many reading tests. Although this approach was developed with the intent of having the child orally read the story passages, adaptations could be made which take into account a variety of expressive modes used by hearing-impaired children while maintaining the semantic and syntactic miscue analysis (Ewoldt, 1981, 1982).

Organization and Presentation

These lists, which are by no means exhaustive, together with listings reported elsewhere (Hasenstab & Horner, 1982; Levine, 1981; Sullivan & Vernon, 1979; Zieziula, 1982) provide a general overview of the types of cognitive, psychoeducational, social-emotional, and adaptive behavior scales being used with hearing-impaired students. There is tremendous variability in the applicability of these tests to the hearing-impaired student and, in particular, to the hearing-impaired developmentally disabled student. When examiners are able to derive norm-referenced and/or criterion-referenced interpretations of the child's performance from such instruments, they are then faced with decisions regarding the organization and presentation of the information.

Ross (1982) suggested that norm- and criterion-referenced information can be organized and presented according to three standards: (1) comparing the child to himself or herself, for example, by looking at gains made since the child's last evaluation; (2) comparing the child to other hearing-impaired children of the same age; and (3) comparing the child to normal-hearing peers. Each of these comparisons, if and when instruments selected allow for them, may be of value to consumers of assessment information, particularly administrators responsible for educational placement and documentation. The organization and presentation of information that is of greater interest to teachers will depend largely on the creative use to which examiners employ the assessment instruments.

Adaptations of Assessment Instruments

As mentioned, a major objective in evaluation is to derive results that are of use not only to administrators, but also to teachers who must develop and implement educational programs. Meeting the needs of teachers is not necessarily incompatible with meeting the needs of administrators. The inclusion of criterion-referenced instruments as one of various objective evaluation techniques would yield performance descriptions that have practical value to teachers. Criterion-referenced tests describe the child's performance relative to some standard of mastery; that is, some set of specific goals in the content area under consideration. Salvia and Ysseldyke (1981) explained:

> Items on criterion-referenced tests are often linked directly to specific instructional objectives and therefore facilitate the writing of objectives. Test items sample sequential skills, enabling a teacher not only to know the specific point at which to begin instruction, but also to plan those instructional aspects that follow directly in the curricular sequence. (p. 20)

By balancing the selection of criterion- and norm-referenced tests in planning assessment strategies, the needs of both administrators and teachers are acknowledged. This strategy also recognizes that "both norm-referenced and criterion-referenced testing have relatively distinct roles to play, and both contribute to our understanding of the child's abilities" (Sattler, 1982).

Whether a test was designed as criterion-referenced or norm-referenced, the outcome of its administration is a "product" description of the child's function rather than a "process" description. That is, in the case of norm referencing, what the child can do at that point in time is compared to what other children of comparable age can do. The concern is how the product of the child's performance compares to that of other children in the same age group. In the case of criterion-referenced measurements, the results may be more descriptive of what specific skills the child has or has not mastered; nevertheless the results are still a product description of where the child stands at one point in time. Assessment strategies would be qualitatively enhanced by gathering "process" information in addition to the "product" results that most tests and observational scales provide.

The aim of process assessment strategies is to discover what supports, cues, and aids are needed to get the child to respond correctly to the items failed. In a sense, the examiner asks, "What do I need to do to teach this task to the child?" and then creatively experiments with test administration until a desired change in performance is effected. Creative, yet planned, alterations in the use of standardized instruments can be employed to answer process assessment questions. What is being advocated here has been recommended elsewhere under terms such as "testing of limits" (Sattler, 1974, 1982), the "zone of proximal development" (Vygotsky, 1978), and "mediated learning experiences" (Feuerstein, 1979).

Sattler's (1982) discussion of testing-of-limits procedures presented the rationale for creative use of standardized instruments.

> [T]here are times at which examiners desire to go beyond the standard test procedures (testing of limits) in order to gain additional information about the child's abilities. These occasions may be infrequent, but when they occur, the information gained from testing-of-limits procedures can be helpful, especially in clinical settings. Any successes obtained during testing of limits, of course, cannot be credited to the child's score. (p. 92)

The aim is not to increase the child's score; on the contrary, Sattler recommended that testing-of-limits procedures not be initiated until standard test administration is completed, so as to guard against the possible inflation of scores that might results from introducing cues and feedback. The aim is to collect information specifying how the child solves problems and what types of support are needed to enhance the child's performance. Possible testing-of-limits procedures include providing extra cues to the child, giving explicit feedback on performance, having the child explain his or her approaches to problem solving, and providing additional time for tests with set time limits (Sattler, 1982).

Vygotsky's (1978) discussion of the "zone of proximal development" also addressed the difference between what is known from a final group-normed test score and what is understood about individual differences in problem-solving and maturational processes. That is, two children of comparable mental ages may differ greatly in their ability to benefit from a teacher's guidance. The difference between the child's independent problem-solving level and the level he or she can demonstrate when given instruction defines the child's "zone of proximal development."

> It is the distance between the actual developmental level as determined by independent problem solving and the level of potential development as determined through problem solving under adult guidance or in collaboration with more capable peers. (p. 86)

By adhering to this conceptualization, examiners alter assessment strategies so as to learn how much aid and what kinds of guidance are needed to move the child from his or her actual developmental level to a next level. In Vygotsky's scheme, "the zone of proximal development defines those functions that have not yet matured but are in the process of maturing" (p. 86); the task of the examiner is to specify what mediation is necessary to reduce the gap between the child's actual level of development and his or her prospective level.

A System of Process Assessment

Perhaps the most detailed description of process evaluation can be found in Feuerstein's (1979) work with Israeli children who were described as culturally deprived, educably mentally retarded, and experiencing various learning disabilities. In more than 30 years of research, Feuerstein developed a system, the Learning Potential Assessment Device (LPAD), designed to measure the degree to which the child profits from being instructed in problem solving. Feuerstein's "Mediated Learning Experience" (MLE)

> is defined as the interactional process between the developing human organism and an experienced, intentioned adult who, by interposing himself between the child and external sources of stimulation, "mediates" the world to the child by framing, selecting, focusing, and feeding back environmental experiences in such a way as to produce . . . appropriate learning sets and habits. (p. 71)

This system includes a test-teach-test model in which the mediations are well planned and designed so that the examiner can systematically answer the process evaluation questions. The child is given the test items and, to the degree necessary, is given several different teaching inputs until the task is mastered.

For the purposes of process assessment, Feuerstein (1979) conceptualized a "cognitive map" that "includes seven parameters by which a mental act can be analyzed, categorized, and ordered—content, modality, phase, operations, level of complexity, level of abstraction, and efficiency—and enables the use of a process oriented approach" (pp. 122–123). The seven parameters serve as guides for analyzing the various aspects of the child's reasoning. The tasks we present to the child are systematically modified along one or more of the seven parameters until an improvement in performance is demonstrated.

Descriptions of Feuerstein's seven parameters of a mental act are summarized in Table 1.

Table 1. Summary of the Seven Parameters of a Mental Act

Parameter	Description
Content	The subject matter dimension, including the familiarity versus unfamiliarity of the subject matter
Modality	The verbal, pictorial, figural, numerical, etc., aspects (and their combinations)
Phase	The input (receiving and collecting the information), elaboration (using information), and output (expression of information) aspects
Operations	The strategies and sets of rules for organizing information, including seriation, classification, logical multiplication, as well as mental manipulations involving analogies, syllogisms, and inferences
Level of complexity	The quantity of informational units involved and the novelty or quality of the items
Level of abstraction	The degree to which the mental act is distanced from the object being acted upon
Level of efficiency	The precision, rapidity, and increased (or decreased) productivity aspects of the mental act

Note. Derived from *The Dynamic Assessment of Retarded Performers* (pp. 122-125) by R. Feuerstein, 1979, Baltimore: University Park Press.

The Feuerstein assessment system has a companion pencil/paper cognitive enrichment educational program entitled Instrumental Enrichment (Feuerstein, 1980). The systems are available only to evaluators and educators who receive special training in their use (Palmer, 1983). Research applying the Learning Potential Assessment Device (LPAD; Feuerstein, 1979) to hearing-impaired adolescents has been initiated (Braden, 1983), as has research using the Instrumental Enrichment program (Martin, 1983). In applying the LPAD to people with impaired hearing, Braden reported that advantages of the system include its use with culturally different hearing-impaired students (such as Indochinese refugees and Mexican adolescents new to U.S. schools and culture) and its ease in translating results for direct use by teachers and educational planners. A reported disadvantage of the system is that it assumes the availability of educational remedial programs not currently available in most educational settings for the deaf.

An example of applying the Feuerstein educational program to deaf education was reported by Martin (1983). In a two-year pilot program applying Instrumental Enrichment to hearing-impaired adolescents, Martin reported cognitive improvements across the following areas: systematic approaches to problem solving, completeness and organization in problem solving, reading comprehension, math achievement, ability to generate several problem-solving strategies, and ability to logically defend their strategies.

The Feuerstein system of process assessment, like testing-of-limits procedures (Sattler 1974, 1982) and Vygotsky's (1978) zone of proximal development, encourages one to view assessment not as an approach to seeking a product statement on the child's level of development but, rather, as a creative means for discovering the process by which a child can be instructed and guided to higher levels of functioning. Assessment strategies that add process evaluation techniques to the product evaluation techniques would offer a qualitatively enhanced description of the child's abilities.

References

Alpern, G. C., & Shearer, M. S. (1980). *Developmental profile II manual*. Aspen, CO: Psychological Publications.

Altepeter, T., & Moscato, E. M. (1982, March). *An equating study of the revised Vineland: Hearing impaired sample*. Paper presented at the meeting of the National Association of School Psychologists, Toronto, Canada.

American Association on Mental Deficiency. (1974). *AAMD adaptive behavior scale, public school version*. Washington, DC: Author.

American Association on Mental Deficiency. (1975). *AAMD adaptive behavior scale*. Washington, DC: Author.

Anderson, R. J., & Sisco, F. H. (1977). *Standardization of the WISC-R performance scale for deaf children*. Washington, DC: Gallaudet College.

Ashurst, D. I., Bamberg, D., Barrett, J., Bisno, A., Burke, A., Chambers, D., Fentiman, J., Kadish, R., Mitchell, M. L., Neeley, L., Thorne, T., & Wents, D. (1977). *Southern California ordinal scales of development, examiner's manual*. Sacramento: California State Department of Education.

Barnett, D. W. (1983). *Nondiscriminatory multifactored assessment: A sourcebook*. New York: Human Sciences Press.

Bersoff, D. W. (1982). The legal regulation of school psychology. In C. R. Reynolds & T. T. Gutkin (Eds.), *The handbook of school psychology*. New York: John Wiley.

Braden, J. (1983). *LPAD applications of deaf populations*. Unpublished manuscript.

Brigance, A. H. (1977). *Brigance diagnostic inventory of basic skills*. North Billerica, MA: Curriculum Associates.

Brill, R. G. (1977). *Brill educational achievement test for secondary age deaf students*. Northridge, CA: Joyce Media.

Connolly, A., Nachtman, W., & Pritchett, E. M. (1976). *Keymath diagnostic arithmetic test manual*. Circle Pines, MN: American Guidance Service.

Diebold, M. H., Curtis, W. S., & DuBose, R. B. (1978). Developmental scales versus observational measures for deaf-blind children. *Exceptional Children, 44,* 275–278.

Doll, E. A. (1965). *Vineland social maturity scale*. Circle Pines, MN: American Guidance Service.

DuBose, R., & Langley, B. (1977). *Developmental activities screening inventory manual*. New York: Teaching Resources.

Dunn. L. M., & Markwardt, F. C. (1970). *Peabody individual achievement test.* Circle Pines, MN: American Guidance Service.

Dunst, C. J. (1980). *A clinical and educational manual for use with the Uzgiris and Hunt scales of infant development.* Baltimore: University Park Press.

Durost, W. N., Bixler, H. H., Wrightstone, J. W., Prescott, G. A., & Balow, I. H. (1971). *Metropolitan achievement test.* New York: Harcourt Brace Jovanovich.

Ewoldt, C. (1981). A psycholinguistic description of selected deaf children, reading and sign language. *Reading Research Quarterly, 16,* 58–89.

Ewoldt, C. (1982). Diagnostic approaches and procedures and the reading process. In R. Kretschmer (Ed.), *Reading and the hearing-impaired individual* [Monograph]. *Volta Review, 84,* 83–94.

Feuerstein, R. (1979). *The dynamic assessment of retarded performers: The learning potential assessment device, theory, instruments, and techniques.* Baltimore: University Park Press.

Feuerstein, R. (1980). *Instrumental enrichment.* Baltimore: University Park Press.

Forcade, M. C., Matey, C. M., & Barnett, D. W. (1979). Procedural guidelines for low incidence assessment. *School Psychology Digest, 8,* 248–256.

Gentry, D., Bricker, D., Brown, E., Hart, V., McCortan, K., Vincent, L., & White, O. (1980). *Adaptive performance instrument.* Moscow, ID: University of Idaho.

Goodman, Y., & Burke, C. (1972). *Reading miscue inventory.* New York: Macmillan.

Haring, N. G., White, O. R., Edgar, E. B., Affleck, J. Q., Hayden, A. H., Munson, R. G., & Bendersky, M. (Eds.). (1981). *Uniform performance assessment system examiner's manual.* Columbus, OH: Charles E. Merrill.

Hasenstab, M. S., & Horner, J. S. (1982). *Comprehensive intervention with hearing impaired infants and preschool children.* Rockville, MD: Aspen Systems.

Hiskey, M. S. (1966). *Hiskey-Nebraska test of learning aptitude.* Lincoln, NE: Union College Press.

Joseph, J. (1979). *Instruction manual for the Joseph preschool and primary self-concept screening test.* Chicago: Stoelting.

Kaufman, A. S., & Kaufman, N. L. (1983). *Kaufman assessment battery for children.* Circle Pines, MN: American Guidance Service.

Leiter, R. G. (1980). *Leiter international performance scale instructional manual.* Chicago: Stoelting.

Levine, E. S. (1981). *The ecology of early deafness.* New York: Columbia University Press.

Lundell, K., Brown, W., & Evans, J. (1976). *Criterion test of basic skills.* Navato, CA: Academic Therapy Publications.

Madden, R., Gardner, E. F., Rudman, H. C., Karlsen, B., & Merwin, J. C. (1972). *Stanford achievement test, special edition for hearing impaired students.* Washington, DC: Gallaudet College Office of Demographic Studies.

Martin, D. S. (1983). *Cognitive education for the hearing-impaired adolescent.* Manuscript submitted for publication.

Meadow, K. P. (1980). *Meadow/Kendall social-emotional assessment inventory for deaf students.* Washington, DC: Gallaudet College.

Office of Education. (1977, August). Education of handicapped children: Implementation of part B of the education of the handicapped act. *Federal Register,* pp. 42,496–42,497.

Palmer, L. L. (1983). Reuven Feuerstein's instrumental enrichment: A program for the teaching of thinking? *Developmentalist, 2,* 5–12.

Raven, J. C. (1956). *The coloured progressive matrices.* New York: Psychological Corp.

Raven, J. C., Court, J. H., & Raven, J. (1976). *Manual for Raven's progressive matrices and vocabulary scales.* London: H. K. Lewis.

Raven, J. C., Court, J. H., & Raven, J. (1977). *Standard progressive matrices.* London: H. K. Lewis.

Ray, S. (1979). *An adaptation of the Wechsler intelligence scales for children–Revised for the deaf.* Natchitoches, LA: Northwestern State University of Louisiana.

Ray, S., O'Neill, M. J., & Morris, N. T. (1983). *Low incidence children: A guide to psycho-educational assessment.* Natchitoches, LA: Steven Ray Publishing.

Ray, S., & Ulissi, S. M. (1982). *An adaptation of the Wechsler preschool and primary scale of intelligence for deaf children.* Natchitoches, LA: Northwestern State University of Louisiana.

Ross, M. (1982). *Hard-of-hearing children in regular schools.* Englewood Cliffs, NJ: Prentice-Hall.

Salvia, J., & Ysseldyke, J. E. (1981). *Assessment in special and remedial education.* Boston: Houghton Mifflin.

Santa Cruz Special Education Management System. (1973). *Behavioral characteristics progression.* Palo Alto, CA: VORT Corp.

Sattler, J. M. (1974). *Assessment of children's intelligence.* Philadelphia: W. B. Saunders.

Sattler, J. M. (1982). *Assessment of children's intelligence and special abilities* (2nd ed.). Boston: Allyn and Bacon.

Smith, A. J., & Johnson, R. E. (1977). *Smith-Johnson nonverbal performance scale.* Los Angeles: Western Psychological Services.

Spragins, A. B., Spencer Day, P., & Blennerhassett, L. (1982). *Intellectual, adaptive, social-emotional, developmental, language, and academic tests used with hearing impaired children.* Workshop materials presented at the American Speech-Language-Hearing Association, Rockville, MD.

Stillman, R. (Ed.). (1978). *The Callier-Azusa scale.* Dallas: University of Texas at Dallas, Callier Center for Communication Disorders.

Stutsman, R. (1948). *Guide for administering the Merrill-Palmer scale of mental tests.* Los Angeles: Western Psychological Association.

Stutsman Ball, R., Merrifield, P., & Stott, L. H. (1978). *The extended Merrill-Palmer scale.* Chicago: Stoelting.

Sullivan, P. M., & Vernon, M. (1979). Psychological assessment of hearing impaired children. *School Psychology Digest, 8,* 271–290.

Uzgiris, I. C., & Hunt, J. (1975). *Assessment in infancy: Ordinal scales of psychological development.* Urbana: University of Illinois Press.

Vygotsky, L. S. (1978). *Mind in society: The development of higher psychological processes.* Cambridge: Harvard University Press.

Wechsler, D. (1967). *Manual for the Wechsler preschool and primary scale of intelligence.* New York: Psychological Corp.

Wechsler, D. (1974). *Manual for the Wechsler intelligence scale for children–Revised.* New York: Psychological Corp.

Zieziula, F. R. (Ed.). (1982). *Assessment of hearing-impaired people: A guide for selecting psychological, educational, and vocational tests.* Washington, DC: Gallaudet College Press.

Part IV

Bridging the Gap between Assessment and Programming

Chapter 13

The Child Psychiatric Viewpoint: A Psychosocial Perspective

Carl B. Feinstein

This chapter will review the functions of a child psychiatrist as they pertain to the hearing-impaired developmentally disabled child. First, the way in which a child psychiatrist approaches evaluation and case formulation will be presented. Second, the principal ways a child psychiatrist can be useful to the interdisciplinary team working with such children will be outlined. Finally, certain critical developmental issues for the hearing-impaired developmentally disabled child will be reviewed, and the child psychiatrist's approach to these issues described.

Orientation and Skills of the Child Psychiatrist

No single discipline or individual can possibly master all the knowledge and techniques involved in the care of the hearing-impaired developmentally disabled child. Unfortunately, for these children, the complex demands for evaluation, treatment, and education frequently lead to fragmented, uncoordinated assessments and interventions by many different specialists. Medical, educational, and vocational rehabilitation specialists, as well as psychologists, audiologists, speech/language pathologists, and social workers are often inclined to treat that aspect of the child's dysfunction which seems amenable to the procedures and interventions specific to their discipline. Further aggravating this problem is the inevitable tendency among specialists to repeat endlessly the fable of the three blind men and the elephant; that is, to assume their observations are definitive and to disregard the observations of other specialists. Complicating this situation is the observation that some specialists overlap in their areas of expertise and compete with each other. Yet, for the hearing-impaired developmentally disabled child or adolescent, an interdisciplinary approach is mandatory.

What role can the child psychiatrist play in this scenario? A review of the professional qualifications and functions of the child psychiatrist is necessary to address this question. First, the child psychiatrist is a medical specialist who is conversant with a wide range of medical diagnoses and treatments relevant to the illnesses and disabilities which the child may experience. Such knowledge may be employed in direct service to the child. More frequently, the child psychiatrist can explain the medical aspects of a child's condition in the team setting and can mediate or coordinate the child's medical, educational, and social management.

Second, the child psychiatrist is a primary resource when serious emotional and behavioral problems occur. Pharmacotherapy, inpatient hospitalization, and evaluation of potential for suicide or violence are all primary psychiatric functions.

Third, the child psychiatrist is a specialist in the evaluation and the treatment of emotional and behavioral disorders in children and adolescents. The psychiatrist is involved in the synthesis of medical, social, and cognitive assessments—both those performed by other specialists and those requested by the child psychiatrist in the course of evaluation and treatment. The child psychiatrist's five years of intensive training in psychotherapy can constitute a unique resource to the team serving the hearing-impaired developmentally disabled client. For many child psychiatrists, psychotherapy is the largest single activity in their practice.

Finally, the core theoretical discipline unique to the child psychiatrist is the study of maturation and development utilizing the biopsychosocial perspective. This orientation of the child psychiatrist, which involves consideration of biological factors, personality traits, and environmental influences, dictates a systematic approach to the problem child that includes the following diagnostic procedures:

1. Gathering information about the parents and family dynamics;
2. Taking a careful developmental history, including medical, cognitive, psychosexual, and social relationship information;
3. Reviewing the child's past and present behavior patterns, both at home and at school;
4. Evaluating the child's mental status, which involves assessment of appearance, activity level, motor coordination, language functioning, intellectual capacities, modes of thinking, emotional state, manner of relating, and fantasy life;
5. Undertaking cognitive or projective psychological testing, as indicated; and
6. Referring for more detailed neurological evaluation, EEG, further physical examination, or laboratory tests as needed to clarify diagnostic issues.

While the range of formal diagnostic entities is too lengthy and complex to review here, an analysis of the child's developmental status is a trademark of the child psychiatrist's diagnostic approach. This "developmental profile" attempts to define at what normative age level the child is functioning cognitively, socially, emotionally, and sexually, and to identify the key environmental factors promoting or impeding the child's developmental progression.

While the practical circumstances in which emotional/behavioral problem solving takes place may preclude obtaining complete information in all these areas, this comprehensive approach remains the goal. There is no child for whom the family history, the developmental history, the elucidation of coping styles and personality traits, cognitive functioning, and the mental status evaluation are irrelevant considerations.

Potential Contributions of the Child Psychiatrist

Given these qualifications and technical orientation, what can the child psychiatrist offer to the professional team working with the hearing-impaired developmentally disabled individual? The possible contributions can be summarized in these broad categories.

- Direct psychiatric evaluation and treatment;
- Regular participation in the interdisciplinary team;
- Supervision and inservice training of direct service mental health staff;
- Prevention of behavioral/emotional problems by influencing institutional policy and programs; and
- Support services to program staff on issues of burnout and morale (see Chapter 18).

Harris (1981) described the role of the child psychiatrist in delivering services to deaf individuals. My views reflect personal experience as a child psychiatric consultant as well as Harris's recommendations.

Direct Psychiatric Evaluation and Treatment

Direct evaluation and treatment are obligatory parts of the child psychiatrist's contribution to the interdisciplinary team. This is the case for two reasons. First, the child psychiatrist can best evaluate and treat those with such serious psychiatric disorders as psychoses and suicidal states. Frequently, these conditions require psychiatric hospitalization and/or pharmacotherapy. In addition, certain other disorders encountered among hearing-impaired developmentally disabled persons—such as attention deficit disorder, severe depressive disorder, and severe anxiety disorder, as well as less severe psychotic conditions—may call for the direct services of a psychiatrist. These services are more effective when provided by a psychiatrist who has regular contact and communication with the team rather than by isolated psychiatric referrals only during crisis situations. This approach also reinforces a *preventive* rather than crisis-oriented mode of operation in the service setting.

Second, it is only by direct clinical experience that the child psychiatrist can become sufficiently familiar with the specific effects of hearing impairment and with the available specialized resources to function effectively as a consultant with this population.

Recent reviews of the prevalence of emotional/behavioral problems in the deaf school-age population remind us, however, that the prevalence of psychiatric disorders is very high for this group, yet the number of child psychiatrists available to provide a significant amount of direct services is extremely limited (Jensema & Trybus, 1975; Meadow & Trybus, 1979). For these reasons, the consultative role of the child psychiatrist is critical and must be carefully tailored to each program so that the psychiatrist's expertise has the greatest possible impact and so that maximum use is made of full-time educational, counseling, and mental health personnel.

Regular Participation in the Interdisciplinary Team

As Matkin has stated (Chapter 5), regular communication among the various professionals providing services to the hearing-impaired developmentally disabled client is essential. Emotional or behavioral problems manifesting themselves in the clinical or school situation all too frequently have their origins in the home life of the child. This is often detected by the professional team; however, the gap between clinic or school and home often proves difficult to bridge. Available information frequently is based on informal, sporadic, and unplanned contacts between various members of the staff and the parents. In those settings fortunate enough to have social workers or family-oriented counselors as part of the team, more information may be available. However, there may be confusion and uncertainty regarding how to use that information in dealing with the child's problems.

In the residential setting, a similar communication gap often exists between the dormitory and the school. Different working hours, separate administrative structures, and different training backgrounds between the educational and dormitory staffs often lead either to a breakdown in communication or to unacknowledged conflict. The child psychiatrist—with emphasis on the whole child, with appreciation of the primary importance of parent-child interactions, and with an orientation towards synthesizing information from diverse aspects of the child's life into one developmental formulation—can function as a catalyst for more effective communication. The psychiatrist may direct the attention of the interdisciplinary team to the contributions of home life dynamics to the school picture and to the impact of emotions or preoccupations developed in one setting upon the child's functioning in another.

The child psychiatrist also contributes to the interdisciplinary team as a case finder. The professional staff, as a result of continuous exposure to the complex problems of large numbers of hearing-impaired developmentally disabled children, frequently becomes habituated to and exhausted by the behavioral and academic difficulties they confront on a daily basis. As a consequence, their threshold for labeling a given child's behavior as problematic is very high. Potentially treatable problems may be overlooked for years because of low staff expectations or because of preoccupation with the handful of children who present the most serious management problems.

Psychiatrists have noted on many occasions that the staff grossly underestimates the prevalence of even major psychiatric disorders among the hearing-impaired developmentally disabled school-age population (Altshuler, 1971). For example, the same children who have been referred to a psychiatrist for crisis intervention may not have been formally reported on surveys by the school administrators as those considered to have emotional/behavioral problems. Underreporting of psychiatric disorder is illustrated in the literature by comparing the prevalence rates for emotional disorders in deaf school-age children reported from national survey data by Jensema and Trybus (1975) and those summarized by Pless and Roghmann (1971) covering all forms of chronic childhood illness or disability. Jensema and Trybus found a prevalence rate for emotional/behavioral problems of 8 percent in the school-age hearing-impaired population and 20.4 percent among the multihandicapped hearing impaired. In sharp contrast, Pless and Roghmann found that 30–50 percent of all chronically ill or disabled children had secondary social and emotional problems.

In addition to this "not noticing" phenomenon, some professionals, particularly educators, are reluctant to assign diagnostic labels. Whereas medical or other clinical professionals see diagnostic formulations as the necessary first step to treatment planning and service delivery, many educators see the process instead as one that assigns social stigma. This attitude often precludes program development and service delivery.

Children with extremely underdeveloped or deviant social skills and children with attention deficit disorder, both treatable problems, often are not conceptualized as needing psychiatric referral by the educational supervisor or specialist. The child psychiatrist in a team setting, therefore, can function to alert the staff to children who have treatable emotional disorders.

Supervision and Inservice Training of the Mental Health Staff

One of the most efficient uses of psychiatric consultation time is to enhance the assessment and treatment skills of the counseling and support services staff in the area of mental health. This consultation may take the form of direct supervision of psychotherapeutic work. Support and supervision of parent counseling and information gathering are particularly important. Continuing education in the form of diagnostic staff conferences or didactic presentations can be used to increase the staff's capacity to identify the various symptoms and syndromes of psychiatric disorder. One caution is that child psychiatrists typically do not have extensive experience with hearing-impaired developmentally disabled children.

For supervision to be effective in this setting, it is first necessary for the psychiatrist to observe and participate in interviews conducted by members of the professional team. Without such direct experience, the child psychiatrist will lack sufficient familiarity with deafness issues, particularly the wide range of communicative capacities and styles among the children and the staff. With such knowledge, the child psychiatrist and the staff members will be alert to the severe limitations of verbally oriented psychotherapy for most deaf children. Activity-oriented therapy may be the only appropriate mode of choice for hearing-impaired clients whose disabilities include severe language delay or disorder regardless of the child's use of an oral or manual mode of communication.

An optimal strategy for teaching interviewing and psychotherapy skills to counselors while simultaneously expanding the psychiatrist's knowledge of issues involved with hearing-impaired developmentally disabled clients is to teach by direct example. The most helpful model of consultation begins with a preliminary staffing conference during which information regarding the various aspects of the child's problem, history, and current functioning are reviewed; clinical hypotheses are generated; and agreement is reached about what topics to pursue in a direct interview with the child.

This staffing conference is followed by an interview with the child or the parent, as appropriate. The interview is conducted by the psychiatric consultant in full and equal collaboration with the counselor or mental health worker. It is made clear to the client that the interview is being conducted by both individuals, although the child psychiatrist may often play the more active role. Interviewing the client with the mental health worker may be far more productive than bringing in an outside interpreter. Not only is a mental health worker familiar with many aspects of the client, but he or she is also conversant with the language and terminology of mental health. In addition, more often than not, the client and family members may be far more at ease in the presence of a familiar and supportive figure.

In those frequent instances when the client's main communication modality is sign language, the mental health worker interprets both from voice to sign and from sign to voice if the psychiatrist requires this assistance. It is preferable, of course, for the child psychiatrist to be fluent in sign language. However, such individuals are extremely rare, and the absence of signing ability should not preclude direct interviewing using the method described above. The essential issue is one of adequately matching the communication method and native language of the client with that used by the mental health worker. A registered sign language interpreter might be used; an interpreter with knowledge in the field of mental health or with training as a supportive team member is ideal. This method not only maximizes the rapport achieved and information obtained in the clinical interview but also serves a valuable training and continuity function.

By directly observing the interviewing techniques and orientation of the psychiatrist, the counselor can augment his or her own skill in this regard. In addition, the counselor develops a perspective about what a psychiatrist can and cannot do in a clinical interview. Such direct observation undercuts preconceptions and stereotypes about psychiatrists that often impair trust and communication between the psychiatric consultant and other professional staff members. Another immediate benefit of this combined interview strategy is that the counselor is fully aware of what happened in the psychiatric interview. This, in turn, greatly facilitates the counselor's own understanding of and future work with the client.

Following the interview, the key members of the team reassemble, and the interview is reviewed and discussed by both the psychiatrist and the counselor. A diagnostic formulation and plan of action are then developed. Using this format, the staff may periodically request a follow-up interview of the child with the same participants. This greatly enhances the child psychiatrist's capacity to assist in the actual counseling by increasing familiarity with the child as well as increasing the counselor's sense of confidence in and collegiality with the psychiatrist.

Harris (1981) made excellent suggestions regarding the selection of the child psychiatric consultant. As he observed, the ideal situation is to establish a collaborative relationship with a child psychiatrist who is closely affiliated with a medical school or teaching hospital. A psychiatrist in such a setting is more likely to be familiar with other problems of medically ill and handicapped children. Furthermore, he or she is likely to have access to high-quality medical specialists and, through those connections, can participate in the development of a medical support system with at least some familiarity with the issues of deafness.

Behavioral/Emotional Problems and Institutional Policy

Influencing institutional policy may offer the greatest long-range benefit to the hearing-impaired developmentally disabled population. In this capacity, the child psychiatrist functions as a champion for incorporating a developmental approach into educational and residential practice. The psychiatrist underscores the importance of addressing emotional issues in the child's program and the promotion of social development as part of the mission of the interdisciplinary team. He or she also continually reminds the professional staff and program administrators of the importance of family influences on the client and of the need to stress communication with families as well as the vital functions of family support and training.

In this role, the psychiatrist is not only involved in the primary prevention of psychiatric disorder, but also in minimizing the tendency of psychosocial trauma to turn disabilities into handicaps. Pless and Pinkerton (1975) have distinguished between the concepts of *disability* and *handicap*. The former is defined as flowing directly from the underlying biologic impairment. The latter refers to the effect of stress on the client, family, or social network, which then leads to a level of adaptation below that person's capability. With appropriate use of psychiatric consultation, the degree of handicap imposed by the combined disabilities may, in fact, be lessened for hearing-impaired developmentally disabled individuals and their families.

The following is a partial list of major issues affecting the client to which the child psychiatrist may contribute.

1. The development of social and emotional support programs for parents, families, or primary caregivers;

2. The incorporation of new knowledge regarding early child development and parent-child interaction into the planning of more flexible and individually tailored early intervention programs;

3. The development of sound practices regarding residential placement and the structuring of residential living, based on understanding the child's need for consistent parenting and the long-range effects of separation from parents at various ages;

4. The structuring of school programs so as to promote social development based on appreciation of the enormous importance of social skills and peer relations in overall psychosocial adjustment; and

5. The planning of school and residential programs for teenagers based on a full understanding of the major psychosocial and sexual issues of adolescence.

Development of Increased Social and Emotional Support for Parents

The danger posed to the hearing-impaired developmentally disabled child by unresolved grief or other maladaptive reactions on the part of the parents is well known in the field. Mindel and Vernon (1971) reviewed in depth some of the most common emotional reactions of parents to the discovery of deafness in their baby. However, awareness of this problem by itself is insufficient. Unless the parents can be helped to work through their grief, and can be successfully encouraged to undertake the many additional efforts required, the result for the child may be catastrophic.

The most common manifestation of a problem in this area consists of a failure on the part of the parents to develop a satisfactory communication channel with their child. In turn, this failure to communicate has profound consequences for every stage of development and greatly increases the likelihood that the child will suffer from social, behavioral, or emotional problems. Therefore, no effort should be spared to reach out professionally to the parents of hearing-impaired developmentally disabled children.

Many factors may influence the parents' choice of a language modality. While the deafness expert has much to offer in the way of counseling with regard to this specific issue, at no time should the professional lose track of the basic principle that any developed modality of communication is better than no communication at all. An active "reaching out" approach to parents on the part of clinical and educational professionals is essential. While this effort may initially be experienced as intrusive by some parents, the cost to the child's future is too great to remain merely passive or observant.

The child psychiatrist may be able to play a useful role in helping parents deal with their reactions to their child's handicap. This may be done using either individual or group therapeutic approaches. Direct psychiatric intervention however should be supported by ready access to other professionals who are equipped to offer direct services to the child, e.g., the audiologist, speech/language pathologist, sign language teacher, or deaf educator. Care must be taken to prevent further alienating the already vulnerable parent by emphasizing the "mental health/mental illness" aspects of the intervention. Parent support groups, in which the psychotherapist is primarily in an educative and facilitative role, are most useful in this regard.

Incorporating New Knowledge into Intervention Programs

In view of the overriding need to help grieving parents and to establish an early channel of communication, there has been a tendency to view the development of the hearing-impaired developmentally disabled child solely as an interaction between the child's handicap and the parents' reactions to the handicap. A standard model of psychological development for the deaf child based on Erikson's stages (Schlesinger & Meadow, 1972) has been generally useful, as has the application of separation/individuation theory (Mahler, 1979) and Freud's (1953) theory of psychosexual stages. These developmental models, however, do not take into account the steadily accumulating data regarding inborn individual differences in temperament and the reciprocal nature of parent/child interactions (Bell & Harper, 1977; Brazelton, 1973; Thomas & Chess, 1977). Without regard for these two factors, however, critical individual differences among children may be overlooked.

It is now generally accepted that infants vary widely in their innate neurobehavioral organization. Brazelton and colleagues developed a highly reliable scale for measuring these differences (Brazelton, 1973). Thomas and Chess (1977) identified nine categories of temperament which are stable and reliably present as early as two months of age. These categories have been applied to several longitudinal studies of children from diverse national, cultural, and class backgrounds.

Thomas and Chess defined temperament as the "how" of behavior, referring to the style or approach with which children sense, react, and interact. Thus, two children may perform a similar task, respond to similar stimuli, or interact socially in distinctly different fashions. The temperament categories identified by Thomas and Chess are activity level, rhythmicity of biological functions, approach or withdrawal to the new, adaptability to new or altered situations, sensory threshold or responsiveness to stimuli, intensity of reaction, quality of mood, distractibility, and attention span or degree of persistence.

Thomas and Chess identified at least three general temperamental groupings of children using ratings of these nine categories of temperament. They label the first general pattern as "the easy child." This child is characterized by regularity, positive approach responses to new stimuli, high adaptability to change, and mild or moderately intense mood which is predominantly positive. A second group, called "the difficult child," is characterized by irregularity in biological function, negative withdrawal responses to new stimuli, nonadaptability or slow adaptability to change, and intense mood expressions which are frequently negative. The third category of child is called "slow to warm up." Children in this group show a combination of negative responses of mild intensity to new stimuli with slow adaptability after repeated contact.

Differences in cognitive styles have also been identified. Kagan and colleagues (1964), for example, identified "reflection vs. impulsivity" as a significant dimension of cognitive style. Nelson (1981) has described three very different patterns of language development in young children: "expressive," referring to children who use speech primarily to describe actions, interactions, and needs; "referential," referring to children whose language-learning strategy is oriented primarily toward naming objects and ideas; and a "combined" language-learning style. It is becoming increasingly clear to child psychiatrists that these temperamental and cognitive patterns must be assessed if one is to properly understand any given child and to tailor an intervention strategy to the particular temperamental and cognitive style of that child.

Along with the increasing recognition that the infant is not a tabula rasa, but rather comes into the world with distinctive tendencies, both cognitive and temperamental, it has also become clear that the direction of influence between parent and child is a reciprocal one rather than one in which the parental style alone determines the interaction. Stern (1977) and Bell and Harper (1977) discussed at length the myriad ways in which the appearance, behavior, and innate interactive and reactive tendencies of the child influence the way the parent responds to him or her.

The most relevant aspect of this reciprocal interaction is referred to as "goodness of fit." As summarized by Thomas and Chess (1977), goodness of fit results when the properties of the environment's expectations and demands are in accord with the child's own capacities, motivations, and styles of behaving. "Poorness of fit" refers to discrepancies and dissonances between environmental challenges and the temperamental characteristics of the child. A parent might be comfortable rearing an infant with one style of temperament and yet have major difficulties with another. For example, a withdrawn, depressed mother, who is "slow to warm up" might do better with an active, positively engaging "easy" baby but might have more difficulty with a more passive, quieter infant. Conversely, a mother with a low stimulus threshold and a need for order might do better with a quieter infant and be more stressed by an active, impulsive child.

These considerations should play a role in early assessment and intervention strategies for the hearing-impaired developmentally disabled child. Take, for example, the young child with a moderate hearing loss. A question might exist as to whether an oral approach could be applied from the earliest age without recourse to teaching sign communication, or whether total communication would be preferable. Usually these decisions are made on strictly "educational" grounds, depending upon the prejudices of the parent and the orientation of the early intervention specialist. However, referring to the concept of "goodness of fit," it would seem that an energetic, nondepressed mother with a reflective, "easy" child would have a much greater likelihood of succeeding with an oral approach than would a depressed, overworked, and irritable mother with a child who is impulsive and "difficult." In this example, assessment of goodness of fit might be the single most valuable consideration guiding the selection of an early intervention approach. These factors, however, are rarely taken into account.

The same sort of consideration might apply to the type of school placement, the structure of the classroom, and the type of instructional method most useful for any given hearing-impaired developmentally disabled child. An educational policy that utilizes one particular approach to the education of all hearing-impaired developmentally disabled children is overlooking the wide range of temperamental and cognitive styles found in such children. Such an approach might be a "good fit" for some children but a "poor fit" for others. For example, a program emphasizing academics, in-seat behavior, and prolonged "listening" to instructional material might work well for the less impulsive, more reflective child with better attentional abilities and less need for motor discharge. The same program would probably work poorly for a more impulsive, action-oriented child with limited attention capacities and a drive toward active expression. Both of these children might have equal cognitive endowments as measured by conventional intelligence tests, yet one might become a "problem child."

Therefore, the child psychiatrist who is prepared to observe, focus on, and communicate to other professionals the importance of these temperamental and "goodness of fit" considerations could play a useful role in the educational team when decisions regarding placement and instructional method are being made.

Understanding the Child's Need for Consistent Parenting

It has been clearly established from clinic practice and in detailed retrospective studies that prolonged separations in early childhood play a causal role in the etiology of depression. This has been extensively reviewed by Bowlby (1980). Depression in children and adolescents often involves manifold related behavioral disturbances and academic problems. Since it has been clearly demonstrated that hearing-impaired developmentally disabled children are already more vulnerable to these problems than others (Jensema & Trybus, 1975), it logically follows that every effort be made to prevent early separation of these children from their parents.

The statistics, as reviewed by Wolk, Karchmer, and Schildroth (1982), remind us, moreover, that it is still not uncommon for deaf children as young as the age of four to be placed in residential settings. Supporters of this practice argue that in geographical areas where educational resources are scarce, the residential setting may be the only way to provide language instruction for the deaf or hearing-impaired developmentally disabled child. For the child psychiatrist this is a dubious and one-sided assertion. How can the 4- to 6-year-old deaf child comprehend the reasons that he or she is suddenly and inexplicably sent away from family and home? It is difficult enough for the hearing child of the same age, with adequate language abilities, to comprehend or accept even short-term, carefully explained separations. The deaf child, however, cannot receive these explanations and, furthermore, is likely to be less mature, more dependent, and more emotionally vulnerable than the hearing child. The residential placement of young hearing-impaired developmentally disabled children should be carefully reviewed. This review should always include child psychiatric consultation.

Given the presence and continued existence of residential programs for young children, however, careful attention must be paid to the structuring of residential life so as to minimize the harmful consequences of disrupted parenting. From the child psychiatrist's point of view, an adequate program would possess the following features:

1. The residential staff should have a high percentage of individuals with special training in early childhood development.
2. Each child should be assigned to a single "special" residence staff person whose work schedule is patterned to provide continuity of care and close familiarity with the child.
3. The ratio of children to residential staff should be very low.
4. A cottage or small group living arrangement is highly preferable as the basic unit of residential life; a large group dormitory for younger children cannot meet the needs of those children for consistent attentive parenting.

The child psychiatric consultant should play an important role in the residential school in structuring both the living arrangements and the school program so as best to support the emotional needs of the younger child.

Helping School Programs Promote Social Development

The school years, both primary and secondary, are crucial ones for the development of social competence. The ability to form and maintain meaningful friendships and to participate in peer group life is acquired in a series of stages beginning in the early school years and extending through high school. The later ability to enjoy social relationships and work cooperatively with other adults depends greatly on how well the individual was able to learn socialization skills in childhood peer group activities. Difficulty with socialization in the school years is a sensitive indicator of emotional disorder and, unless overcome, a good predictor of emotional disorders in later life.

Peer group life is essential in helping children individuate and become more independent of their parents, providing a new network of social support. Children use peer group participation as a vehicle for role and gender identity formation. Through peer group activities, children learn "the traffic rules of life," develop concepts of fairness and unfairness, and acquire the ability to delay gratification in exchange for longer term social rewards.

Children learn socialization from their peer group experiences in two primary settings: the neighborhood and the school. Deaf children in general and hearing-impaired developmentally disabled children in particular, however, are likely to suffer major experiential deprivation in the social sphere in both settings, what Altshuler (1971) refers to as a "deficit in general experience."

The deficit in social experience for the hearing-impaired developmentally disabled child is often profound. Its early roots lie in the frequent absence of a satisfactory communication channel between parents and their children. This is particularly the case for the many families in which the parents have no sign language skills, yet the child's only effective means of communication is through signing. When these children enter latency and turn toward their peers, many have had only the most scanty experiences with pleasurable, verbally mediated social interactions. In their neighborhoods, these children are frequently isolated from peer social contacts for lack of a common communication mode or language.

School, where the children are surrounded by peers who sign, is, in effect, the only setting where peer social contacts employing language can take place. However, inadvertent deprivation in social experience at school often occurs as a by-product of the great stress placed on academic remediation. Classroom time is structured so that "active teaching" by the teacher is favored over the encouragement of expression by the students. As Craig and Holman (1973) stated, "In schools for deaf children . . . creative and concrete student activity is frequently skipped over in order to get to the business of education."

In its extreme form, such an emphasis on academics results in the child being moved from one structured classroom setting to another from the moment of arrival at school, with brief breaks, until the end of the school day. School, the only setting in which these children have the opportunity to develop social skills, thereby suppresses the opportunities for such experience.

The viewpoint of the child psychiatrist is that education in social skills must be given a much higher priority in programs for the hearing-impaired developmentally disabled child. Without substantial opportunity for formal and informal social experience in the school, the child is deprived of an asset, social competence, which is of the greatest importance to later adaptation. Educators often have difficulty with this issue. Time provided for children to socialize informally is too easily viewed as taking away from time needed to develop academic competence. Ultimately, no child will become highly motivated to achieve academically unless meaningful social identifications and social rewards in the form of peer respect reinforce academic success.

The child psychiatrist, therefore, as a participant in the interdisciplinary team, functions as an advocate for training and experience in socialization in the school setting. Such socialization is a vital component of the overall educational program.

Helping the Teenager Cope with Psychosocial Problems

According to Erikson (1963), the core developmental task of adolescence is "identity versus identity confusion." It seems clear, however, that hearing-impaired developmentally disabled children are likely to carry into adolescence unresolved issues from other developmental stages. For example, the child dealing with communicative isolation and other disabilities is likely to have unresolved problems from the earlier developmental crisis of "autonomy versus shame and doubt."

To understand how these issues affect the child, it is necessary to review the elements that need to be present in the psychosocial milieu of adolescents to ensure healthy identity development. According to Zinn (1979), the development of a secure sense of self depends on the teenager's experiencing both an appropriate, balanced set of expectations for increasing autonomy on the one hand, and the opportunity to practice autonomous functioning on the other. The consolidation of a strong identity also requires the availability of different role models or the opportunity to experience a variety of social selves.

The key points of vulnerability in the identity formation of the hearing-impaired developmentally disabled adolescent are summarized in three words from Zinn's formulation: opportunity, expectation, and experience. Disability may limit the opportunities for a teenager to participate in social situations, appropriate work environments, or in other situations which might challenge or promote development of self-care skills. A deficit in experience may then develop, leaving the hearing-impaired developmentally disabled youngster deficient in the skills necessary to enter into social, work, or self-care activity. The expectations of significant others, whether it be the attitude of peers, school authorities, or parents, may directly affect the opportunities for experience either by discouraging the adolescent from trying or by limiting growth-inducing activities.

Zinn described the two essential features of the social environment and milieu necessary to foster secure identity development in adolescents.

1. The environment must be supportive but not intrusive or infantilizing.

2. The environment must provide graded opportunities to master increasingly demanding situations. The failure to provide opportunities leads to feelings of unsureness and untestedness. On the other hand, excessive, unrealistic situations or demands are potentially devastating to self-esteem. (pp. 157, 168)

Data from the Boston longitudinal study of Vaillant (1981) indicated that the capacity to work in the teenage years is a powerful predictor of adult mental health. Evidence of adolescent mastery of work skills was a more important predictor of later healthy adjustment than other powerful variables, including parental education, social class, and growing up in a multiple-problem family.

What are the implications of these principles for educational policy regarding hearing-impaired developmentally disabled adolescents? First and foremost, they mandate a basic change in the philosophy of education for these youngsters. The high school program must not be judged solely in terms of its educational activities. The view which stresses academics as an end in itself neglects the overwhelming need to prepare the youngster for the very difficult adaptive challenges that face him or her as an adult. Those challenges include finding and keeping a job in a constricted labor market and developing the necessary skills to negotiate the activities of daily living. Even for those children for whom the degree of handicap is so severe as to preclude full independent living, these are still the primary challenges faced at the end of school.

In view of these considerations, high school for the hearing-impaired developmentally disabled youngster should be geared toward practical preparation for adult living. Comprehensive prevocational and vocational training throughout the school years is essential. Not only must relevant work skills be taught, but the student must have the opportunity to practice those work skills in a series of experiences beginning with the more sheltered and progressing in incremental steps toward work placements that approximate real life. This incremental approach is necessary for development of the social skills required to function in the workplace.

Some of these skills are (1) overcoming feelings of shame and avoidance regarding communication (e.g., asking or writing questions, risking the use of impaired speech, etc.); (2) finding some way of interacting with other workers, including hearing people;

(3) learning to tolerate the discipline of the workplace; and (4) most of all, dealing with the shame-inducing or anxiety-provoking situations that inevitably arise in the work arena.

Skills of daily living, which are becoming a more important part of the curriculum of many special education programs, must be stressed even more and should include practical exercises of graded difficulty outside of the school environment. High-school-age hearing-impaired and developmentally disabled students must learn how to turn to each other for psychological support, as they will surely need it when they leave the relatively supportive cocoon of the special school. Social skills must be systematically promoted by providing frequent opportunities for informal and more organized social interactions. School is likely to be the last daily opportunity these youngsters will have to receive support in the development of social competence.

In summary, the child psychiatrist in the interdisciplinary team can be a spokesperson for the incremental training of real life competencies in hearing-impaired developmentally disabled adolescents without which shame, avoidance, and progressive social withdrawal will greatly impede the already limited opportunities that these youngsters will confront in later life.

References

Altshuler, K. Z. (1971). Studies of the deaf: Relevance to psychiatric theory. *American Journal of Psychiatry, 127*(11), 1521–1526.

Bell, R. Q., & Harper, L. V. (1977). *Child effects on adults.* Hillsdale, NJ: Lawrence Erlbaum.

Bowlby, J. (1980). Loss: Sadness and depression. In J. Bowlby (Ed.), *Attachment and loss* (Vol. III). New York: Basic Books.

Brazelton, T. B. (1973). Neonatal behavioral assessment scale. *Clinics in Developmental Medicine,* No. 50.

Craig, H., & Holman, G. (1973). The "open classroom" in a school for the deaf. *American Annals of the Deaf, 118,* 675–685.

Erikson, E. (1963). *Childhood and society.* New York: Norton.

Freud, S. (1953). Three essays on sexuality. In J. Strachey (Ed. and Trans.), *The standard edition of the complete psychological works of Sigmund Freud* (Vol. 7). London: Hogarth Press. (Original work published 1905)

Harris, R. (1981). Mental health needs and priorities in deaf children and adults: A deaf professional's perspective for the 1980s. In L. Stein, E. Mindel, & T. Jabuly (Eds.), *Deafness and mental health.* New York: Grune and Stratton.

Jensema, C., & Trybus, R. (1975). *Reported emotional behavioral problems among hearing impaired children in special educational programs: United States, 1972–73* (Series R, No. 1). Washington, DC: Gallaudet College Office of Demographic Studies.

Kagan, J., Rosman, B. L., Day, D., Albert, J., & Phillips, W. (1964). Informative processing in the child: Significance of reflective attitudes. *Psychological Monographs, 18*(1).

Mahler, M. S. (1979). Separation-individuation. In M. S. Mahler (Ed.), *The selected papers of Margaret S. Mahler* (Vol. II). New York: Jason Aronson.

Meadow, K., & Trybus, R. (1979). Behavioral and emotional problems of deaf children: An overview. In L. Bradford & W. Hardy (Eds.), *Hearing and hearing impairment.* New York: Grune and Stratton.

Mindel, E. D., & Vernon, M. (1971). *They grow in silence.* Silver Spring, MD: National Association of the Deaf.

Nelson, K. (1981). Individual differences in language development: Implication for development and language. *Developmental Psychology, 17*(2), 179–187.

Pless, I. B., & Pinkerton, P. (1975). *Chronic childhood disorder: Promoting patterns of adjustment.* Chicago: Year Book Medical Publisher.

Pless, I. B., & Roghmann, K. J. (1971). Chronic illness and its consequences. *Journal of Pediatrics, 79,* 351.

Schlesinger, H., & Meadow, K. (1972). *Sound and sign.* Berkeley: University of California Press.

Stern, D. (1977). *The first relationship: Infant and mother.* Cambridge, MA: Harvard University Press.

Thomas, A., & Chess, S. (1977). *Temperament and development.* New York: Brunner/Mazel.

Vaillant, G. E. (1981). Natural history of male psychological health: Work as a predictor of positive mental health. *American Journal of Psychiatry, 138,* 1433–1439.

Wolk, S., Karchmer, M. A., & Schildroth, A. (1982, April). *Patterns of academic and non-academic integration among hearing-impaired students in special education* (Series R-9). Washington, DC: Gallaudet College Center for Assessment and Demographic Studies.

Zinn, D. (1979). A developmental preventive approach to problems of psychopathology in adolescence. In J. Noshpitz (Ed.), *Basic handbook of child psychiatry* (Vol. 4). New York: Basic Books.

Chapter 14

Content and Process in Curriculum Planning

W. Scott Curtis and David Tweedie

Those who work with hearing-impaired developmentally disabled children are well aware of the considerable amount of time and planning that goes into the evaluation of the child's liabilities and assets. The detailed effort made to determine hearing, vision, motor, adaptive, and intellectual abilities is well documented in earlier chapters. It is of equal importance that we, as professionals, also evaluate the curriculum to which the child is exposed once the personal evaluation is so carefully completed. The meaningfulness of evaluation, for educational purposes, would be lost if the child were placed in a generic curriculum that was not finely tuned to the needs of his or her disability group and personal prognosis. The following material is designed to assist in the evaluation and refinement of curricula for the hearing-impaired developmentally disabled child.

Needs and Rationale

The curriculum has several major roles to play in education. First, the curriculum is a structure or an organizational scheme that serves as a guide to the establishment of more specific learning goals. In this sense, the curriculum is a map which the teacher can use to guide the child's learning—a map of territory traveled before by other teachers and pupils and one which has been improved as each new class succeeds or fails to reach its destination.

Curriculum and Schedule

The curriculum is related to but different from the class schedule, with which it is sometimes confused. The schedule tells when something will be focused on as a learning task while the curriculum tells which skills or activities will be learned. Schedule is related to curriculum in an important way. If a major curricular component is, for example, self-care skills, the quality of the program and the success of the child may be determined by when a specific activity will be studied or practiced. For example, if the integration of the program is so effective that the child has learning experiences for shoe tying in the classroom, the home, the dormitory, and the recreation program, then greater learning will occur than if the activity were taught in one environment only. Clearly, the scheduling of the learning experiences that are identified in the curriculum can change the frequency of opportunity, the frequency of adult involvement, the generalization opportunity and, therefore, the outcome for each child on each curricular item.

Curriculum and the Individualized Education Program

Curriculum and schedule also have an important and close relationship to the Individualized Education Program (IEP), which consists essentially of the operational subcomponents of the curricular categories. For example, the curriculum in most programs for the hearing-impaired developmentally disabled student will call for self-help (activity of daily living) skills which have many operable subcomponents, such as dressing, toileting, eating, etc. The schedule will tell when each is to be studied or practiced, and the IEP will specify for each child the specific activity he or she is to learn. The special value of the IEP to the curriculum and schedule is that it is the smaller, more operable unit of the system, the component which can be most easily measured as a quantifiable achievement and developed for a particular student. Curriculum, IEP, and schedule work together but have different important roles for classroom planning.

The evaluation of the extent to which a curriculum is desirable or appropriate calls for reviewing it within the context of those other programmatic factors which integrate with it. Van Etten, Arkell, and Van Etten (1980) suggested several important considerations, including the availability of assessment procedures to monitor the curriculum, type of data management procedures, clarity of behavioral strategies, and approach and format, which derive from the orientation of the curriculum to developmental or other systems.

Tymitz-Wolf (1982) clarified the role of the goals and objectives in curricular plans. Her checklist for evaluating the appropriateness of these plans is shown in Table 1 on the following page.

The relationship between schedule and curriculum is discussed by Lund and Bos (1981), who suggest seven considerations for reviewing the potential effectiveness of a schedule for implementing a curriculum.

- Does the schedule allow time for meeting each student's IEP goals?
- Is the length of time for each component appropriate for the students?
- Does the sequence of events provide for a variety of learning experiences?
- Does the sequence flow in a logical progression?
- Do the components vary from one-to-one to group activities?
- Are transitions between activities planned to minimize confusion?
- Does the schedule provide a stable routine?

The guidelines offered by Lund and Bos for evaluating scheduling of the curriculum and the Tymitz-Wolf checklist for evaluating goals and objectives provide the reader with valuable strategies for curricular selection and implementation.

In addition to providing a structure which specifies the broad learning components of the program, the curriculum is the first line of communication among the teacher,

Table 1. Checklist for Evalution of Goals and Objectives

1. Does the goal statement refer to target areas of deficit? **OR** Have I written a goal which is unrelated to remediation needs described in present level of performance and assessment information?

2. Given the assessment data, is it probable that this goal could be achieved in a year (i.e., annual period for the IEP)? **OR** Is the goal so broad that it may take two or more years to accomplish?

3. Does the goal contain observable terms with an identified target area for remediation? **OR** Have I used words which fail to accurately describe the problem area or direction I am taking?

4. Have goals been written for each area of deficit? **OR** Do I have dangling data (data which indicate a need for remediation but have been overlooked)?

5. Is the scope of the objective appropriate? **OR** Have I written any objectives that encompass the entire year, thus making them annual goals?

6. Do the objectives describe a subskill of the goal? **OR** Have I failed to determine the hierarchy needed to teach the skill?
   - Did I simply rephrase the goal statement?
   - Did I describe a terminal skill, but only less of it?

7. Are the objectives presented in a sequential order? **OR** Have I listed the objectives in random order, unrelated to the way the skill would logically be taught?

8. Do the objectives show a progression through the skill to meet the goal? **OR** Do the objectives emphasize only one phase of a particular skill?

9. Does the objective contain an appropriately stated condition? **OR** Have I failed to describe the exact circumstances under which the behavior is to occur?
   - Have I described irrelevant or extraneous materials?
   - Does the condition refer to an isolated classroom activity?

10. Does the objective contain an appropriately stated performance using observable terms? **OR** Is the mode of performance (e.g., oral) different from the desired goal (e.g., written)?

11. Does the objective contain an appropriately stated standard? **OR** Is the standard unrelated to the assessment information and level of performance?
    - Am I using the performance statement as a standard?
    - Am I using percentages when the behavior requires alternative ways to measure?
    - Have I chosen arbitrary percentages?

Note. From "Guidelines for Assessment IEP Goals and Objectives" by B. Tymitz-Wolf, 1982, *Teaching Exceptional Children, 14*(5), p. 200. Copyright 1982 by Council for Exceptional Children. Reprinted by permission.

the school administrators, the child, the parents, the institutional support staff, and related professionals such as speech/language pathologists. All these significant individuals must perform their duties in a unified manner if the child is to succeed. There must be agreement on what is being taught (the curriculum) and who has the various responsibilities for its achievement. A new vocabulary word or sign, for example, ought to be made known to all personnel seeing the child in varied settings so that it can be reinforced through the curricular activities in class; practiced at home, in the residence, and in the recreational program; and integrated into the speech and language therapy plan. Although consistent and constant application and reinforcement of curricular items are goals of any educational program, they are especially critical to the instruction of the individual with hearing impairment and developmental disability.

Another significant function of a curriculum is that it subtly classifies the nature and extent of the child's strengths and limitations so that the educational team can perceive the functional level of the child and make some prognosis about his or her future. The curriculum that includes self-help skills and perceptual motor training is obviously developed for a purpose very diffferent from one that includes spelling, algebra, and science. Since the hearing-impaired developmentally disabled child does not receive the customary grade level placement, the child's curriculum level serves as a necessary and clear indicator of his or her achievement level in the school.

Another value of the curriculum is that it facilitates placement. A curriculum that is clearly defined and in print makes it easier for placement staff and parents to choose a school, institution, or program appropriate to the individual child's needs as revealed through a diagnostic evaluation. When the curriculum is obscure or poorly defined, parents are left with labels that are misleading or meaningless, such as "deaf-blind class" or "program for emotionally disturbed deaf children," to assist them with their placement selection. Many authors have explained the need to place hearing-impaired developmentally disabled children on the basis of needs and abilities rather than diagnostic labels (Tweedie & Shroyer, 1982), but this requires clearly defined curricula.

In view of the stated benefit of the well-defined curriculum, one would expect that curriculum development for the hearing-impaired developmentally disabled student would be well delineated at this time. Not so. Curriculum development follows the development of classes for special groups of children, and the development of classes follows the development of new categorical labels. The diagnostic entity, hearing-impaired developmentally disabled, has only recently emerged, and even within the past few years it has had conflicting definitions (see Chapters 1 and 2). It is not surprising, then, that specific curricula for hearing-impaired developmentally disabled children are not readily available. There are many traditional categories offering long-standing training programs, i.e., deaf retarded, emotionally/behaviorally disturbed deaf, etc., which also do not yet have a variety of well-developed curricula. As late as 1961, Ewing and Ewing suggested the need to segregate the severely and profoundly deaf from the partially deaf saying, "It cannot be good for them to mix with children more severely handicapped by deafness than they are. . . . " (p. 139). At that late date they noted with approval the initiation of special classes for the mentally retarded deaf and the deaf-blind with the recommendation that classes for the cerebral-palsied deaf be developed. Twenty years later, we have classification and classroom grouping problems yet to be resolved.

It should have been relatively easy to justify the need for curricula for hearing-impaired developmentally disabled individuals on the basis of numbers of children receiving or needing appropriate services. The figures are available in this book (Chapter 3) and speak for themselves. But there is an additional basis for considering the problems of curriculum selection for this group of children: It appears to be easier to relabel the children's problems than to change the curriculum in significant ways.

Perhaps the need to review the curricula for these children was most recently made clear by the conflict during efforts to formulate legislation (Crosby, 1982) and the problem of defining hearing-impaired developmentally disabled for that legislation. During the discussions some people argued that the hearing-impaired developmentally disabled were those children who had been previously identified under such labels as deaf-blind, retarded deaf, emotionally and behaviorally disturbed deaf, cerebral-palsied deaf, and, sometimes, multihandicapped deaf. Others argued that programs (and curricula) for those groups were already in existence and that the new term was to identify those children who "fell between the cracks" of these diagnostic labels.

In most cases, educators agree that these children's problems are early in onset, profound in nature, and long term in duration. Due to the lack of definitively validated curricula for such children, we have chosen to present examples of curricula for the various dyads of disorder which clarify what is taught to deaf children who have one or more other handicaps of early origin, severe nature, and long duration. The curricula reviewed are preceded by a discussion of factors that influence curriculum selection and are followed by a discussion of problems impeding curricular effectiveness.

One fact stands out clearly when reviewing curricula within the definitive areas of severe, long-term, early diagnosed disorders: There are more similarities among curricula than there are differences, even though the areas of disability for which the curricula are designed differ widely. It would appear that beyond a certain level of handicap, the children's needs and behaviors become more homogeneous even though their diagnostic categorization becomes more heterogeneous.

A curriculum is essentially a superordinate-subordinate paradigm wherein the major domains of learning are identified and divided into increasingly smaller and more operable units which eventually reach the applied level of an activity to be performed by a child and teacher in the classroom. An example of the hierarchy might be:

Level 1	Curricular domain	Self-help skills
Level 2	Long-term objectives	Feeding self
Level 3	Short-term goals	Eating with a fork
Level 4	IEP activity	Grasping fork
Level 5	Support activity	Occupational therapy for manual dexterity

Klein, Pasch, and Frew (1979) provided several examples and an extensive discussion of the levels of curricular detailing. Figure 1 outlines the continuing subcategorization which they described.

EXPLANATION

In order to manage money efficiently, individuals must be able to distinguish between necessities and luxuries and make the appropriate decisions regarding budgeting of personal finances.

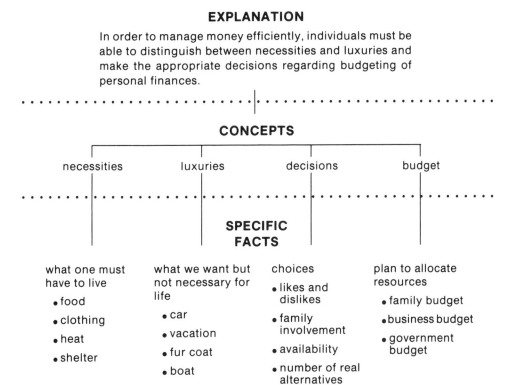

CONCEPTS

| necessities | luxuries | decisions | budget |

SPECIFIC FACTS

what one must have to live	what we want but not necessary for life	choices	plan to allocate resources
• food	• car	• likes and dislikes	• family budget
• clothing	• vacation	• family involvement	• business budget
• heat	• fur coat	• availability	• government budget
• shelter	• boat	• number of real alternatives	

Figure 1. Levels of curricular detailing. From *Curriculum Analysis and Design for Retarded Learners* (p. 164) by N. Klein, M. Pasch, and T. Frew, 1982, Columbus, OH: Charles E. Merrill. Copyright 1982 by Charles E. Merrill. Reprinted by permission.

This chapter is concerned with Levels 1 and 2 of the curricular hierarchy. Level 3 addresses individualized instruction and is child-specific. The curriculum sets only the framework for the broad areas in which development must be guided and training undertaken. Task analysis is then carried out to determine the components of long-term objectives which become short-term goals and serve as the basis for development of the child's Individualized Education Program. The IEP design makes it possible for a specific child to succeed. When the child cannot achieve with usual special educational techniques, a support base is built by specialists in specific behavioral domains, such as occupational therapy, physical therapy, speech/language pathology, etc. These treatments are often a critical part of the curriculum, especially with developmentally disabled children. When the child is hearing impaired, then the speech/language pathologist presumably will be included in the educational plans for communication development.

Choosing Curricular Items

Wilson (1981) identified four models for choosing curricular items. Some items will be chosen because they fit the developmental expectations we have for children. A second group of curricular items will be selected because of their utility to the child. A third group will relate to the findings of task-analysis studies that indicate the problems with which the child must cope. A final group will be based on prosthetic needs, to help the child overcome sensory and motor handicaps. Wilson reviewed several specific curricular programs which need not be discussed further here. They include the Portage Guide to Early Education, the Illinois Programs, Systematic Instruction for Retarded Children, the Marshall Town Project, the Right-to-Education Child, the Teaching Research Curriculum for Moderately and Severely Handicapped, the Behavioral Characteristic Progression, and several language-specific curricula.

To which major needs of the hearing-impaired developmentally disabled population should curricula be addressed? A long-term study of severely multisensory handicapped children was conducted by Curtis and Donlon (1978). They listed 19 behavioral characteristics of severely and profoundly handicapped children which transcend the etiology of disabilities. When the objective of education is normalization, the goals they suggested for curricula can be summarized as follows:

1. Improve the children's ability to care for themselves and respond to grooming so that they appear more typical than untypical;
2. Identify developmental areas which can be aided and focus efforts on those;
3. Increase self-help skills;
4. Develop the values and concepts of reward and punishment as part of the child's behavior control system;
5. Improve the child's ability to function in increasingly larger classes with fewer teachers;
6. Improve the child's ability to function with a reduced amount of supervision;
7. Increase the child's skills and opportunities for interacting with peers;
8. Develop the child's ability to engage in new and divergent activities while reducing willingness to engage in old repetitive tasks;
9. Develop a strong, active, and healthy physical education program;
10. Normalize acting out and disruptive behaviors;
11. Develop a curriculum that can benefit from the many professional groups acting on the child in a "team approach;"
12. Focus the curriculum on life skills in addition to academic skills;
13. Set curricular goals that seek placement in a less isolated educational environment;
14. Because testing is a complex problem, arrange a curriculum that can be evaluated by an observational or informal system;
15. Give special attention to teaching the child to learn on his or her own a skill that does not come naturally;

16. Utilize a curriculum that progresses from trainability to educability;

17. Develop a curriculum that forces occasional trial opportunities (realistically) in a less restrictive educational environment;

18. Create a curriculum that does not rely too heavily on rote practice and token reward systems; and

19. Arrange the scheduling of the curricular components to arouse the mental and physical vigor of the children.

These goals, based on child study, will change as definition, age, service delivery system, and other factors are altered. Some of the directions of change have been forecast. In a survey of trends in the field of deaf-blind education, Tweedie and Baud (1981) reported several trends that may have a positive effect on future curriculum development for hearing-impaired developmentally disabled children. They conclude:

- A greater emphasis will be placed on vocational training.
- Improved teaching material will be developed.
- Socialization skills will receive greater emphasis in the programming.
- Increased attention will be given to the development of leisure time activities.
- There will be an increase in sensory integration training.
- Communication technology will increase.
- Program accountability will receive greater emphasis.
- Orientation and mobility skills will receive greater emphasis.
- Adaptive equipment will become more readily available.
- Sex education programs will increase.

Because the majority of these items are concerned with larger variables rather than details of the curriculum, it seems that curricular growth in the direction of life involvement and adaptation to the environment will result in greater change than such traditional specifics as self-care and mobility. Some of these projected changes may be due to the fact that a large group of children from the rubella epidemic of the 1960s are now reaching adulthood, and the problems of adulthood for the hearing-impaired developmentally disabled are being seen in crisis proportions for the first time.

Examples of Curricula

If one curriculum for the hearing-impaired developmentally disabled child were clearly definitive, a review such as this would not be necessary. Curricula vary and are often incomplete or unsatisfactory for reasons discussed at the conclusion of this chapter. Consequently, the educational planner is obligated to study programs from several sources. First, there are specific curricula for hearing-impaired developmentally disabled, multihandicapped deaf, and deaf-blind children which are directly pertinent. Second, there is a plethora of curricula prepared for the severely and profoundly handicapped, trainable retarded, and multihandicapped that have much in common with each other and with curricula which are deaf-specific. Third, some aspects of curricula for such specific disorders as blindness, brain injury, and learning disabilities have been developed and are relevant.

Crosby (1982), in a discussion of implementation of the developmental model, described six domains that curriculum and all other services must address in meeting the needs of the developmentally disabled population. The six domains are motor development, sensory development, cognitive development, communicative development, social development, and affective development. These six categories are a basic superstructure around which specific curricula vary in only moderate dimensions.

Curricula appear to have two features of major importance. The first is the domains of knowledge, which usually include the items in column A of Table 2. The second includes the items in column B, and might be called performance areas. The best curricula do not confuse the two categories but display a matrix showing how each element of column A interacts with each of column B and vice versa.

Table 2. Elements of Curricular Planning

Knowledge	Performance
Communication domain	Activities of daily living
Adjustment domain	Social adaptation
	Personal adjustment
Learning domain	Academic performance
Motor domain	Recreational skills

Hearing-Impaired Developmentally Disabled Curricula

Appell (1982) presented a curriculum for early education of the severely handicapped hearing-impaired child with the following components:

- Intersensory coordination and stimulation,
- Communication development,
- Motor development,
- Adaptive development, and
- Affective development.

Within each of these major components, she specified subcomponents consistent with a comprehensive curricular taxonomy.

Underlying her curricula are three important premises upon which the preschool curriculum is built: (1) a theoretical foundation in cognitive theory, (2) normal developmental principles, and (3) continuing evaluation. The most unique specific component of her structure is the emphasis on body awareness through tactile and kinesthetic activities—a goal sometimes omitted from other curricular schemes.

Mavilya (1982) suggested five major curricular categories: self-care activities, basic skills (sensorimotor skills), communication skills, occupational skills, and recreational skills. The author made two points generally not mentioned. First, language and communication should be developed in a natural environment; second, language education is dependent on memory development. Both of these concepts are reasonable features of any curricular component, not just language learning.

Restaino (1982) described a curriculum having developmental objectives for the young deaf child with special learning disabilities. She identified five broad objectives, including gross motor development, sensorimotor integration, visual analysis, attention and memory, and conceptualization. The program she described is identified as the Cooperative Research Endeavors in the Education of the Deaf (CREED) V curriculum. It offers the teacher a system of developmental objectives and procedures. The curriculum proposes six important assumptions relevant to teacher and school planning for the learning-disabled deaf child.

1. The same developmental sequence is followed as for other children.
2. A lack of prerequisite skills particularly hinders development.
3. Special attention to the structuring of his or her learning environment is needed.
4. Opportunities to learn outside the classroom are fewer than for other children.
5. More failure has been experienced than for most children.
6. The population is not homogeneous. (pp. 180–182)

Funderberg (1982) also considered the problems of the learning-disabled hearing-impaired child and suggested six special needs which the curriculum must meet: "memory problems, uneven learning skills, perceptional problems, motor problems, language problems, and attention and hyperactivity problems" (p. 62).

Brill (1974) reported guidelines for the development of an educational program for the slow-learning deaf child which include (1) the use of concrete stimulus materials, (2) vivid and attractive materials, (3) practical materials aimed at adult usefulness, (4) teaching to strengths rather than weaknesses, (5) a program that promotes a feeling of success, and (6) physical participation by the student in the learning process.

These considerations can certainly be applied more broadly to all hearing-impaired developmentally disabled children as a means of assessing the relevance of curricula to the children's needs. In addition, although most of these issues are met in the normal course of curricular planning, for the hearing-impaired developmentally disabled population, the special area of perceptual problems should focus the reader's attention on the importance of discriminating between sensory and perceptual levels in the child's input channels.

Donlon and Burton (1976) developed a curriculum for severely and profoundly handicapped children which grew out of research on the deaf-blind. They described programs for developing body image, experience with objects, tactile stimulation, olfactory and gustatory training, visual stimulation, movement in space, self-care skills, communication, socialization, and play. The authors focused on the earliest aspects of behavior which clearly precede the usual curricular structure of the preschool group.

This very early educational program blends nicely with curricula developed for deaf multihandicapped children at the California School for the Deaf at Riverside, the Colorado School for the Deaf and Blind, and the Kendall Demonstration Elementary School at Gallaudet College.

Sailor (1982) made a strong appeal for the delivery of curricula in the home and school environments, as opposed to delivery in an institutional setting. He described a matrix contrasting critical functions of the child's adaptation (eating, toileting, mobility, communication, and hygiene) with the setting in which the function is addressed by the teacher and practiced by the child. The settings include school, vocational areas, recreation, domestic, and community. The stress in his approach is on the mastery of a curricular item across the variety of locations in which the child must function. One could extend his idea to say that the achievement of the curricular goal may not be related as much to what the child learns as to how well this learning is applied in the variety of life circumstances.

Generic Severely/Profoundly Handicapped Curricula

The following curricula were not developed for the hearing-impaired developmentally disabled population per se, but for severely handicapped young children. Because these curricula for the trainable multihandicapped have been under development for a much longer time, the advantages of modifications through use may assist in selection of the most applicable features for programs for the hearing-impaired developmentally disabled.

The Los Angeles Unified School District (1981) prepared an Extended Skills Curriculum for preschool developmentally handicapped children. It is a highly preacademic program, with its major categories being reading, writing, oral language, mathematics, health education, music, art, mobility training, home economics, prevocational training, physical education, and science. Within those categories are components of value to a fundamental program plan. For example, although the first item of the curriculum is reading, which may seem high level for many children with impaired hearing and developmental disabilities, there are eight subtopics of that item. They are tracking, visual closure, visual discrimination, figure ground, decoding, vocabulary, study skills, and comprehension. This hierarchy for visual training is then developed through an extensive task analysis outline. The program is comprehensive in many ways and well developed in its presentation.

Perhaps Kissinger's (1981) sequential curriculum for the severely and profoundly mentally retarded/multihandicapped is one of the most fully stated traditional program displays. The major components and subcomponents presented in Table 3 are discussed in each identified area.

McCormack and Chalmers (1978) focused on the very early aspects of cognitive instruction with a detailed list of activities for matching, sorting, constructing, recognizing, identifying, remembering, and sequencing. These particular activities, treated in other curricula as parts of several categories, are presented by these authors as skills to be learned across curricular components. For example, sorting can be part of visual, auditory, and daily living activities. The notion that the children need certain basic skills prior to moving very far in any one curricular category is not without merit and reminds us of the very basic level at which the curriculum starts.

Table 3. Sequential Curricula

Sensory Development	Motor Development	Activities of Daily Living
Tactile Development	Gross Motor Development	Eating and Drinking
Reacts to tactile stimulation	Head control	Special problems
Explores objects tactually	Rolling	Eating
Matches objects tactually	Creeping and crawling	Self-feeding with a spoon
Auditory Development	Sitting	Using knife and fork
Identifies source of sound	Standing	Drinking
Discriminates sounds	Walking	Table manners
Reproduces sounds	Running	
Visual Development	Jumping and hopping	Toileting
Visually attends	Moving to music	Establishes a pattern of elimination
Visually tracks objects	Wheelchair mobility	Eliminates on toilet
Visually indentifies objects		Indicates toilet needs
	Fine Motor Development	Performs toileting procedures
	Reach	
	Grasp	Dressing and Undressing
	Manipulation	Undressing
		Dressing
		Appearance and clothing care
		Washing and Bathing
		Bathing
		Hand washing
		Hair care
		Nasal Hygiene
		Oral Hygiene
		Toothbrushing
		Oral care
Receptive Language	Awareness of People	Attending Skills
Identifies source of sound	Awareness of self	Attends to environment
Discriminates sounds	Awareness of others	Interacts with environment
Expressive Language	Play Activites	Attends to objects
Expresses self nonverbally	Basic Social Skills	Preacademic Skills
Vocalizes		Coordinates eye and hand movements
		Visually discriminates
		Auditorally discriminates
		Relates memory to environment

Note. From *A sequential curriculum for the severely and profoundly mentally retarded/ multihandicapped* (pp. XI-XIII) by E. Kissinger, 1981, Springfield, IL: Charles C. Thomas. Copyright 1981 by Charles C. Thomas. Reprinted by permission.

A program for severely handicapped students developed for the Madison (Wisconsin) Metropolitan School District (1978) divided curriculum into five domains: (1) domestic, (2) vocational, (3) recreational, (4) community functional, and (5) interactional (nonhandicapped). The last two categories are important and not often emphasized. They require that the severely handicapped have an opportunity to participate in community activities and learn to participate with the nonhandicapped.

Van Etten, Arkell, and Van Etten (1980) divided their curriculum for the severely and profoundly handicapped into three major stages: (1) sensory and sensorimotor development; (2) motor development; and (3) prevocational, vocational, and leisure skills. The first stage is concerned with early basic discriminatory and awareness activities that maintain and develop the child's contact with the learning environment. Stage 2 is typical of the traditional curricular areas of gross and fine motor development, self-help skills, communication, social and interpersonal skills, and cognitive skills in both preacademic and early academic activities. Stage 3, involving vocational and leisure activities, has often received the least attention.

Klein, Pasch, and Frew (1979) identified many of the components of curriculum already mentioned but suggest two—applications of basic skills to daily life and applications of appropriate reasoning and judgment in environmental mastery—which should draw the teacher's attention to the important problem of making the curriculum useful to children in daily life. Since immediate applicability of school learning to life does not always receive attention in curricula for nonhandicapped children, continuing reminders of the need for this kind of integration are important when planning for the hearing-impaired developmentally disabled child.

Antash (1977) divided major curricular components somewhat differently in the PUSH (Program Unlocking the Severely Handicapped) curriculum. His four major categories are (1) acquisition of body skills, (2) acquisition of concrete concepts, (3) acquisition of abstract concepts, and (4) acquisition of self-organization. This latter category is unique. Its subcategories include

- approaching and exploring an unfamiliar object or situation;
- choosing and executing actions to obtain a desired end;
- acting appropriately in environmental situations;
- using functional objects appropriately;
- performing routine actions at the appropriate time;
- acting appropriately in social situations; and
- using previously learned skills in new situations.

Other Related Curricula

When disabilities are severe and complex, there are many special aspects of learning that do not fit into the usual curricular structure. Examples include the problems of mobility training for the blind, the special problems of the cerebral palsied, and the unique problems of educational planning for the emotionally disturbed.

Orientation and mobility training for the multihandicapped deaf are required as the degree of visual loss becomes severe. Signorat and Watson (1981) described the steps involved in orientation and mobility training. The training begins in early childhood with motor training in such activities as balance ability and body awareness. The program also includes environmental awareness, stressing the special needs of the deaf child to develop and enhance his or her awareness of the physical world. This phase of the program requires the development of concepts inherent in spatial localization and form/function relationships, such as a vocabulary for right and left and other locatives. A third component of the training is an orientation referencing system; that is, a map-making concept that allows the child to become aware of alternative routes and the goals of mobility. Other program features include solo travel, route planning, and auditory training for mobility safety.

Lyndon and McGraw (1973), also concerned with the orientation and mobility of the visually handicapped, observed that the teaching of many subjects dealing with mobility was often hindered by the delayed general concept development of their students. Their suggestions about body image, gross motor movement, postures, tactile discrimination, sound, facial expression, and time and distance are comprehensive and practical. In addition to a detailed listing of teaching materials, techniques, and work area description, the authors presented thoughtful guidelines to draw the teacher's attention to the effects of these factors on a child's concept development.

Tretakoff's (1969) program recommendations showed a close similarity between curricula for hearing-impaired developmentally disabled children and curricula for retarded blind persons. In addition to frequently noted categories of curriculum, he added (1) the ability to deal with such cognitive problems as divergent and convergent thinking, creativity, memory, problem solving, and evaluation; and (2) the ability to deal with such affective problems as receiving attention, trust, motivation, independence, and achievement.

An experimental prevocational project concerned with multihandicapped young adults was described by Martino and Perla (1976). Their work, which serves to remind us that hearing-impaired developmentally disabled children will become adults, has five specific objectives.

1. Job-oriented academic skills in math, reading, language, social skills, and vocational concepts;
2. The development of a resource room with learning stations focused on specific prevocational activities;
3. Opportunities for the student to learn how to express affective concerns;
4. Enhanced student integration with the general deaf populations; and
5. Counsel and support of the student and vocational personnel involved.

Millham, Fannin, Brewer, and Caccamise (1974) described another prevocational program for retarded deaf students in the 7- to 17-year age group. Their program includes (1) a five-phase language and conceptual training program for the students, (2) a family counseling program involving group meetings, and (3) a communications training program for the parents.

Stewart (1982) discussed curriculum for severely emotionally disturbed hearing-impaired students. He pointed out that the curriculum must allow opportunities for old, patterned noncoping behaviors to be replaced by more appropriate response patterns. Although not a curriculum, the following guidelines for developing positive coping behaviors were recommended:

1. Identify the behaviors and reinforcing patterns that maintain maladaptive behavior;
2. Identify rewards for desirable behaviors;
3. Plan activities which eliminate maladaptive behavior and promote more positive behavior; and
4. Systematically evaluate progress.

An additional and important reference is Cruickshank's *Cerebral Palsy: A Developmental Disability* (1980). Curricular adaptation for problems of severe motor disorders is discussed in detail. Cruickshank (1967) also presented a comprehensive view of the needs of brain-injured children and outlined the educator's role in meeting the special problems associated with perceptual motor handicaps that result from childhood neurologic problems. He showed how these problems ultimately affect the developmental sequence. Although a curriculum as such is not presented, much of the value of this work lies in the innovative environmental controls suggested for shaping the child's learning environment. Chapters dealing with visual motor materials and activities, abstract concept development, and related teaching materials are detailed and amenable to adaptation for the hearing-impaired developmentally disabled child.

Guidelines for Choosing a Curriculum

Over the last few years, a number of curricula have been developed primarily for use with hearing-impaired students in both residential and mainstream environments and for multihandicapped students. Few curricula, however, have been designed specifically to meet the needs of hearing-impaired developmentally disabled children. As we have seen, those that have been developed are frequently adaptations of curricula used with such other disability groups as the deaf-blind or the physically disabled.

Because so many curricula could be adapted for programs serving hearing-impaired developmentally disabled children, 15 guidelines are useful for minimizing haphazard curriculum selection and maximizing an appropriate program-to-curricula match.

1. The curriculum must be flexible enough to be adapted to heterogeneous groups of hearing-impaired developmentally disabled children.

    Most programs providing such services more often than not serve students with varying and compounding disabilities. A curriculum that is not modifiable to meet the needs of such heterogeneous groups will need to be supplemented from other curricula or perhaps discarded.

2. The abilities and competencies of the teachers charged with carrying out the curriculum must be realistically evaluated.

    Instructional personnel must have inservice training and coursework in areas appropriate to varying aspects of the curriculum. Appropriate selection of curricular activities calls for individuals well trained and experienced in working with hearing-impaired developmentally disabled students. People unfamiliar with needs of this group may have expectation levels that are too high or too low and thus may be unprepared to set realistic goals for each of the children.

3. The physical plant must meet the space and activity needs of the curriculum.

   The learning environment must be modified to meet the needs of students who are physically impaired or whose additional sensory disabilities warrant an environment suitable for their unique needs. Hearing-impaired students with other disabilities may need an environment that provides reduced sensory stimulation and/or one without physical barriers that would inhibit their mobility from one activity area to another.

4. Support staff should be available as needed to meet both intracurricular and extracurricular aspects of the program.

   To fully implement a curriculum, such support staff as residential living supervisors and teacher aides will, in all probability, be necessary to individualize a program. The support staff must be trained to meet the needs of this unique population.

5. The services of speech/language pathologists and other nonteaching professionals should be considered as part of the curriculum and not "ancillary services" as they are typically regarded.

6. The curriculum should be adaptable to the primary receptive and expressive communication mode of each child in the class.

   One must be concerned with whether or not the concepts identified in the curriculum can be modified to meet communication needs of the hearing-impaired developmentally disabled student. Does the curriculum take into consideration the instructional needs of the students, permitting them to use any of the varied modes for learning and expression?

7. The curriculum should be appropriate to the children's developmental level.

   Can the students progress through the curriculum stages in such a way that successful and meaningful experiences are provided as well as experiences that challenge their creativity and cognitive abilities? If the material being taught is on an inappropriate developmental level for the student, then boredom, confusion, or lack of progress may result. Great care must be taken to ensure that concepts, skills, and abilities taught are relevant to the everyday lives of the students.

8. The materials associated with the curriculum should be appropriate for the auditory and visual acuity and processing of the children in the class.

   In any class of hearing-impaired developmentally disabled students, one can expect to find individuals with varying auditory and visual acuity and processing abilities. Thus, appropriate assessment and evaluation of curricular activities using these modalities must be accomplished prior to assuming that all children in a class can benefit. For example, reception of connected discourse through sign language, or understanding a printed or graphic visual display, requires the processing of complex information. Existence of the required abilities should not be assumed; it should be assessed through a hierarchy of activities designed to reveal the congruence of the materials with the child's abilities.

9. The curriculum should accommodate the needs of physically disabled students.

Can the curricular activities be modified to meet the needs of those with gross or fine motor disabilities? Can students who are wheelchair bound and/or have other perhaps more subtle motor problems benefit from activities designed for children without these limitations? Special equipment purchase or modification may be necessary to ensure that children with such physical limitations can benefit from the activities specified in the curriculum.

10. The curriculum should contain alternatives which take into account possible additional health problems of the children.

Children with developmental disabilities frequently experience health problems or may need continuing medication, either of which may require modifications in the educational programming. The instructor should be aware of each student's medication needs and of possible side effects that could impede that student's progress. Similarly, the teacher must also be aware of medically indicated restrictions of physical activity. Unless an appropriate match is made between the physical vitality of the student and the curricular experiences, the teacher will not be able to predict if one is adversely affecting the other. Therefore, a curriculum that takes into account the possibility of such limitations is the preferable choice.

11. The social and emotional development of the student should constitute a part of the curriculum.

Consequently, the choice of curriculum should be predicated on its inclusion of those skills and functions best learned at home or in the dormitory under the supervision of the family caretakers or residential living staff.

12. The curriculum should provide opportunities to learn to manage increasingly difficult life situations.

Learning to deal with frustrating situations can be a positive aspect of a curriculum. If the curriculum is appropriately challenging, frustrating situations will naturally arise; they must be dealt with so that continued self-esteem results. Acting-out behaviors may be more prevalent in this population; thus, the curriculum should address strategies for behavior management and the channeling of energy in a positive direction.

13. The curriculum should ensure the transferability of learned skills to daily living and real-life problems and situations.

The curriculum selected or developed should be concrete, encompassing real-life situations. Activities should relate to the everyday experiences of home or dormitory life. For example, language lessons can relate to such everyday experiences as recent visits to a community event. Another example is role playing, which may assist the student to choose the appropriate behavior for a specific real-life situation.

14. The curriculum should foster the skills needed to succeed in a less restrictive environment.

    The term "least restrictive environment" evolved from Public Law 94-142. This concept should be thought of in terms of moving a student from an environment modified to meet personal needs to a less structured environment in which the successful student will be able to participate and function appropriately. Least restrictive should not connote brick and mortar; it should imply levels of independence and participation on an equal basis. The curriculum should guide the student from dependence to as much independence and decision making as is possible. Least restrictive certainly includes increasing interaction with nonhandicapped peers.

15. A curriculum should include procedures for regular evaluation of student progress and confirmation of both short- and long-range goals.

    The curriculum should include a method for assessing the movement of the student through its stages or be adaptable for such evaluation procedures. It should provide appropriate breadth and depth for students capable of higher stages of functioning. Evaluation of progress through the curriculum must be reviewed within a framework of overall assessment information and decisions regarding appropriateness of placement.

Implementation Concerns for the Curriculum Development Planner

Clearly, many developments still need to occur in the design and refinement of curricula in order to meet all the contingencies arising for such a heterogeneous group of handicapping conditions as occur in the hearing-impaired developmentally disabled population. Unfortunately, even the best available curricula will not always provide maximal success for every child. The following are some factors that impede the effective use of curricula.

Tweedie and Baud (1981) surveyed teachers of deaf-blind children to determine factors that might improve or worsen the education of deaf-blind children. The findings appear particularly apropos for the hearing-impaired developmentally disabled population as well. Identified problems, in order of probability of occurrence, were:

1. Decreased emphasis on academic skills;

2. A teacher training emphasis on severe and profound handicaps rather than specialization in the area of deaf-blind education;

3. Integration of deaf-blind students into classes for severely and profoundly handicapped children;

4. Fewer residential programs;

5. Increased class size;

6. Higher teacher attrition (see Chapter 17); and

7. Decreased individualized instruction due to mainstreaming.

If these trends are realized, then each can clearly be seen as a factor limiting curricular effectiveness. If all were to occur, the result would be fewer but larger classes; some of the severely multihandicapped deaf children would be mainstreamed on the basis of expediency or assumed cost reduction, while others might be improperly placed, as in the past, in classes for the severely and profoundly mentally retarded. In this eventuality, the majority of hearing-impaired developmentally disabled children might never encounter a curriculum specifically designed for their problems.

Despite these predictions of future problems by informed members of the profession, some current problems have notably interfered with curricular implementation for a long time.

Curriculum and Institutional Setting

When a child has more than one handicapping condition, a special challenge is placed on the curriculum planning team. For example, is a deaf retarded child different from a retarded deaf child? This may seem a small semantic difference, but, in reality, it may have a profound effect on the child's educational placement and thus determine the curricular focus and the subsequent reinforcement of newly acquired skills. If the child is placed in a class for the retarded in a school for the deaf, she or he will likely encounter certain predictable extracurricular language, communication, and adaptive life-style patterns. Most of the children in the school for the deaf will have manual or oral communication skills in common and will thus be able to share a wider variety of ideas and feelings. If the same child were placed in a class for deaf children in a school for the retarded, she or he would probably have more difficulty communicating outside the classroom; even the support staff might not be able to communicate freely with such a child. The curriculum in the two situations might be quite comparable, but the cognitive and affective aspects of the curricular learning experiences will not be as equally reinforced in both settings. Therefore, the educational setting in which the curriculum is delivered is of considerable importance to the hearing-impaired developmentally disabled student.

Teacher Certification Laws

One of the barriers to real improvement in services is teacher certification laws. There is no specific certification for those teaching hearing-impaired developmentally disabled children. A common pattern is for a teacher to be certified in one disability area, such as mental retardation. With a minimum of additional training, perhaps only three courses, such a teacher can obtain a second certification in, for example, the area of deafness. However, a teacher so trained and certified is unlikely to have the knowledge and skills one would desire in a professional working with hearing-impaired developmentally disabled youth. Certification for teaching the multihandicapped is even less adequate. Such certification does not exist in some states. In others, the requirements are so generic that they do not provide the knowledge and skills necessary for dealing effectively with hearing-impaired developmentally disabled people. The net effect is that while government, with one hand, is supporting the establishment of high-quality programs, it is creating a major obstacle to such quality programming with the other hand, in the form of its teacher certification laws.

Curriculum and Teacher Training

Few, if any, teachers are prepared to undertake a curriculum designed for the hearing-impaired developmentally disabled child with complete training in all areas of importance: motor development, sensory development, cognitive development, communicative development, social development, and affective development. The limited training each teacher will bring to curriculum implementation may differ depending upon the type of exposure the training institution provides or the practicum teaching experiences that have been encouraged. The major distinction to be considered is whether the teacher received a broad exposure to the range of programs and educational methods available across disability domains, or whether he or she was programmed in a highly doctrinaire system that rejected consideration of alternate approaches required by the individual hearing-impaired developmentally disabled child.

The differences between aural/oral and manual communication orientations, skills, and philosophies are well known and documented. Yet, there are many other contrasts of equal importance to be considered. Not all of the educators fully understand and make use of such systems as the Tadoma methods, American Sign Language, or Signed English. They differ in the orientation they take to total communication, use of natural gestures, or speech training. Dealing with hearing-impaired developmentally disabled children demands that the teacher have a flexible attitude toward curriculum adaptation to fit the requirements of programs and individual children.

Similar difficulties arise when teachers are trained with a particular educational orientation and are employed at a school in which the administration believes in a different orientation. In the areas of emotional disturbance or social adjustment management, the teacher may have an orientation to an iconoclastic system, such as Wood's (1975) developmental therapy program, or to a rational adaptive orientation, such as Strain's (1980). If the teacher is trained in one system and required to work in the other, curriculum adaptation problems may occur.

In the case of educational approaches to mental retardation, the most identifiable dichotomy in teacher orientation is between orientation to specific token learning systems and orientation to more rational adaptive systems such as a Piagetian approach. When a curriculum is based on one of these models and the teacher's training is in the other, problems and adjustments are predictable.

When dealing with blind children in the hearing-impaired developmentally disabled population, the teacher may have a background that is heavily oriented to low-vision programs, or the teacher may have been trained to teach compensatory skills and focus on Braille and tactile learning experiences. The choice has important implications for long-term placement of the child.

Some teachers trained in the area of motor disabilities may have studied in a context of medical and electromechanical control of the motor problem, while other teachers may have studied perceptual/motor training such as Cruickshank (1967) described. Even within this latter area, wide differences in philosophical orientation exist.

There have always been and probably always will be highly divergent educational approaches and philosophies for each of the major problems of these children. Different philosophies will lead to variations in teacher training and institutional (or school) curriculum. Effective continuity of the curriculum will depend on adequate inservice training not only for teachers but for all "significant others" who interact with children in a prescribed program. As newly trained teachers arrive with new ideas, curricular modification will always occur.

Curriculum and Communication Modality

It is generally recognized that the goal of language development will be stressed in curricula for all categories of exceptionality. At the functional level, the importance of an agreed upon language development approach is most important. In addition, the communication modality through which the child will convey language is a curricular consideration of great importance. The curriculum will undoubtedly have some goals for language development and some for communicative modality development. It should be recognized that, aside from the curricula delivered by the teacher in the classroom, there will probably be other specialists, such as speech/language pathologists and audiologists, who will also be planning a language and expressive modality treatment program. A mechanism must be created for the coordination of language and communication modality training within the curriculum and extracurricularly.

The population is quite heterogeneous in its range of communication modalities. Expressive systems include speech, picture boards, Bliss symbolics, spelling gloves, electronic speech synthesizers, the Tadoma methods, natural gesture, signing, manual spelling, Braille, opticon, and some very personalized programs. Few who read this list will be skillful in all or even several of the possible alternatives they will encounter or should be able to offer.

However, the fact remains that the success of the communicative modality program both within the curriculum and extracurricularly will depend on the degree to which the teachers, speech/language pathologists, parents, and support staff are able to use and reinforce the system needed for each child. And, it seems safe to say, the effectiveness of communicative modality usage will influence the success of the language curriculum which, in turn, will no doubt determine the speed and depth of cognitive and social learning. The competence of the teachers and significant others in the use of the child's most useful communicative modality cannot be overstressed as a basis for the implementation and generalization of the curriculum.

The Value of Very Early Intervention

Most of the research on programs for hearing-impaired developmentally disabled children stresses the value of early intervention. Appell (1982) reviewed several of the studies and concluded, "delayed intervention, that is, waiting until the severely handicapped hearing-impaired child is three years old, contributes to feelings of incompetence for both the infant and the caregiver" (p. 183). Although the value of early intervention has not been well documented for its effect on later life success, the value of the preparation of children for "school-age" curricula seems well supported.

Population Distribution

In rural and less populated areas of the country, the opportunity to group children homogeneously diminishes. To provide services at all, children are often grouped with those who live nearby rather than those who have the same needs and disabilities. When this happens, the flexibility of the curriculum is tested to its limits, and the competencies of the teachers are constantly challenged. This limitation has, of course, been a factor in developing residential institutional programs that bring together children for more homogeneous grouping. In the past decade, a national mood supporting de-institutionalization and mainstreaming has joined a conflict not yet resolved over the relative merits of homogeneous classes in residential institutions versus heterogeneous classes in the home community. Each approach has value, and the problem obviously needs careful study. In the meantime, this educational/philosophical dilemma can produce situations in which some children will be placed in programs with less than ideal curricula.

Parent Involvement

The curriculum is clearly associated with "the school" in the minds of families. It is sometimes seen as a plan etched in stone, a map, with the teacher as the guide. The family must come to know that, for a child who is severely, profoundly, or multiply disabled, the curriculum is related to the development of all life skills. Family involvement is critical to reinforce and practice daily living skills with the child. The curriculum will be most successfully accomplished when the family is involved in this generalization of curriculum to life activities.

References

Antash, A. (1977). *PUSH: A program guide for severely multiply handicapped children.* New York: Meeting Street School.

Appell, M. W. (1982). Early education for the severely handicapped/hearing impaired child. In R. Campbell & V. Baldwin (Eds.), *Severely handicapped/hearing impaired students.* Baltimore: Brookes.

Brill, R. (1974). *Education of the deaf: Administrative and professional developments.* Washington, DC: Gallaudet College Press.

Crosby, K. (1982). Implementing the developmental model. In J. Gardiner, L. Long, R. Nichols, & D. Laguilli (Eds.), *Program issues and developmental disabilities.* Baltimore: Brookes.

Cruickshank, W. (1967). *The brain injured child in home, school or community.* Syracuse: Syracuse University Press.

Cruickshank, W. (1980). *Cerebral palsy: A developmental disability.* Syracuse: Syracuse University Press.

Curtis, W., & Donlon, E. (1978). *Meeting the needs of the school aged child.* Paper presented at the AAMD Special Training Institute, Denver, CO.

Donlon, E. T., & Burton, L. (1976). *The severely and profoundly handicapped: A practical approach to teaching.* New York: Grune and Stratton.

Ewing, I. R., & Ewing, A. W. G. (1961). *New opportunities for deaf children.* London: University of London Press.

Funderburg, R. (1982). The role of the classroom teacher in the assessment of the learning-disabled hearing-impaired child. In D. Tweedie & E. Shroyer (Eds.), *The multihandicapped hearing impaired* (pp. 61–74). Washington, DC: Gallaudet College Press.

Kissinger, E. (1981). *A sequential curriculum for the severely and profoundly mentally retarded/multihandicapped.* Springfield, IL: Charles C. Thomas.

Klein, N., Pasch, M., & Frew, T. (1979). *Curriculum analysis and design for retarded learners.* Columbus, OH: Charles E. Merrill.

Los Angeles Unified School District, Division of Special Education. (1981). *Extended skills curriculum.* Los Angeles: Author.

Lund, K., & Bos, C. (1981). Orchestrating the preschool classroom. *Teaching Exceptional Children, 14*(3), 120–125.

Lyndon, W. T., & McGraw, M. L. (1973). *Concept development for visually handicapped children.* New York: American Foundation for the Blind.

Madison Metropolitan School District. (1978). *Curricular strategies for developing longitudinal intervention between severely handicapped students and others and curricular strategies for teaching severely handicapped students to acquire and perform skills in response to naturally occurring cues and correction procedures* (Monograph, Vol. 3, Part 1). Madison, WI: Author.

Martino, S., & Perla, R. (1976). Crossing the frontier: An experimental education program for multiply handicapped deaf students. *Journal of Rehabilitation of the Deaf, 10*(3), 1–18.

Mavilya, M. (1982). Assessment, curriculum, and intervention strategies for hearing-impaired mentally retarded children. In D. Tweedie & E. Shroyer (Eds.), *The multihandicapped hearing impaired* (pp. 113–123). Washington, DC: Gallaudet College Press.

McCormack, J. E., & Chalmers, A. J. (1978). *Teaching sequences: Early cognitive instruction for the moderately and severely handicapped.* Champaign, IL: Research Press.

Millham, J., Fannin, A., Brewer, D., & Caccamise, F. (1974). A program for mentally retarded deaf children and their families. *Journal of Rehabilitation of the Deaf, 8*(1), 43–58.

Restaino, L. (1982). A curriculum development project for the multihandicapped hearing-impaired child ten years later. In D. Tweedie & E. Shroyer (Eds.), *The multihandicapped hearing impaired* (pp. 162–182). Washington, DC: Gallaudet College Press.

Sailor, W. A. (1982). Commentary response, chapter 14. In R. Campbell & V. Baldwin (Eds.), *Severely handicapped hearing impaired students.* Baltimore: Brookes.

Signorat, M., & Watson, A. (1981). Orientation and mobility training for the multiply handicapped deaf. *Teaching Exceptional Children, 14*(3), 110–115.

Stewart, L. G. (1982). Developing the curriculum for severely disturbed hearing-impaired students. In D. Tweedie & E. Shroyer (Eds.), *The multihandicapped hearing impaired* (pp. 124–134). Washington, DC: Gallaudet College Press.

Strain, P. S. (1980). Social behavior programming with severely emotionally disturbed and autistic children. In B. Wilcox & A. Thompson (Eds.), *Critical issues in educating autistic children and youth*. Washington, DC: Bureau for Education of the Handicapped.

Tretakoff, M. I. (1969, March). *Proceedings of the regional institute on the blind child who functions at a retarded level*. New York: American Foundation for the Blind.

Tweedie, D., & Baud, H. (1981). Future directions in the education of deaf-blind multi-handicapped children and youth. *American Annals of the Deaf, 126,* 829–834.

Tweedie, D., & Shroyer, E. (Eds.). (1982). *The multihandicapped hearing impaired*. Washington, DC: Gallaudet College Press.

Tymitz-Wolf, B. (1982). Guidelines for assessing IEP goals and objectives. *Teaching Exceptional Children, 14*(5), 198–201.

Van Etten, V., Arkell, C., & Van Etten, C. (1980). *The severely and profoundly handicapped: Programs, methods, and materials*. St. Louis: C. V. Mosby.

Wilson, A. (1981). Curriculum selection for deaf blind severely handicapped. In *Understanding and educating the deaf blind/severely and profoundly handicapped* (pp. 133–182). Springfield, IL: Charles C. Thomas.

Wood, M. (1975). *Developmental therapy*. Baltimore: University Park Press.

Chapter 15

Selection of Augmentative Communication Systems

Howard C. Shane

Professional attention to people with severe communicative disorders has increased in recent years. Two principal factors have contributed to this escalated interest. First, there has been unparalleled professional optimism about the ability of severely handicapped individuals to achieve communicative competency through a means other than oral speech. Underlying this view has been a growing professional realization that current knowledge and techniques will not lead to all people becoming oral communicators. At the same time, innovative technological advances (including computer assistance) and applications of sign language offer avenues of expression heretofore unavailable to people with serious speech impairments. Thus, some segments of the professional community have begun to explore and accept alternative or augmentative communication solutions to the professional dilemma about remediating severe communication problems.

A second explanation for the growing awareness of the problems associated with severe speech impairment stems from attitude changes regarding handicapped citizens within society itself. Historically, large institutions were the most common living and educational arrangements for mentally retarded and congenitally physically disabled individuals. When habilitative professionals were available in these settings, they were typically few in number or lacked adequate training and instructional methodology to effect positive change in the communicative behaviors of their clientele. Recent ideological shifts and resultant legislation, however, have led to a general movement by society to deemphasize use of large residential facilities and to educate all people, regardless of their handicapping condition, within the community. As a result, considerably more people with serious speech impairments are seeking and receiving services in community-based clinics, schools, and hospitals. This increased demand for professional services, coupled with the potential to incorporate technology into meaningful treatment, has led to the current optimistic climate for developing the communicative potential of those with serious speech impairments.

In 1981, the American Speech-Language-Hearing Association published a position paper on nonspeech communication (Ad Hoc Committee, 1981; see Appendix). In that position statement, augmentative communication procedures were described as methods designed to supplement whatever vocal skills the individual may have. Figure 1 is a schematic diagram of the three components requisite for any individual (speaking or nonspeaking) to achieve communicative competence: a technique, a symbol set/system, and communicative interactive behavior. As shown in Figure 1, the technique or the means to transmit ideas can be of two types, aided and unaided. The term *unaided* refers to methods of transmission of ideas that do not require any physical assistance. Manual gestures or signs, expression through facial or body movement, and speech itself are examples of unaided techniques. The term *aided* refers to techniques that require use of some physical object or device. Communication boards or advanced microprocessor-based communications systems are examples of aided communication techniques.

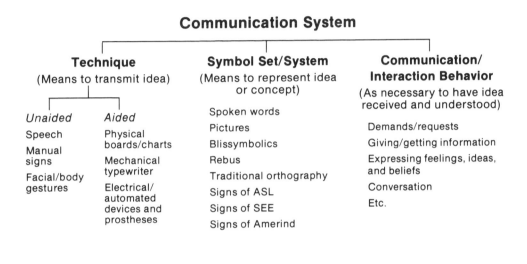

Figure 1. Communication system. From "ASHA Position Statement on Nonspeech Communication" by the Ad Hoc Committee on Communication Processes for Nonspeaking Persons, 1981, *Asha, 23,* p. 578. Copyright 1981 by American Speech-Language-Hearing Association. Reprinted by permission.

The second aspect of a communication system, the symbol set, is used to represent ideas and concepts. Thoughts and ideas are expressed through this symbol set whether transmitted through the medium of a physical device or through movement of some part of the human anatomy. Several symbol-set options are noted in the middle column of Figure 1.

Finally, for a communication system to be fully functional, it must allow for interactive communication. A communication system, therefore, must minimally provide the expressor with the means to give or seek information, to make demands on others, and to express feelings and beliefs, as well as to perform other communicative functions.

The Election Decision Process

The purpose of this chapter is to provide criteria upon which to base the decision to employ an unaided (e.g., manual sign language) or an aided (e.g., communication board) technique for a child requiring augmentative means to support communication.

Thus, the focus will be principally with the clinical decision making that surrounds the first component of an augmentative communication system—the technique or the means to transmit ideas. For the person who is nonspeaking, hearing impaired, and developmentally disabled, the clinician must choose between an augmentative or a supplemental system. For our purposes, the reader should assume that the person under clinical consideration exhibits a communication problem severe enough to warrant introduction of a supplemental communication strategy. Shane and Bashir (1980) referred to the process of determining candidacy for an augmentative communication system as the "election decision process." Once it is determined that supplemental procedures will enhance an individual's overall communication, a second level of decision making occurs to determine whether an aided or unaided procedure is most appropriate. This second level of decision making has received virtually no attention in the clinical literature.

The decision to employ an augmentative or supplemental communication procedure should be based upon a critical review of the candidate's current communication abilities and future potential for intelligible speech production. Ideally, the decision is arrived at jointly by a team of professionals knowledgeable about supplemental communication methods and about the people with whom the candidate lives, works, socializes, and learns. Families and some professionals are often reluctant, however, to introduce an augmentative communication system. Typically their hesitation relates to a fear that such a system will inhibit further speech development, believing that the user will become dependent upon the augmenting technique at the expense of trying to improve or initiate speech. As a result, augmentative communication techniques have become a treatment procedure of last resort and not an early intervention procedure.

It is this writer's clinical impression that the introduction of a supplemental procedure serves to facilitate rather than inhibit speech production and that early intervention of this kind has a prophylactic effect overall. In addition, the considerable frustration associated with early failure to produce speech is often reduced by the use of the supplemental communication method, which, in turn, prevents development of other maladaptive behaviors and fosters the individual's capability to benefit from speech therapy.

To summarize, when speech failure is leading to frustration and an apparent performance discrepancy between expressive communicative potential and current expressive abilities, a supplemental communication strategy should be considered. Families and professionals should be aware, however, that such approaches are meant to augment and not to replace speech. In fact, the reality of clinical practice suggests that combined methods are often used to promote communicative competence in the person who is nonspeaking.

This chapter is structured so as to add to the clinician's store of personal knowledge on the topic of system selection by identifying user-specific and environmental factors that must be considered in employing one technique over another.

Criteria for System Selection

In the early days of augmentative communication systems, fairly naive criteria were used to determine an appropriate system for a particular user. One rule of thumb, for example, was that if a person could walk, then he or she should use sign language (an unaided approach). A second rule of thumb was that if a person had cerebral palsy, then a communication aid (aided approach) was appropriate. These criteria for decision making, though simplistic by today's standards, do acknowledge the need to consider the individual's motor capabilities in prescribing a communication system. Clearly missing from these criteria are a number of additional factors which we now recognize as critical to prescribing a system that is relevant to the user. These factors include consideration of the individual's cognitive abilities; the different environments in which the system will be used; and the attitudes of various family members, friends, and teachers who will support the user in employing the system.

Factor 1: Extremity Motor Control

The first factor to consider in testing various system options is the person's upper extremity motor control abilities viewed in conjuction with his or her level of language comprehension. At what level does the person comprehend language? How easily and successfully can the person move his or her upper extremities for communicative purposes? Is control of the upper extremities sufficient to allow the system in question to be usable for expressive communication? In essence, does the person have enough control of the upper extremities to equalize or bring together any existing gap between language comprehension and production abilities? If so, a sign system or other gestural system could be warranted, based at least on this aspect of motor control ability. In this case, the gestural system selected must be one that allows the individual to communicate expressively on a level commensurate with his or her comprehension abilities. For a child who comprehends at a 5-year-old level, for example, the professional would want to choose an expressive communication technique that would allow the child to reach the 5-year level. In essence, the level of comprehension serves as the standard to which one attempts to raise production.

How does one examine upper extremity control for use of a manual sign system, such as American Sign Language (ASL)? The method that follows is a procedure described by Shane and Wilbur (1980). In their investigation, Shane and Wilbur used a motor task analysis of ASL comprising 63 distinct handshapes, locations, and motions as suggested by Stokoe, Casterline, and Croneberg (1965). Using a several hundred word initial signing lexicon proposed by Fristoe and Lloyd (1980), each lexical entry was analyzed according to the 63 distinct motor factors. Table 1 (next page) contains a summary of the most common motor movements.

An examination of the table shows that the need to produce a flat hand, for example, occurs with 30 percent of the signs in that vocabulary and presumably in American Sign Language in general; the ability to extend the index finger is needed for 26 percent of ASL signs; a curved hand appears in 17 percent of signs; a fist in 14 percent; and touching the thumb in 5 percent. When trying to determine an individual's ability to benefit from ASL as an unaided communication technique, one might conclude that if a person could not accomplish these five motor components individually, then, assuming the additive nature of these criteria, he or she would be unable to perform approximately 90 percent of the signs of American Sign Language.

Shane and Wilbur also found (Table 1, next page) that the movement of putting one's hands against one's chest occurs in 37 percent of the signs of ASL; that a hands-together movement is required for 32 percent of the signs; and that movement of

Table 1. **Summary of Motor Components Used in 5 percent or More of Analyzed Core Vocabulary**

Motor Component	Percentage of Occurence
Location	98.9
Chest	37.0
Hand	32.9
Face	29.0
Handshape	92.8
Flat hand	30.2
Index finger	26.2
Curved hand	17.0
Fist	14.4
Thumb touch	5.0
Motion	99.1
Linear	52.8
Handshape	11.3
Rotate/twist	9.2
Repeat	7.3
Circular	7.3
Arc	5.6
Hold	5.3

Note. From "Potential for Expressive Signing Based on Motor Control," by H. C. Shane and R. B. Wilbur, 1980, *Sign Language Studies, 29,* p. 339. Copyright 1980 by Linstok Press. Reprinted by permission.

hands in the vicinity of the face is required for 29 percent of the signs. It seems that similar criteria and procedures are needed and should be developed to ascertain the user-appropriateness of gestural systems other than ASL, such as American Indian Hand Talk (Amerind; Skelly, 1979).

Factor 2: Motor Speech Involvement

A second motor-related factor to consider when assessing a person's candidacy for an aided or unaided system is the presence of a motor speech condition which includes either dysarthria or apraxia of speech. Although these conditions relate to the oral motor system, their confirmed presence nevertheless has possible consequences for upper extremity motor control.

Dysarthria is defined by Darley, Aronson, and Brown (1969) as a collective name for a group of speech disorders resulting from disturbances in muscular control over the speech mechanism due to damage to the central or peripheral nervous system. It designates problems in oral communication due to paralysis, weakness, or in-coordination of the speech musculature. Apraxia of speech, on the other hand, is an articulatory disorder resulting from brain damage in which the programming or motor planning of articulatory movements is impaired. Clinically, it is imperative, first, to determine the presence of a motor speech condition and, second, to differentially diagnose between a dysarthria and an apraxia of speech. This differentiation has obvious treatment implications. More specifically, knowledge of the nature of the motor speech condition leads to selection of varying treatment procedures.

Presence of the more extreme or severe form of speech apraxia or dysarthria (referred to as anarthria) quite often results in the clinical decision to introduce an augmentative communication system (Shane & Bashir, 1980). This decision occurs because a severe motor speech condition typically requires intensive therapeutic efforts to produce noticeable oral speech gains. Quite often, the introduction of an augmentative communication system allows effective expressive communication to take place while speech therapy is ongoing. For many people, the frustration often associated with an inability to speak is thus ameliorated by the introduction of a supplemental communication system.

The presence of dysarthria can act as a "red flag" indicating that the upper extremities, like the motor speech system, are plagued by paralysis, weakness, or incoordination of varying degrees of severity. Symptomatically, this can translate, at one end of the continuum, into a mild interference with fine motor control (which may appear as clumsiness) or, at the other end of the continuum, into an inability to achieve accurately any discernible handshape, location, or motion configuration. The presence of an apraxia of speech presents a different clinical issue. Because a speech apraxia disrupts motor planning in the child or adult, the effects of a more generalized apraxic involvement may be manifested in difficulty with movement sequences performed by the upper extremities. Thus, the presence of a motor speech disorder might suggest the presence of a motor control problem that may adversely influence the movement of the upper extremities. The latter may stem from neuromuscular weakness or motor planning difficulty.

Bashir, from the Boston Children's Hospital Medical Center, often says that one's mouth does what one's hands do. It follows that the person with a dysarthria or an apraxia of speech may very well have some apraxic involvement of the limbs and some upper extremity motor control difficulties as well. In clinical examination of the dysarthric or apraxic person, one wants to examine the clarity and precision of observable gestures and attempt to ascertain the extent to which the person uses gestures to communicate. Many of the nonspeaking children that we see use gestures much more effectively than they use oral speech. The presence of cerebral palsy certainly affects our thinking about a person's use of upper extremities to equalize his or her comprehension-production gap. In addition, the presence of apraxia—whether limb apraxia, truncal apraxia, or developmental apraxia of speech—may result in a person using sign in much the same way that he or she executes speech, or executing speech in much the same way that he or she executes other motor movement, that is, with possibly poor organization, planning, and delivery.

Factor 3: User Characteristics

A third factor to be examined is user-related characteristics. These range from the personal preferences of the user to the presence of environmental supports that increase the user's receptivity to the system and the likelihood that it may be comfortably employed across environments and with people with whom the user interacts.

Picture Oriented. Some candidates, for example, are picture oriented; they spend a lot of time with pictures that arouse their interest. They match them, look at them for extended periods of time, and derive meaning from them. The child who is picture oriented is often found to develop his or her own "spontaneous" communication aid using magazines and family albums to communicate special events or to request items or services. For that child, it would make sense to think about a communication aid, since he or she is already showing that such a method will be successful.

Gesture Oriented. Other people are, conversely, gesture oriented; they have a tendency or talent to invent very complex gestures to communicate needs or ideas. For the child who has developed a gestural inventory, one might want to encourage use of a more formal gesture or sign language system as a natural extension to the spontaneous gestural inventory.

Previous Exposure. In addition to examining the candidate's particular orientation or communication style, one must examine his or her previous exposure to and success or failure with various system options.

Many individuals arrive at our clinic with a successful history of communication aid or sign language use. Other children, who may have had several years of solid instruction in learning sign language, show little signing capability for the amount of time and instruction invested. Examining a child's history and experience with communication system options helps the clinician decide whether previous methods have or have not reaped lasting positive results. This writer's clinical experience has shown that, even in one clinical session, some students may demonstrate marked potential for a communication technique other than the one previously taught.

One example is J. D., a 5-year, 5-month-old boy with a diagnosis of moderate mental retardation, severe language disorder, and suspected dysarthria. For the previous two years he had been involved in a total communication signing classroom with five other children of a similar skill level. He reportedly comprehended 12 functional signs, produced 3 signs (eat, drink, and toilet), but used only 1 sign (eat) spontaneously.

We exposed J. D. to a $12'' \times 18''$ communication aid containing $1\frac{1}{2}''$ concrete line-drawings of 20 familiar items. He immediately demonstrated recognition by pointing to each item upon request. After a 20-minute training session he was able to spontaneously request 10 different items and comment on an ongoing activity.

Availability. Another user-related factor to consider in weighing system options is aid availability, including its size, power source, and physical accessibility. The author has seen many communication aids that are so heavy and immobile that they are "available" only to a person who spends a great deal of time in a wheelchair. Many lightweight aids are similarly unavailable because they are too awkward to carry or fold.

Certainly, our hands are our most useful, flexible communication aids. For this reason, the unaided sign system is preferred over all other systems because of its availability across people and environments. For the child who has proficient use of his or her hands, perhaps the closest aided option to use of the hands alone is a communication aid that either is small or can be folded to fit into a pocket. These aid characteristics ensure its availability for the majority of the user's interactive needs. Availability is a critical concern when selecting an aid(s) appropriate to the child's academic, social, and personal self-care needs.

Familiarity. How familiar are the child's parents, teachers, and playmates with the communication aid in question? This is a critical user-related factor. Today, most people are aware of or familiar with sign language, and many people—both human service professionals and otherwise—are being exposed to automated communication aids. Anyone who watches the children's television program "Sesame Street" will observe a considerable amount of signing; and while this author has yet to see a communication aid on television, he suggests that the time to introduce one is certainly here.

Willingness. The willingness of the listener to employ a communication aid or technique is a user-related factor closely associated with listener familiarity. Many people will tell you that they are willing to introduce a particular system into one or more domains in a child's life; however, the clinician must be careful to ascertain the exact nature and extent of that willingness before selecting a system. At the same time, good clinical work can help shape this willingness.

Preference. Another factor to consider is the preference of the person who will be employing the system (the communicator) and the preferences of the people who will be receiving the communication (friends, family, teachers). All things being equal, user and listener receptivity to a particular system is the critical determinant in choosing one system over another. The professional will often hear, for example, that sign language is not indicated for a certain child because no one in his or her environment appreciates what the signs mean. Oftentimes, this statement is enough to suggest that people significant to the user will not learn signing or take the time to become competent in its use. Without such cooperation from significant people in the user's environment, system success is far from guaranteed.

A "User" Community. Hearing-impaired developmentally disabled children eventually become hearing-impaired developmentally disabled adults. Another major consideration, then, is the availability of a user community in which the adult can feel at home. Despite the unquestionable value of, for example, voice-synthesis communication boards for communication with the hearing/speaking majority of society, these are still very artificial and uncomfortable for constant communication because of rate, language level, etc. Sign language, to a degree even in simplified forms, carries a unique advantage in that there is an existing user community to which the hearing-impaired developmentally disabled adult may be able to relate more naturally and spontaneously than any currently available device permits. Clinicians and families must not be allowed to lose sight of the fact that children do not long remain children, and their communication world will not remain limited to family and school forever. Being able to integrate socially into a minority language community of signers can be far more supportive of adult development than can always clumsy and always limited interaction with a larger world not attuned to device-using for ordinary day-to-day communication interaction.

Training. Training is another factor requiring consideration in deciding between an aided and an unaided technique. Training relates not only to instruction of the user but also refers to the intensity of training required for listeners in the environments in which that user will reside, socialize, be educated, and work. Generally speaking, the fewer people one needs to train, the better.

Secondary Benefits. Another area of consideration is the potential for positive benefits secondary to communicative competence. For example, a communication aid often is an ideal bridge between a child's academic curriculum (especially the reading program) and his or her symbol system. Specifically, one can use the aid to augment reading activities. Creative use of a communication aid may have other far-reaching effects. If one views the communication aid as an integral part of the school experience, then material being introduced as part of the curriculum can be incorporated into the communication aid program. Thus, the child would have an opportunity to demonstrate understanding of a lesson by selecting vocabulary specific to that lesson on the communication aid. Symbols designating size concepts (e.g., big/little) placed on the communication aid can help the user demonstrate recognition of the concept during instruction; they may also be incorporated into daily experiences where their use will be generalized.

The more typical the symbol set that the nonspeaking person uses, the more likely it is that the individual may be integrated into a more typical academic setting. If signs are a person's only symbol set, for example, it may be extremely difficult to mainstream that individual into a more typical educational environment. On the other hand, being able to express one's self through the alphabet may have the opposite positive effect. One option is to employ a symbol set that serves the person on his or her communication aid and also assists the person in learning signs. Employing pictured signs as the symbol set on the communication aid could facilitate learning of the actual sign being taught simultaneously.

The potential for voice output from a communication aid is a significant advantage that an aided technique has over an unaided technique. Voice offers the user the distinct advantage of communicating with people unable or unwilling to comprehend the meaning of signed expressions or graphic symbols. In addition to audience expansion, vocal expression increases one's opportunities to interject, to communicate in the dark, and to get attention from a distance.

Rate. Rate of expression is another factor that enters into the decision of whether to employ an aided or an unaided technique. The fact that one can communicate through sign at rates comparable to a normal speaking rate gives signing the advantage in this category. The rate of expression using communication aids, although increasing with microprocessor-based assistance, generally remains below 30 words per minute.

Perceptions by Others. The final user-related factor to consider is the effect the system's use will have on other people's perceptions of the user. Will he or she be perceived as being similar to and acceptable by other people or different from them in a negative way by virtue of using the technique in question? This factor, considered in Wolfensberger's (1972) philosophy of normalization, is a crucial determinant in system selection. The chosen system should not only increase the user's communicative competence but also present a valued perception of the user in the eyes of people with whom he or she interacts. No system should increase social barriers between the speaker and the listener. The clinician should attempt to prescribe those systems that will maximize the user's opportunities for desired social integration.

Multiple System Use

It is not unusual to find a situation in which several communication systems are used in order to optimize interaction. The selection of multiple communication strategies requires both a willingness on the part of the user to shift communication modes and a competence by the instructor to teach multiple approaches.

In this regard, a kind of assertiveness training can be extremely useful; the user of an atypical system then takes the initiative in a communication situation, explaining briefly the nature of the problem and how the communication is to proceed.

Another critical point is not to permit oneself as clinician, or the client and his or her family, to adopt unnecessarily an either/or approach to communication systems. A severely retarded hearing-impaired child may be limited to using a single approach despite its many restrictions and disadvantages. Another individual with motor limitations but good general intelligence, however, may well be able to learn several systems: signing for interaction in a deaf community or school for the deaf and using a speech-output device for interaction with unfamiliar hearing people.

We should remember that the use of multiple languages or communication systems is a daily fact of life for much of the human population of the world. We must guard against allowing our tendency toward single-language chauvinism to interfere with aiding a client to master a multiple systems approach where this can enlarge his or her options and opportunities.

Some Actual Selection Cases

The following cases exemplify aided versus unaided system selection as a function of personal abilities and environmental considerations. In all cases, decision making is dynamic and reflects changing performance characteristics of the user and/or adjustment in expectations or desires of significant people in that individual's life.

Case 1: Steven

Steven is a thin, somewhat aloof boy with Down's syndrome, who was seen at the chronological age of 9 years, 1 month for his initial communication consultation. The purpose of the evaluation was to determine any physical basis for his lack of expressive speech and whether sign language training should be continued. The evaluation was requested by Steven's parents.

Social history is significant for early deprivation and multiple residences. His current foster placement is with his former teacher and her husband. (Three years after the initial evaluation he was legally adopted.)

By formal and informal language comprehension measures, Steven showed a scatter of abilities between 2- and 4-year-old level. Expressively, his vocal repertoire consisted of several unintelligible noises. No intelligible vowels, consonants, or words were reported or observed. His oral structure was notable for extremely poor dentition, a persistent open mouth posture, and a flaccid tongue. Steven had a history of middle ear infection, including a fluctuating mild to moderate conductive hearing impairment. He refused to cooperate for either gross motor or oral imitation. According to his mother, however, he learned through observation and could easily perform the handshape, motion, and location motor requirements of the upper extremity motor control screening test. According to his foster mother, "He seems to lack the desire to speak." Steven had never received any speech or language therapy.

Steven's initial exposure to a supplemental communication system occurred six months prior to this evaluation when sign language was tried. This unaided system was initiated by his mother (then his teacher), who had read that sign language facilitated speech production in children who are nonspeaking. He quickly learned to use 12 functional signs spontaneously. During this evaluation, he spontaneously signed "bathroom" (to request his desire to use the toilet), "bus" (to label the picture of a bus), and "more food" (to request an additional cracker). Despite Steven's initial successes with sign language, his current classroom teacher had not supported the unaided programming efforts, suggesting that it would inhibit Steven's speech development. No other children in the school used any type of augmentative communication system.

Additional relevant competencies identified during this first evaluation included Steven's ability to associate objects and actions with concrete line-drawing representations. (By report, however, he had never been interested in any form of pictographic information, including pictures from magazines, photo albums, or picture books.) Also, he had a 25-word sight vocabulary consisting mainly of function words such as *exit, bathroom,* etc.

The resulting recommendations included (1) beginning individual speech/language therapy and (2) continuing and expanding unaided programming efforts. The first recommendation stemmed from the absence of any previous formal speech therapy. Recommendation number two was based on several user-related factors.

1. Adequate upper extremity motor control to equalize the existing gap between expressive and receptive ability;
2. Demonstrated success with an unaided system;
3. Gestural orientation as evidenced by self-invented gestural communication;
4. Obvious family willingness to utilize an unaided system (it was believed at the time of this evaluation that the attitude of the academic environment toward the introduction of a supplemental communication system could be changed); and
5. A nonpicture-oriented child, as evidenced by a lack of interest in pictorial stimuli.

A second evaluation held approximately six months later revealed continued opposition to sign language instruction by the school personnel. Speech therapy had been initiated, but no appreciable differences were reported or observed. Steven was more cooperative during his second visit and demonstrated considerable imitative skills. Although no formal sign training was taking place at school or at home, Steven continued to invent new signs weekly. Also, he continued to employ previously learned signs to request goods and services. At school, Steven was gaining proficiency in matching written words to pictures and objects.

Discussion with the teacher revealed, as expected, opposition to sign language, but interest was expressed in a communication aid as a "viable communication system."

From this conversation it became evident that the teacher's preference for an aided system stemmed from an unfamiliarity with unaided systems, a belief that sign language would inhibit speech, and a belief that the teacher and his staff would need less training to introduce and support an aided communication system. Although the family continued to prefer an unaided method, their desire for Steven to receive formal instruction with some supplemental system led them to support trial use with an aided communication system. Subsequent recommendations included:

1. Speech therapy should be continued.
2. A portable communication aid should be developed for school and home. It was urged that the system be used throughout the day in both environments and reflect Steven's needs, preferences, and lifestyle. A host of specific recommendations regarding overall board size, target size and arrangement, symbol set/system, and teaching strategies were made.
3. Sign language or gesturing should not be discouraged.

At the third evaluation held six months later, it was revealed that there was initial opposition at the school to the communication aid recommendations. However, Steven began to develop considerable frustration in school, apparently because of his restricted expressive communication abilities. As a result, he broke into tears during one particularly difficult incident. At this point, members of the academic environment recognized the importance of a supplemental system and, the following day, introduced his first communication aid. Unfortunately, that communication aid contained an inappropriate symbol set system (words written in standard alphabet exclusively). Although the teacher finally perceived the need for the communication aid, he insisted that the symbol set be alphabetic. However, other features of the communication aid's design adhered to the prescribed format. During the session, Steven, who had been exposed to this aid for four months, evidenced considerable difficulty using the aid as a communication tool and locating vocabulary contained upon it. In addition, although he made no appreciable gains in speech, self-invented gestures continued to expand.

It should be noted that the school had been and continued to be in violation of Steven's Individualized Education Program. However, due to the mother's previous employment in the school system, the family was reluctant to engage in any activity that would be perceived as hostile. As a result, the recommendation at this time strongly urged implementation of all previous recommendations, especially with regard to symbol set and teaching strategies. School personnel were also reminded that sign language remained an option and one that would probably lead to considerable communicative success.

Four months later, and 16 months since the initial evaluation, the fourth evaluation was held. It was reported that Steven continued to prefer to gesture/sign at home and essentially used it exclusively with his family. A few graphic symbols were added to his communication aid, mostly representing important toys or food. Recommendations included:

1. Increase the amount of vocabulary represented by graphic symbols;
2. Increase communicative functions which the communication aid can convey;

3. Train appropriate school personnel in communication aid use through this clinic.

The fifth evaluation session was held five months later. At that time Steven continued to demonstrate difficulty locating information on his communication aid and refused to use it at home. It was also questionable whether the aid was being used for more than labeling common objects at school. The mother also reported that frustration associated with communicative failure was increasing at home. At this time, she admitted that Steven "definitely wants to sign!" Also, he was scheduled to return to the same classroom with the same teacher during the next academic year.

Twenty-one months following Steven's initial evaluation (where the unaided communications system approach seemed clearly indicated), that recommendation was restated. This restatement, however, followed considerable loss of programming time due largely to an academic setting unwilling to implement the appropriate service. The unwillingness and preference of the academic setting shaped the course of Steven's augmentative communication training for a considerable period of time.

Steven was subsequently placed in a language-based classroom outside of his local community (following a short but emotional confrontation with the local school district). His new teacher, competent in sign language instruction, encouraged its use and expansion. In addition, the parents received formal sign language instruction. Correspondingly, there has been a marked improvement in communication ability and a decrease in Steven's frustration associated with communication failure. Currently (six months since the fifth evaluation) Steven has an expressive vocabulary of approximately 200 signs. He uses the signs to initiate conversation, to request goods and services, question others, comment, demand, and command. Although he occasionally signs three-word expressions, the majority of his expressive attempts are one or two words.

Case 2: Marie

Marie was seen for a communication evaluation at the chronological age of 11 years, 1 month. The purpose of the evaluation, initiated by her parents and teacher, was to consider the adequacy of sign language as an augmentative communication system. She was moderately to severely mentally retarded, ambulatory, although having cerebral palsy (spastic type) and a seizure disorder. Her hearing was normal bilaterally.

Receptively, on formal language evaluation measures, she was functioning at the 20- to 26-month level. Expressively, she was able to say "ma" for mother. She rarely gestured to express herself. She currently enjoyed and reportedly always had delighted in examining catalogs, magazines, and photograph albums.

Marie lived at home with her parents and older sister and attended a small, structured, language-based classroom with six other children. All of her classmates were considered nonspeaking, and sign language instruction was provided on an individual basis and used throughout the school day. Parents of all children in the program were provided with a sign language instruction booklet and attended bimonthly sign language seminars. Both the classroom teacher and aide were competent signers.

During the 18 months Marie attended this class, she learned to spontaneously employ only two signs, *eat* and *drink*. She used these signs interchangeably. Marie was characteristically quiet, yet sociable, throughout the evaluation session. She did not request through sign (spontaneously or through prompting) any of the preferred food or drink items brought to the session by her parents. Evaluation of Marie's upper extremity motor control revealed slowness and difficulty in achieving target precision for the handshape and location movements considered necessary for manual expression. Marie was presented with a 5″ × 7″ photograph of a candy bar. After three trials in which her index finger was physically guided to the picture, followed by receiving a candy reinforcer, she spontaneously requested several more pieces. When other photographs of salient auditory (e.g., radio, toy piano) and visual (e.g., wind-up toys) objects were provided, Marie generalized the pointing/requesting behavior to these items. This occurred when the representations were presented singly or in groups of five. She also demonstrated the ability to associate objects with iconic (i.e., highly pictographic) line-drawing representations. Discussion with the parents and the classroom teacher revealed that although they preferred an unaided approach, they were willing to utilize any method that enhanced Marie's expressive potential.

Based on Marie's behavior, it was recommended that a communication aid be developed on a trial basis. Actual programming was preceded by several instructional sessions on the development and use of a communication aid. The aided communication recommendation was based on several factors.

1. Previous exposure to and training in the unaided system (despite an apparently competent and intensive effort) were essentially unsuccessful.

2. Marie's upper extremity motor control (related to the existence of the neuromuscular condition) did not seem capable of supporting expressive communication.

3. She appeared to be picture-oriented.

4. She did not appear to be gesture-oriented.

5. Members of both academic and residential environments seemed willing to support the recommendation.

A second evaluation held three months later revealed that Marie immediately learned to use the communication aid as an expressive communication tool. The teacher readily introduced the supplemental communication system into her existing classroom model. In fact, other children in the classroom, following instruction, learned to comprehend some of Marie's expressive communication efforts. But several difficulties arose associated with the communication aid.

1. Although Marie was willing to use the communication aid when it was left stationary on her desk (in school) or kitchen table (at home), she refused to carry it.

2. Reduction of the size of the pictures and placement of more than seven on a single display seemed to create visual/perceptual difficulties.

3. Marie preferred to use a crooked rather than extended index finger to point.

Recommendations at this time were aimed at the emerging perceptual and motor difficulties (including improving aid portability) while continuing to expand the vocabulary and use of the communication aid.

Case 3: Peter

Peter was seen for a communication evaluation at the chronological age of 3 years, 5 months. The purpose of the evaluation was to select an augmentative communication system and assist with educational placement and programming. Peter had an athetoid type of cerebral palsy affecting his four extremities, and he spent the majority of his day in a nonelectronic wheelchair. He was severely dysarthric, and his speech was unintelligible even to familiar listeners. In addition, he had a severe bilateral sensorineural hearing loss for which he wore bilateral body aids. Amplification brought his hearing sensitivity for the speech frequencies within the moderate loss range. Because of the severity of his hearing impairment and physical involvement, intellectual and receptive language levels were only estimates at that time; they suggested that he was functioning approximately 1½ to 2 years below his chronological age. He was curious, extemely observant, and frequently attempted to imitate observed gross motor movement. He attempted to use some gestures to express himself. Because of his severe neuromuscular involvement, however, those gestures required context and familiarity to be comprehended. He was unable to produce any of the handshape configurations thought necessary to become a competent user of American Sign Language. Peter recognized photographs of family members and could associate line drawings with objects. Following a short training session held during the evaluation, he learned to associate several ASL signs with their referents.

In light of this information, a communication approach that incorporated both aided and unaided systems was recommended. More specifically, it was recommended that Peter attend a total communication preschool classroom for hearing-impaired children.

Receptive language training should focus on sign language instruction. Because he was incapable of expression through sign, an aided system should be provided for expressive output. The symbol system contained on his communication aid should comprise photographs (to request significant people) and pictured signs (photocopied from a sign language booklet) for other vocabulary items.

The cases portray those factors that can influence the selection of an augmentative communication system. It is unfortunate that in the first example, that of Steven, unusual family relationships with the academic environment allowed the school to negatively influence communication progress for such an extended period. For the second child, Marie, teachers and parents immediately changed an ineffective expressive communication system for one that was more closely aligned with her presenting abilities and needs. Introduction of the aided method meant a change in orientation by the academic staff who had already developed an effective unaided program for other children. For Marie's parents, it meant adjustment to still another augmentative communication system. Peter (case 3) had a unique set of problems that necessitated a dual system combining principles and procedures from both aided and unaided options.

References

Ad Hoc Committee on Communication Processes for Nonspeaking Persons. (1981). ASHA position statement on nonspeech communication. *Asha, 23,* 577–581.

Darley, F. L. Aronson, A. E., & Brown, J. R. (1969). Differential diagnostic patterns of dysarthria. *Journal of Speech and Hearing Research, 12,* 246–270.

Fristoe, M., & Lloyd, L. (1980). Planning an initial expressive sign lexicon for persons with severe communication impairment. *Journal of Speech and Hearing Disorders, 45,* 170–180.

Shane, H. C., & Bashir, A. S. (1980). Election criteria for the adoption of an augmentative communication system: Preliminary considerations. *Journal of Speech and Hearing Disorders, 45,* 408–414.

Shane, H. C., & Wilbur, R. B. (1980). Potential for expressive signing based on motor control. *Sign Language Studies, 29,* 331–348.

Skelly, M. (1979). *American Indian gestural code based on universal American Indian handtalk.* New York: Elsevier North Holland.

Stokoe, W., Casterline, D., & Croneberg, C. (1965). *A dictionary of American Sign Language on linguistic principles.* Washington, DC: Gallaudet College Press.

Wolfensberger, W. (1972). *The principle of normalization in human services.* Downsview, Ontario: National Institute on Mental Retardation.

Appendix
ASHA Position Statement on Nonspeech Communication

The following position statement, drafted by the Ad Hoc Committee on Communication Processes for Nonspeaking Persons, was adopted as an official policy statement of the American Speech-Language-Hearing Association by its Legislative Council in November, 1980 (LC 15-80). 1980 committee members included: Billie Ackerman, ex officio; David R. Beukelman; Faith Carlson; Carol Cohen; Pam Elder; Suzanne Evans-Morris, public representative; Rich Foulds, public representative; Macalyne Fristoe; Linda F. Goodman; Debrah Harris; Arlene Kraat, public representative; Lyle Lloyd; Judy Montgomery; Howard Shane, chairman; Franklin G. Silverman; Barbara Sonies; Ronnie Wilbur, public representative; Gregg Vanderheiden; James Viggiano, public representative; and David Yoder, Vice President for Clinical Affairs.

WHEREAS, the Executive Board of the American Speech-Language-Hearing Association (ASHA) established an Ad Hoc Committee on Communication Processes for Nonspeaking Persons, and

WHEREAS, one of the committee's charges was to develop a position statement for ASHA relative to its role in serving the communication needs of the more than 1½ million nonspeaking persons, and

WHEREAS, such a paper has been developed and published in the April, 1980 issue of *Asha* for peer review, and

WHEREAS, revisions of the position paper have been made to be in compliance with the ASHA Code of Ethics and the Council on Professional Standards in Speech-Language Pathology along with other membership concerns; therefore

LC 15-80. RESOLVED, That the position paper on Nonspeech Communication be adopted and disseminated in the same manner as have other position papers.

Recently, there has been a rapid and dramatic increase in the quality and quantity of services available to severely handicapped persons. Diversification of the provision of services to persons with multiple or severe handicaps has resulted in the expansion of professional competencies required of service providers. This situation has become particularly acute in those instances where professionals are assuming the responsibility of developing comprehensive service delivery programs for heretofore unserved or minimally served populations. One such group of individuals includes children, adolescents and adults who are nonspeaking and who usually exhibit to some degree neurological, emotional, physical, or cognitive handicaps. It is encouraging that programs and services are now being made available to these persons, and that many advances have been made recently regarding the types of communication programs and systems which are available to them. Provision of effective and beneficial services and programs, however, depends upon the competencies of professional service providers. Although numerous professions will be included in the provision of communication services to the nonspeaking individual, speech-language pathologists should be primarily responsible for the development of treatment and intervention programs as such. Speech-language pathologists must have thorough working knowledge of and training in topic areas related to communication development for persons for whom speech may not be the primary mode of expression. There are a number of issues and concerns which relate to the development of such competencies in the speech-language pathologist. Issues of concern related to the design, implementation, and evaluation of communication programs for nonspeaking persons include: (1) terminology and delineation of client populations; (2) historical perspective related to service delivery in this area; (3) delineation of components involved in service delivery; (4) the role and professional responsibility of the speech-language pathologist in the provision of services; (5) impact of service needs on personnel preparation and the development of professional competencies; (6) professional ethics related to service delivery; and (7) current research and interprofessional activity needs.

Terminology

Numerous terms have been used to label the nonspeaking population, the methods used to improve their communication, and the intervention programs which have been used. The most frequent labels that are, and have been, used to describe the population include: severely speech impaired, speechless, nonoral, nonvocal, nonverbal, aphonic, and nonspeaking. Operationally we are discussing a group of individuals for whom speech is temporarily or permanently inadequate to meet all of his or her communication needs, and whose inability to speak is not due primarily to a hearing impairment. In order to provide consistency with regard to terminology, the population under consideration will be referred to as nonspeaking persons. It is recognized that, although some of these individuals can produce a limited amount of speech, the speech exhibited is not adequate to meet all of their communication needs.

In order to provide effective communication systems for individuals whose speech is not fully functional a number of communication techniques have been developed which are in widespread use. Terms often used interchangeably to describe such communication techniques and programs include: nonoral, manual, nonvocal, gestural, nonspeech, nonverbal, alternative, assistive, augmentative, supplementary, aphonic, prosthetic, and aided.

These communication techniques are seen as augmentative in that they are designed and utilized in such a manner as to supplement whatever vocal skills the individual may possess. The term augmentative will, therefore, be used to refer to this general classification of procedures which include both aided and unaided communicative techniques.

The term *augmentative communication system* will be used to refer to the total functional communication system of an individual which includes: (1) a communicative technique; (2) a symbol set or system; and (3) communication/interaction behavior (see Figure 1 [p. 271]).

The term *unaided* will be used to refer to all techniques which do not require any physical aids. Manual, gestural, manual/visual, sign, or facial communication as well as oral speaking are considered *unaided communication* techniques (see Figure 1).

The term *aided* will be used to refer to all techniques where some type of physical object or device is used. Techniques which use communication boards, charts, and mechanical or electrical aids are considered *aided* communication techniques.

Symbols and symbol systems refer to the means to represent ideas and concepts. Examples of symbol sets/systems include spoken words, pictures, Blissymbolics, Rebus, traditional orthography, signs of American Sign Language, signs of Signing Exact English, and signs of Amerind (see Figure 1).

It should be recognized and cautioned that these "definitions" are generic and that speech-language pathologists should describe and provide specific detail regarding the etiology of the nonspeaking condition when referring to clients and to the specific type of communication technique and intervention program used.

Historical Perspective on Service Delivery

Historically, nonspeaking persons were placed in a speech treatment program or not given treatment because oral speech did not appear to be feasible. Some pioneering efforts were made by a small number of speech-language pathologists and others in the development and use of communication boards for the severely physically handicapped and in the use of manual signs with hearing, mentally retarded persons.

Recent technological advances in the development of augmentative communication aids and systems have offered new options for the nonspeaking population. In addition, augmentative communication systems have been developed, and/or applied differently, to effect communication with this population. The combined use of these communication techniques and symbol systems has been found to be effective in augmenting residual speech skills and providing communication access.

Given the state of the art regarding the development and use of communication techniques, there is no nonspeaking person too physically handicapped to be able to utilize some augmentative communication system. Therefore, the speech and language professional is now faced with increasingly diverse program and treatment options for nonspeaking persons and she/he must develop the competency necessary to serve these clinical needs.

A large, previously untreated population exists. Recent prevalence figures indicate that there are over one million children and adults who are nonspeaking as a result of neurological, physical, emotional, or cognitive disability. The development of effective communication systems is a current unmet need of these persons, a need which will become the primary responsibility of speech and language professionals. For example, recent legislation (PL 94-142) mandates the development and implementation of effective educational programs for all handicapped persons under 22 years of age. As a result, many nonspeaking persons are currently being enrolled in educational programs. Their success depends upon the acquisition and demonstration of competent communication skills. The above factor alone will dramatically increase the number and diversity of nonspeaking persons on the speech and language professional's caseload within an educational setting. Another factor which will affect provision of service involves recent advances in the development and use of communication techniques and symbol systems.

Recent rapid advances in the development of augmentative communication systems have been fortunate for nonspeaking persons. At present, there is a critical need to supplement the speech and language professional's current knowledge of basic speech, language, and communication processes with training specifically dealing with the development and implementation of augmentative communication systems.

Components Involved in Service Delivery

1. Assessment to Determine the Need and Appropriateness of an Augmentative Communication System or Systems:

In order to determine the need for the development and use of an augmentative system, and the intervention entry point, the nonspeaking person should be assessed with regard to physical, sensory, emotional, and cognitive ability; speech and language skills; correct seating and positioning; general communication skills; communication needs (conversational and written) for social, emotional, educational, and/or vocational purposes; family needs; and nature and quality of supportive services.

2. Selection and Development of an Effective Augmentative Communication/Interaction System or Systems:

Once the need for intervention has been decided, specific exploration related to selection and development of augmentative systems, which can provide the individual with the most effective and functional communication, needs to be explored. This involves consideration of unaided and aided communication techniques. In addition to determining the physical expressive means, an appropriate symbol system through which communicative messages can be formulated and expressed needs to be developed. This involves consideration of symbol

3. Developing Interactive Skills:

Once an augmentative communication approach has been selected, the nonspeaking person will need to be provided with training in skills which will enable him/her to utilize the augmentative technique and symbol system in such a manner as to be able to achieve communicative competence as defined by the message-receiving community. This training includes: use of appropriate technique and selected symbols, strategies for developing effective communication interaction, as well as the training of persons who interact or potentially will interact with augmentative communication system users.

4. Follow Up and Ongoing Evaluation:

Appropriate implementation should include continual evaluation of the communication/ interaction effected by the system, appropriate alteration of the system and communication strategies if indicated, and preparatory training for future use of different or more complex systems.

Role of the Speech-Language Pathologist

Depending upon the particular needs of the client, the interdisciplinary evaluation team may include any or all of the following: speech-language pathologist, physical therapist, occupational therapist, educator, medical specialists, audiologist, psychologist, seating and fitting specialist, engineer, social worker, vocational counselor, vendors, third party agent, extended family and friends, primary caregivers, and the client.

The central role in initiating and coordinating the services of this team should be taken by the person most likely to initiate the recommendation for an augmentative communication system, based on his/her evaluation of the client's oral motor peformance, language competence, and communication needs. Further, the person needs to possess the knowledge of language development and communication interaction which will be essential to the client's success in augmentative communication. In most cases the speech-language pathologist would be the person who best meets these requirements.

Therefore, the professional role of the speech-language pathologist in providing services to nonspeaking persons includes:

1. Assessing, describing, documenting, and continually evaluating the communication/interaction behaviors and needs of these persons;

2. Evaluating and assisting in the selection of the various communication techniques in order to develop an effective repertoire of communicative modes;

3. Developing speech and vocal communication to the fullest extent possible;

4. Evaluating and selecting the symbol systems for use with above selected techniques;

5. Developing (and evaluating the effectiveness of) intervention procedures to teach the skills necessary to utilize augmentative systems in an optimal manner;

6. Integrating assessment and program procedures with family members and other professional team members;

7. Training of persons who interact with the nonspeaking individual; and

8. Coordination of augmentative communication services.

In addition to the above, another primary role of the speech-language pathologist is that of client advocacy. Although there is continual increase in the use of nonvocal communication modes, there remains, for the most part, a knowledge/experience gap in terms of the general public's acceptance and understanding of these modes. Successful communication development programs necessitate that speech-language pathologists help clients to develop effective skills with which to interact with both speaking and other nonspeaking persons in their community. In order to achieve this, and in order to help clients secure financial support for needed communication prostheses, clinicians must be able to serve as client advocates—educating their co-workers and communities about nonspeech communication in general and their client's needs in particular.

Personnel Preparation

Current training should provide speech-language pathologists with competency in the areas of basic speech, language, and hearing processes. Training in competency areas specifically related to the development and use of augmentative communication systems has not been incorporated into most programs. This latter training should include the development of competencies specifically related to:

1. Assessment procedures for determining augmentative communication system candidacy and selection of system components;

2. Assessment of prelinguistic communicative interaction strategies in nonspeaking persons;

3. Knowledge of currently available aided and unaided techniques;

4. Knowledge of available symbol options;

5. Knowledge of the nature of augmentative communication in interaction with speaking and nonspeaking persons;

6. Development and evaluation of communication intervention programs specifically designed to teach nonspeaking persons those skills needed in order to achieve communication competence via augmentative communication techniques;

7. Knowledge of the effect of appropriate seating and positioning on the user's control of the speech mechanism and on a nonspeaker's communication techniques; and

8. Advocacy and funding procedures.

Professional Ethics Related to Service Delivery for Nonspeaking Persons

The revised Code of Ethics of the American Speech-Language-Hearing Association effective January 1, 1979, stresses the professional responsibility of speech-language pathologists and audiologists in providing services. For those individuals who serve nonspeaking persons and recommend augmentative communication systems, several fundamental rules of ethical conduct are particularly relevent:

Training

"Individuals shall maintain high standards of professional competence. . . . Individuals must neither provide services for which they have not been properly prepared, nor pemit services to be provided by any of their staff who are not properly prepared"* (Principle of Ethics II, Ethical Proscription 1).

Few education and training programs include instruction or clinical experience in augmentative communication. Therefore, speech-language pathologists and audiologists who lack formal training in nonspeech communication must assume responsibility for continuing education by reading, attending meetings and workshops, seeking consultation, and other means of increasing their knowledge and competence about this aspect of habilitation.

Services

"Individuals shall hold paramount the welfare of persons served professionally. Individuals shall use every resource available, including referral to other specialists as needed, to provide the best-service possible"* (Principle of Ethics I,A).

If a speech-language pathologist or audiologist is unable to adequately assess and instruct clients in the use of augmentative communication systems, the client should be referred to a specialist who can provide appropriate services. Furthermore, it appears to us that the speech-language pathologist has the obligation, despite his/her own bias with regard to speech and an augmentative communication system, to inform the individual and his/her family about the existence of those systems and the available options for communication.

"Individuals shall honor their responsibilities to the public, their profession, and their relationship with colleagues and members of allied professions. . . . Individuals should strive to increase knowledge within the profession and share research with colleagues . . . establish harmonious relations with colleagues and members of other professions . . . inform members of related professions . . . as well as seek information from them"* (Principle of Ethics V, Professional Propriety 3, 4).

Speech-language pathologists and audiologists who are knowledgeable about augmentative communication have a professional responsibility to share information which will benefit communicatively handicapped individuals. Providing nonspeaking persons with augmentative communication devices necessitates interdisciplinary cooperation. Therefore, it is imperative that parents, physical therapists, occupational therapists, psychologists, teachers, physicians, and other specialists involved in providing service to a nonspeaking person be provided and share information about augmentative communication systems.

Dispensing of Products

"Individuals shall maintain objectivity in all matters concerning the welfare of persons served professionally. Individuals who dispense products to persons served professionally shall observe the following standards:

1. Products associated with professional practice must be dispensed to the person served as part of a program of comprehensive habilitative care.

2. Fees established for professional services must be independent of whether a product is dispensed.

3. Persons served must be provided freedom of choice for the source of services and products.

4. Price information about professional services rendered and products dispensed must be disclosed by providing to, or posting for, persons served a complete schedule of fees and charges in advance of rendering services, which schedule differentiates between fees for professional services and charges for products dispensed.

5. Products dispensed to the person served must be evaluated to determine effectiveness (Principle of Ethics IV, A).

In order to dispense augmentative communication devices, speech-language pathologists and audiologists must observe the ethical principles stated above. In addition, they should have an adequate knowledge of various types of devices in order to make a judicious evaluation and recommendation. Ideally, several communication devices should be available to permit a nonspeaking person to use a device prior to the selection and purchase of one.

Current Research and Interprofessional Activity Needs

Attention to the needs of nonspeaking persons has grown so rapidly that the "consumer market" and client population are currently overwhelmed with the variety of aided and unaided techniques and program options available and with the lack of substantive information regarding the use, applicability, and effectiveness of each. As a result, service delivery programs are being implemented in an unorganized fashion and many clients' needs are not being met or are being met in an inappropriate manner. Therefore, critical research needs and questions are:

1. What are the most effective strategies for
   a. symbol acquisition;
   b. learning to use aided and unaided techniques; and
   c. facilitating interaction?

2. Considering the physical, cognitive, linguistic, and communication parameters of the nonspeaking person, which available augmentative systems best meet his/her needs?

3. If clinical observations regarding increase in vocalizations following exposure to augmentative communication systems are correct, why is this so?

4. What is the role of iconicity in the learning of a symbol system?

5. How can spontaneous communication be encouraged?

6. Which factors, singly or in combination, make a person high risk for not becoming an oral communicator?

7. How can interaction best be fostered between speaking and nonspeaking persons?

8. What are effective means of increasing rate of communication by augmentative communication systems users?

9. Does the language development of users of augmentative systems parallel that of normal language development?

In addition, the Committee sees the need for:

1. Greater investigation and use of electronic and computer-assisted systems; and

2. The development of tests and procedures for assessing the communication abilities of the nonspeaking population.

As regards future interprofessional activities, there is a need to develop some vehicle/organization which can

- provide a "common ground" for written and verbal communication between professionals from the diverse disciplines which serve nonspeaking persons;

- assume an active role in advocating and providing for the nonspeaking client's communication needs; and

- disseminate information in the area to professionals, parents, and nonspeaking persons.

Chapter 16

Career Education and Vocational Training Issues

Robert R. Lauritsen and David R. Updegraff

Efforts to provide parity for deaf people in the United States have deep historical roots. Among the most chronicled events were the establishment of the American Asylum for the Education of the Deaf and Dumb (now the American School for the Deaf) at Hartford, Connecticut, in 1817; the founding of Gallaudet College in 1864; the establishment of what is now the National Association of the Deaf in 1880; the beginnings of the Vocational Rehabilitation Program in 1920 as a result of the high numbers of wounded veterans of World War I; the Fort Monroe Conference in 1959; the establishment of the National Technical Institute for the Deaf in 1965; the founding of the Model Secondary School for the Deaf in 1965 and the Kendall Demonstration Elementary School in 1971; the beginnings of the Regional Education Programs in 1968–69; the adoption of Section 504 of the Rehabilitation Act in 1973; and the passage of the Education for All Handicapped Children Act, Public Law 94-142, in 1975.

Services for deaf people have further improved in the past decade. Some examples of improved services are found in the fields of postsecondary education, training of interpreters, and the establishment of interpreter referral services. In the early 1970s, the six federally funded postsecondary programs served most deaf students who wished to continue their education and who met entrance criteria for those institutions. Those programs were Gallaudet College, the National Technical Institute for the Deaf at Rochester Institute of Technology, California State University at Northridge, Seattle Community College, St. Paul Technical Vocational Institute, and Delgado College.* However, *A Guide to College/Career Programs for Deaf Students,* published by Gallaudet College and the National Technical Institute for the Deaf (Rawlings, Trybus, & Biser, 1983) listed more than 100 postsecondary programs for deaf students. In the early 1970s, there was just a handful of programs training interpreters. In the mid-1980s, there were 10 federally funded interpreter training programs and an additional 40 that were locally or state funded. In the early 1970s, there were no formally established interpreter referral services. In the early 1980s, there were more than 150 interpreter referral services with a national organization, the Council of Referral and Interpreter Service Providers (CRISP), in the development stage. Membership in the Registry of

---

*In 1983, Delgado College lost its federal funding; the University of Tennessee was funded to begin a program for deaf students.

Interpreters for the Deaf grew from a charter membership of 100 members in 1964 to more than 4,300 members in 1983. Services were also initiated at the state and local levels. Services for deaf people who are senior citizens were becoming more common throughout the United States. At least 14 states had state commissions or councils for deaf persons. The state of Minnesota legislated a Regional Service Center network that provided a single entry point for all deaf and hard-of-hearing persons into human service delivery systems.

These increases in services took place despite economic swings. As will be discussed in this chapter, however, a significant group of hearing-impaired people has been minimally affected by these service increases: those who are hearing impaired and developmentally disabled. Our advocacy with and for those people is incomplete without a massive effort to close this service gap. Today's changing technologies, coupled with changes in the workforce, are major factors that must be considered if deaf people are to continue to maintain and improve their present levels of achievement in general, and if hearing-impaired developmentally disabled people are to be provided with the services they need to attain the levels of independent functioning of which many are capable. Coping with change can best be accomplished by the human factor; in other words, our leaders must recognize that change is ubiquitous, and they must create the tools and apply them for the benefit of individuals who are hearing impaired and developmentally disabled.

This chapter will attempt to show that the education and training of hearing-impaired developmentally disabled people requires changes proportionate to the rapid changes in skills required to survive in the community, in the workplace, and in society. Hearing-impaired developmentally disabled people need improved support service systems and increased understanding on the part of their communities. Both must be provided by the professionals who serve this population.

Definition and Size of the Population

It is estimated that approximately 15 million people in the United States have some degree of hearing loss. Of this number, more than 1,750,000 are thought to have severe to profound hearing loss (Schein & Delk, 1974). Services are focused on those with severe to profound losses, for very good reasons.

- It is a more easily identifiable group.
- As a population of hearing-impaired people, it has needs which are readily recognizable.
- Individual members of this group tend to identify with each other within a deaf cultural milieu.

The largest number of people with hearing loss have impairments that are of mild to moderate degree. This group of people has needs for services different from the needs of those with severe to profound losses. For example, people with mild or moderate losses tend not to require the service of sign language interpreters, although some may need oral interpreting at times. People with mild or moderate hearing loss tend to

- identify with the broader hearing society rather than with other hearing-impaired people;
- rarely bind together in the community; and
- generally lack a state or federal rallying point for legislative or social action purposes.

Ongoing needs for the hard-of-hearing include attention to the use of residual hearing; alertness to medical breakthroughs; availability of career, personal adjustment, and related counseling services; and support services on the job, in education, and in public gatherings.

Limitations imposed by mild or moderate hearing loss are frequently hidden and are not obvious to the casual observer. People with mild or moderate hearing loss constitute a significant population which historically has been underserved. Case findings by skilled professionals can identify those individuals who can profit from human service delivery system. Functional definitions, as opposed to more rigid stereotyped definitions, should be considered when eligibility for services from human service agencies is indicated. Although this chapter will focus primarily on people with severe to profound hearing losses, the information presented is applicable to some extent to people with mild or moderate hearing loss who also have developmental disabilities.

The model demonstration program conducted under the auspices of the Administration on Developmental Disabilities at the University of Arizona (Stewart, 1978) provided a tentative estimate that the size of the hearing-impaired developmentally disabled population was approximately one million. This was a tentative estimate because of the method used at arriving at the figure, which was based on 1970 census data (see Chapter 3 for demographic data). Many hearing-impaired developmentally disabled people have more than one developmental disability, resulting in some possible duplication of count. Further, an accurate census can be obtained best by a state-by-state census of the target population, which has not been done.

Whatever data base on deafness is reviewed, the reality remains the same: Significant numbers of hearing-impaired people have one or more secondary disabilities. In addition, it is well known that hearing impairment of early onset strongly influences language development and that delayed language acquisition is directly related to an individual's career education and vocational needs.

Special Education: The Critical Years

Special education is a term used to cover educational efforts at the preschool through 12th grade levels on behalf of handicapped children and youth. The special education needs of handicapped youth are well known to authors of federal and state legislation, educators, health care providers, and others in the human service delivery system. The impact of early, profound hearing impairment continues to present one of the most difficult challenges in special education. The education of the deaf is frequently referred to as the most special of all areas of special education. Education of the deaf must become even more specialized when additional handicapping conditions exist.

The added caveats for the education of hearing-impaired youth are the communication barriers imposed by early hearing impairment. The impact upon language development is devastating. As noted throughout the literature, the addition of other disabilities to hearing impairment results not in a simple additive effect, but rather in a multiplier effect, usually unquantifiable and of unknown complexity.

The numbers of multihandicapped school-age children are great. Karchmer (see Chapter 3) estimated that more than 30 percent of school-age deaf children have additional serious handicapping conditions. The directory issue of the *American Annals of the Deaf* (1983) reported that approximately 20 percent of the students in 1,325 programs serving hearing-impaired children in the U.S. were multihandicapped. These numbers are probably underestimates for three reasons.

- Some institutionalized children may not be reported.

- There are still hearing-impaired developmentally disabled youth in the U.S. who are misdiagnosed and not reported.

- Some programs may not report hearing-impaired developmentally disabled children who are not served in a special program.

Educational lags created by early hearing loss have not been ameliorated by the best efforts of trained, dedicated teachers. Achievement profiles of hearing-impaired high school graduates simply do not compare favorably with those of hearing high school graduates. The evidence becomes even more dramatic when information about career selection of secondary school graduates is examined. Few students entering postsecondary education have made career decisions, and the majority of students lack information upon which to make informed career decisions. This reinforces the need for early and structured career education programming in the elementary and secondary schools serving hearing-impaired youth.

The overwhelming majority of hearing-impaired students entering postsecondary training require preparatory training to become eligible for the rigors of education at that level. One need only look at the preparatory programs that are offered at Gallaudet College, the National Technical Institute for the Deaf, St. Paul Technical Vocational Institute, and other postsecondary programs to find clear evidence that hearing-impaired students require extended study time beyond high school to reach a level at which they are ready to handle postsecondary education. One of the primary roles of special education programs is to prepare hearing-impaired developmentally disabled students with such basic skills as they are able to master.

The stress on basics is found in Recommendation A of the 1983 report of the National Commission on Excellence in Education, *A Nation at Risk: The Imperative for Educational Reform,* which said:

We recommend that state and local high school graduation requirements be strengthened and that, at a minimum, all students seeking a diploma be required to lay the foundations in the Five New Basics by taking the following curriculum during their 4 years of high school: (a) 4 years of English; (b) 3 years of mathematics; (c) 3 years of science; (d) 3 years of social studies; and (e) one-half year of computer science. For the college-bound, 2 years of foreign language in high school are strongly recommended in addition to those taken earlier.

Another study, *High School: A Report of Secondary Education in America* (Boyer, 1983), prepared under the auspices of the Carnegie Foundation for the Advancement of Teaching, offered further focus on the needs of education. This report lists as its first priorities the teaching of language and the need to develop the capacity to think critically and communicate effectively through the written and spoken word. The Carnegie report is basically a call for literacy. The national commission's report, the Carnegie report, and others clearly state the need to reshape the condition of education in the U.S.

The Five New Basics and the Carnegie report make inherent assumptions about the learning process and needs of the general population. But there remain significant portions of the U.S. populace for whom these goals will not be realized because of learning disabilities and delays. Public policy in the U.S., as stated in the laws that provide for special education and rehabilitation, needs to be kept in focus; and the accommodations and gains that have been made for those students who cannot attain the goals set forth in the National Commission and Carnegie reports need to be not only preserved but also improved. Hearing-impaired developmentally disabled individuals have the same rights as other citizens and will continue to need special educational and training accommodations provided for them by governing bodies.

For more than 100 years, one of the answerable questions about the education of the deaf that has been debated in the U.S. is, Can good secondary school vocational programming eliminate the necessity for postsecondary programs? The answer is clearly and unequivocally, No. Good secondary vocational programming is essential but will not replace the need for quality postsecondary programming. One need only examine the academic attainments of secondary school graduates from schools and classes for hard-of-hearing and deaf individuals to find dramatic evidence of the need for further education and training. The academic attainments, reading skills, and computational skills of secondary school graduates who have impaired hearing have not changed appreciably over the years.

What is required to maintain good vocational programming? Simply answered, good vocational programs require state-of-the-art instruction, equipment, and facilities. Even the most cursory knowledge of computer technology clearly indicates that this is a technical field undergoing change at an unprecedented rate. Within a few decades, this field has successfully miniaturized its equipment from computers that required a facility of warehouse proportions to the often more powerful microcomputers found in the home or office of today. Applications of computer technology are invasive in nearly all vocational technical areas. Graphic arts is computer based; newspapers, magazines, and other printed materials utilize highly sophisticated word processors coupled with typesetters. The metal trades responsible for manufacturing automobiles, refrigerators, microwave ovens, and other commodities use million-dollar CAD-CAMS (Computer Assisted Design/Manufacturing Systems). The rapid advance of technology from strictly the instructional, equipment, and facility standpoint makes it impossible for local secondary schools and residential schools to keep pace. This rapid change also makes it difficult for many postsecondary programs to keep pace. Many hearing-impaired developmentally disabled students would be better off if their secondary programs provided them with structured training in work attitudes, socialization skills, and basic academic skills to facilitate their entry into the job market and their job retention rates. Many employers today prefer to train their own new employees in the employers' ways of working. Preparation to accept and benefit from such training would surely help students.

Before the advent of extensive mainstreaming, when the majority of hearing-impaired students were in residential schools, the matters of referring students to vocational rehabilitation and informing students about postsecondary education were relatively easy tasks. Mainstreaming of the majority of hearing-impaired students in day schools and day classes throughout the country has created a situation in which hundreds of hearing-impaired youth are graduating from secondary school with minimal, and in some cases no, knowledge about postsecondary training opportunities available to them. Despite the best efforts in publishing and disseminating *A Guide to College/Career Programs for Deaf Students,* there are still students who are unaware of these opportunities. Renewed efforts should be undertaken with teacher preparation programs, vocational rehabilitation agencies, parent groups, and local and national organizations to ensure that each and every hearing-impaired student graduating from high school, and his or her family, has career information available. A national clearinghouse known as HEATH (Higher Education and the Handicapped) is located at the American Council on Education, Washington, D.C., and can assist in information dissemination.

Perspectives on Career Education Needs

The career education needs of the hearing-impaired developmentally disabled population should be addressed from the perspective of a school-based program that begins in the very early school years and progresses through secondary school. Such a program should provide for the roles and relationships of the school itself, the parents, and the child's community. Hearing-impaired developmentally disabled children present a number of severe career-related problems over and above those presented by children who have hearing impairment as a single disability.

Undoubtedly, the most severe career-related problem is the inability to acquire fluency in the language of their society. This text focuses on the hearing-impaired developmentally disabled in the U.S., where that language is English. In the information age in which we are living, lack of fluency in the primary mode of information transmittal is a near fatal career-related difficulty. Compensatory tools must be provided to individuals in this group to assist them to overcome the employment handicaps imposed by their disabilities.

The term "career education" has been used in U.S. education since about 1971. It was coined by the commissioner of education in the U.S. Office of Education, Dr. Sidney Marland (Hoyt, 1975). In 1974, Public Law 93-380 was passed, making career education a congressional mandate. Later that year, the Office of Education published an official policy paper on career education. Dr. Kenneth Hoyt was appointed director of the newly established Office of Career Education in the Office of Education. His writings on career education were prolific and were the main element solidifying the concept of career education in the schools.

Career education is defined as "the totality of experiences through which one learns about and prepares to engage in work as part of her or his way of living." Concomitant definitions are (1) for *career:* "the totality of work one does in his or her lifetime;" (2) for *education*: "the totality of experiences through which one learns;" and (3) for *work*: "conscious effort, other than that involved in activities whose primary purpose is either coping or relaxation, aimed at producing benefits for oneself and/or for oneself and others" (Hoyt, 1975).

This is not the place for an exhaustive history of the career education movement in U.S. education. Suffice it to say that thousands of school districts throughout the country implemented career education programs through the 1970s and early 1980s. Many of these programs continue to assist young people to prepare for the world of work or for further study upon graduation from secondary school. Unfortunately, much of the federal funding for career education has ceased, halting many programs that were dependent on federal dollars.

The major movement in implementing career education in programs for hearing-impaired people began in 1978 with the establishment of the National Project on Career Education (NPCE), a joint project of Gallaudet College and the National Technical Institute for the Deaf. The NPCE grew out of the expressed need of several state residential schools for the deaf for training their faculties in career education. The project produced a training manual in career education concepts and practices and, between 1979 and 1982, provided training to teams of teachers, counselors, and administrators from 60 programs in all parts of the country. The teams of NPCE-trained career educators returned to their schools and, in most cases, provided training to their school faculties. The NPCE initiated a newsletter to maintain the networking among programs begun during the training cycles. Even though the project itself is now officially terminated, the newsletter and the network continue to be active, sharing information about new program directions and related materials. Two offshoots of the training program for teachers, counselors, and administrators are a career awareness summer program for students and a career education training program for parents of hearing-impaired students.

There are several key concepts in career education which should flow through and enliven the curriculum of a school or program serving hearing-impaired developmentally disabled students (Updegraff & Egelston-Dodd, 1982). These concepts are

- self-awareness,
- educational awareness,
- career awareness,
- economic awareness,
- decision making,
- beginning competency,
- employability skills, and
- attitudes and appreciations.

These are eight key elements in a comprehensive career education model. Activities can be structured at any age and maturity level to assist hearing-impaired developmentally disabled students to acquire necessary understanding and skills in each of these areas. There are at least two ways to go about this in a school program. The least expensive and least disruptive to a school's curriculum is to infuse career-education-related activities into each area of the curriculum. This facilitates the teaching of career concepts at the same time that academic concepts are being taught, thus linking school and career in a manner not successfully done in most curricula. The second approach is to "add-on" to the curriculum special courses that convey the career-related material. A number of studies have indicated that the infusion approach tends to lead to greater understanding and higher level skills among students. However, common sense also tells us that highlighting these concepts in separate courses may also have benefits for students, particularly those nearly ready to enter the workforce or those who want to continue their educational preparation for work.

Figure 1 displays graphically how the eight elements should be sequenced in an infused curriculum. The elements are presented in developmental stages, indicating the recommended period of time each should be emphasized. For example, from birth to about Grade 6, self-awareness and educational awareness are the two critical concepts to convey. In Grades 11 and 12, the preparation stage, the critical concepts are decision making and beginning competency. The model also conveys the importance of the three environments in which career education concepts should be taught: the home, the school, and the community.

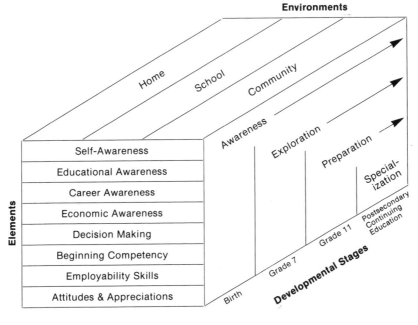

Figure 1. Career development model. From *Trainers Manual: Career Education and Planning Skills* (p. T-5-2) by Model Secondary School for the Deaf/National Technical Institute for the Deaf National Project on Career Education, 1980. Reprinted with permission. Based on Comprehensive Career Education Model (Ohio State University, as modified by Dr. Victor Galloway).

Graduation or school-leaving is the passport to adult status in society. For hearing-impaired developmentally disabled people, some transitional programming is necessary to assist them to cope with the myriad decisions which accompany this transition; these include postsecondary education choices, career choices, job seeking, marriage, independent living, or long-term sheltered employment. However, secondary schools do not universally provide transitional programs, particularly in programs in which hearing-impaired students are mainstreamed fully or partially with hearing students. In most states, the transition phase is dependent upon the availability of vocational rehabilitation services. Where these services are less than optimal or are absent, or in situations in which school personnel do not have regular contact with the rehabilitation counselors for their students, chaos results for the individual and family.

Numerous secondary schools have sought counsel from postsecondary institutions, examining ways in which secondary curricula can be modified to better suit the needs of students. The National Project on Career Education, discussed earlier, came about in part because of such requests (Updegraff, Steffan, Bishop, & Egelston-Dodd, 1979).

Gallaudet College and the National Technical Institute for the Deaf both have legislative mandates to provide such information, as do other postsecondary programs, such as the Regional Education Programs supported under Section 625 of the Education of the Handicapped Act. Although helpful information has been exchanged, there has yet to appear any universal, magical cookbook approach to improve secondary curricula for transition of the hearing-impaired developmentally disabled school-leaver. More extensive and systematic utilization of career education programming would help students accomplish the transition process.

Perspectives on Vocational Needs

Vocational needs may be addressed from a number of perspectives. These perspectives include a three-pronged approach to the vocational needs of deaf people, with an equal emphasis on special education, rehabilitation, and postsecondary education. Within this overall perspective, the central question that emerges is, What are the vocational needs of hearing-impaired developmentally disabled people?

Guidance in responding to this question comes from the report of the planning group for the National Workshop on Independent Living Skills for Severely Handicapped Deaf People (Ouellette & Lloyd, 1980). This workshop, supported in part by the Rehabilitation Services Administration, identified the following topics:

- Basic assessment of independent living skills
- Health/hygiene
- Social/personal behavior patterns
- Job practices
- Money management/budgeting
- Family responsibilities
- Community awareness
- Legal awareness (p. 19)

Participants in the workshop also presented a description of six levels of independent living.

Level 1: lives in an institution

Level 2: lives at home (dependent)

Level 3: lives at home (semi-independent)

Level 4: lives alone

Level 5: skilled

Level 6: professional (p. 20)

The workshop group focused on needs of those described by Levels 1–3. People fitting the descriptions for Levels 1 and 2 are clearly unemployable. Those at Level 3 are typically capable of menial employment. People at Level 4 are basically employable but have poor work records and high absenteeism, may read and understand simple words, may possibly drive, and may have left high school with only a second-to-fourth grade achievement level. Levels 5 and 6 comprise those individuals who will most likely be self-reliant through life. The evidence shows that the majority of deaf people need ongoing specialized services. While there is a great need in the U.S. to provide the previously mentioned Five New Basics and literacy for students, significant numbers of deaf people are struggling for survival skills and lack clearcut programs to assist them in attaining these skills.

The contrasts between the ringing words of the Five New Basics, the call for literacy, and the needs of the hearing-impaired developmentally disabled are great. Yet the goal of education, whether for the academically inclined or for the individual learning survival skills, is the same: achieving human dignity. The pathways to dignity for these two diverse groups are not the same. We are still searching for creative, effective ways of serving the less able.

Vocational Rehabilitation Services

The 66th Congress created the federal-state partnership for vocational rehabilitation in 1920. The intent of Public Law 66-236 was to extend to civilians some of the rehabilitation services that were available to veterans of World War I. The philosophy was that civilian workers injured on the job could easily be returned to productive work by rehabilitation services. Through the years, vocational rehabilitation has expanded in scope and sophistication to provide services to millions of U.S. citizens each year. The system is still striving toward perfection. There are still thousands of families with disabled young people that do not know about rehabilitation services and their impact. The goal of vocational rehabilitation is to provide the services needed by handicapped people to obtain and retain jobs appropriate to their skills and interests. Services provided in search of this often elusive goal may include counseling, medical evaluation, social-psychological evaluation, assistance with purchase of assistive devices, work evaluation, work adjustment training, postsecondary career training, job placement, and follow-up services. These are valuable services that are the birthright of U.S. citizens, and they need to be extended to all in need of them. Vocational rehabilitation professionals have demonstrated that the provision of these services is cost-effective and an investment in the future of the U.S. and its disabled citizens.

For the hearing-impaired developmentally disabled individual, the services of vocational rehabilitation are especially critical. Professionals in vocational rehabilitation have the expertise to coordinate experts from a variety of fields to focus on the needs of the individual. Numerous residential schools across the country have developed exemplary relationships with vocational rehabilitation agencies; some include on-campus offices. The changes brought about by Public Law 94-142 and by the swing away from residential school placement toward the mainstreaming of hearing-impaired students in public school programs have created a gap in referral services. This gap must be closed. Personnel serving mainstreamed hearing-impaired students in public secondary schools must develop relationships with vocational rehabilitation agencies. Such relationships can be especially meaningful in helping individuals formulate substantive educational plans.

A critical issue that needs to be examined is that of the individual's access to appropriate postsecondary rehabilitation programs. With rehabilitation dollars limited, students/clients are being urged and, in some cases, forced to remain in their home states for postsecondary education or rehabilitation programs. This is untenable if the home state lacks appropriate facilities and resources to meet the individual's needs. Students with special learning needs should not be placed in watered-down or splintered programs because of state boundaries or financial restraints. Ideally, every student deserves the opportunity for optimal programming, regardless of that program's location or cost.

In very broad terms, there are three categories of secondary school graduates or school-leavers. The first group includes higher functioning individuals who are able to matriculate at one of the federally funded postsecondary institutions or other postsecondary education programs. The second broad category of deaf students contains those who are likely to be active clients of rehabilitation counselors over an extended period of time. Many of these individuals can profit from postsecondary education in goal-oriented technical/vocational programs. Individuals from this category will typically profit from work evaluation programs to fine-tune their career selection and direction. Many people from this group will seek rehabilitation services and related counseling services throughout their lives.

The third category is deaf individuals with developmental disabilities. They are classically the under-served and difficult to define population. Individuals in this group often do not achieve independence and typically require life-long support. Postsecondary education is often an impossible dream. Many will not profit from traditional vocational rehabilitation services. Members of this group may be found in institutions, long-term sheltered workshops, group homes, and half-way houses, and, unhappily, some are sheltered away from society by their families. Numerous individuals in this group have parents who have invested their lives in seeking solutions for their child who is now an adult or soon to become an adult in a society which has no place for him or her. Language skills for members of this group fall far below the third-grade level and most often are at the level of word recognition; writing skills are below the survival level; money management skills are near absent; and speech and speechreading skills are virtually nonexistent. Members of this group may display such additional disabilities as visual impairment, mental retardation, epilepsy, cerebral palsy, orthopedic problems, and mental and emotional problems. Yet within the group are also some who have normal or above-average intelligence. The social, vocational, and psychological problems of these youngsters may seem insurmountable. However, professionals with actual case experience are aware that, given the proper services, many of these people can move from dependence to independence. Several of the major obstacles that prevent more widespread success stem from attitudinal barriers on the part of society, overrestrictive rules and regulations that do not permit massive attacks on the problems, and lack of appropriate funding to provide the resources and programs needed.

The three broad categories of deaf high school graduates or school-leavers are not numerically equal, though hard and fast figures for a numerical breakdown remain elusive. The best information available indicates that the smallest category contains those students who go on to postsecondary institutions. The second and third categories constitute the majority and the population that remains underserved.

The Labor Market of the Future

The U.S. has become a high technology, information-based society. Attention has been focused on high technology corridors, such as those in California, North Carolina, Louisiana, and Massachusetts. Other states are attempting to bring in high technology industries. The U.S. economy has become inextricably bound with the world economy. One-sixth to one-fourth of products produced anywhere in the country are bound for the world market. The impact of foreign countries on the local market place is readily apparent when shopping for clothing, a television, an automobile, or other commodities. The hearing-impaired population is not isolated from these changes. Sheltered workshops in the U.S. compete with the national labor markets of Mexico, Taiwan, and Korea for jobs that were traditionally subcontracted locally. Futurists state that the workforce will become bimodal, with high technology as one growth area and service occupations as a second growth area. Tens of thousands of citizens have been adjusting to change in the workplace in the past few years. It is self-evident that such change will continue.

Projects with Industry (PWI) is a recent undertaking of the Rehabilitation Services Administration. The PWIs are proving to be excellent change agents for providing creative and innovative methods for assimilating handicapped individuals into the workforce. Futurists, economists, the business sector, and government are providing road maps for the future. Hearing-impaired people, along with the general population, can plan and prepare for the future using these road maps. The need for basic skills will never disappear from the workplace. A renewed emphasis on the basics will help to prepare hearing-impaired developmentally disabled persons for their places in high technology.

However, it must be recognized that many hearing-impaired developmentally disabled people will not develop the skills necessary to compete successfully for jobs in high technology industries. There are routinized jobs in those industries that will be appropriate for hearing-impaired developmentally disabled people, but there will probably be strong competition for such jobs.

Even in this era of high technology, there are many jobs that do not require the skill levels required in high technology industries. Writing in *The Futurist,* Bolles (1983) points out that the jobs that increased the most during the 1970s were in familiar occupations, not in high technology, except for computer operators. Jobs like roofers, teachers' aides, receptionists, mining workers, and business repair services increased in the range of 71 to 190 percent. Other jobs are expected to remain fairly constant or to increase slightly; these include construction workers, clothing workers, food service workers, repair workers for various kinds of equipment, health workers, and in general, "people who are good with their hands, good with their eyes, and good with their minds to do the things that have always needed doing in civilized society" (p. 8). Such jobs do, however, require the kind of basic skills discussed in this chapter. We must assist hearing-impaired developmentally disabled persons to acquire these skills.

Selected Service Options

There are at least two major options for providing cost-effective programs for serving hearing-impaired developmentally disabled people. The first is the establishment of a national resource center. Precedents for such a center are Gallaudet College, the National Technical Institute for the Deaf, the Helen Keller Memorial Center, and other select specialized facilities. A second option is the establishment of regional centers for serving this population. Precedent for regional centers can be found in the Discretionary Programs of the Education of the Handicapped Act. Both options provide the same benefits although the method of service delivery would be different. Several benefits would accrue with the establishment of one national center or a series of regional centers.

1. A concentration of people with similar disabilities would eliminate feelings of isolation and create a critical mass of students/clients. This is viewed as essential to the provision of training/rehabilitation programs from both the student/client's and the staff's points of view. From the student's point of view, a critical mass permits development of friendships, communication with other students in a common native language, and positive self-image.*

   From the staff's point of view, a critical mass permits the organization of programs of adjustment, work evaluation, prevocational training, vocational training, job-readiness training, job seeking skills training, job try-out, job placement, and follow-up.

2. A concentration of the resources of staff, facilities, and dollars would permit trained and qualified staff to develop innovative, creative approaches to the

---

*Placement in a mainstreamed setting separated from peers commonly results in poor self-concept and feelings of isolation among hearing-impaired developmentally disabled individuals. During periods of intensive service delivery, therefore, an environment that supports camaraderie and free communication will typically foster self-esteem and significantly greater progress.

complex problems of the students/clients. Appropriate facilities would concentrate self-assistance aids such as TDDs, special alarm systems, architectural design, and adaptive equipment appropriate for this population. Such
centers would therefore be cost-effective.

3. The opportunity for research to seek ways to improve educational and
   rehabilitation practices suitable and effective for hearing-impaired developmentally disabled people would be available. Depending upon the location,
   affiliation with an established research center would be an additional cost-
   effective measure.

4. Dissemination of information to elementary, secondary, and postsecondary
   schools and to rehabilitation agencies and organizations would be facilitated.

5. Previously unserved and underserved individuals would have equal opportunity and access to the rehabilitation process.

It is common for those techniques that have been successful with deaf students/
clients to have crossover advantages for other handicapped and special populations. One
example is the use of notetakers in postsecondary education. Formalized programs of
notetaking were not part of the U.S. education scene in the late 1960s. In the 1980s,
notetakers are a commonplace educational support service for students with a variety of
handicapping conditions and students who are learning English as a second language. A
federal effort to provide ongoing services for hearing-impaired developmentally disabled
people might be a program designed first to serve this population but with spinoff
benefits for other populations.

The implementation of one national or several regional programs for hearing-
impaired developmentally disabled people might be accomplished with favorable
interpretations of existing legislation or with new congressional legislation.

Essential components of programs for hearing-impaired people include work evaluation and prevocational and vocational training. Work evaluation, also known as vocational assessment or evaluation, is a relatively new professional discipline. Professional
training is available as a full major in this field at Auburn University, the University of
Arizona, the University of Southern Illinois, and the University of Wisconsin–Stout.
Over the years, work evaluation techniques have been applied with deaf clients in a
variety of rehabilitation centers, including the projects for multihandicapped deaf
people of the late 1960s and early 1970s which were unable to continue after the
expiration of federal funding. *Deaf Evaluation and Adjustment Feasibility: Guidelines for the
Evaluation of Deaf Clients* (Watson, 1976) provided a comprehensive overview of the
potential impact of vocational evaluation.

In 1981, the University of Arkansas Rehabilitation Research and Training Center
on Deafness and Hearing Impairment, RT-31, was established with three priorities:
adjustment, employment, and vocational evaluation. In October 1982 the center con-
vened a national symposium on Innovative Research and Practice in Evaluation, Adjustment Training, and Employment Services for Hearing-Impaired Persons.
Publications covering the three topic areas are available from the center. The publication

on vocational evaluation is recommended reading and provides current evaluation methodologies for the three broad categories of deaf people discussed earlier.

Vocational evaluation provides hands-on, pragmatic assessment that, when appropriately designed, is the cornerstone of rehabilitation programs and select postsecondary education programs. Vocational evaluation leads to prevocational training by identifying potential areas of training on an individual basis. Once these areas are identified, prevocational training can take place. Prevocational training provides job sampling and job development. Typically, it deals with very basic fundamentals, including basic arithmetic skills, language development, work nomenclature, and training in daily living skills. Prevocational training may also be vocational training for some people because of learning limitations. Such training may last from a few weeks to a few months, depending upon the individualized plan for each person.

Ideally, vocational training should occur in an established facility that has demonstrated ability to serve hearing-impaired students. The support service model at the St. Paul Technical Vocational Institute is viewed as a model program providing a broad range of support services. These services include a preparatory program, counseling, interpreting, notetaking, and tutoring, provided by a staff trained to serve deaf individuals. No compromises should be made in the provision of vocational training for deaf individuals; they have the same right to quality education that hearing people have. Vocational evaluation, prevocational training, and vocational training are essential services that in part secure the future for hearing-impaired developmentally disabled people.

The Federal Role

Historically, there has been a disparity in funding available for the three broad categories of deaf individuals. The first group, those who have the ability to succeed at the postsecondary level and enter the professional ranks, have received the most federal assistance through the programs of Gallaudet College and the National Technical Institute for the Deaf. Regional postsecondary education programs are also covered under federal legislation, but with a different set of rules, regulations, and funding levels. These programs tend to serve people from the first and second groups. Interpreter training programs are also legislated with separate rules, regulations, and funding levels; these programs tend to be most beneficial to members of the first and second groups, who utilize the services of interpreters to a greater extent than members of the third group.

During the 1960s and early 1970s, federal grant support was available for services to multihandicapped deaf people, but these programs were phased out at the expiration of federal funding. In the early 1970s, federal legislation for multihandicapped deaf people was attempted, but there was not sufficient momentum to carry the bill through the entire legislative process. Eugene W. Peterson, director of the federally funded grant program for multihandicapped deaf people (housed at the Crossroads Rehabilitation Center in Indianapolis during the 1970s), has written and lectured on what he terms, "The Two Sides of Habilitation/Rehabilitation Services for the Deaf" (Peterson, 1981). He presented dollar figures demonstrating that the lack of substantive services for multihandicapped deaf people is much more costly in the long run than providing habilitation/rehabilitation services up front. By 1983, however, there still was no federal grant money earmarked for this group of clients. Federal funding differences are dramatic for the three broad categories of deaf people discussed above. For fiscal 1984, Gallaudet College and the National Technical Institute for the Deaf combined had an authorized ceiling of approximately $80 million; four regional postsecondary education programs were to be funded at not less than $2 million; and 10 interpreter training programs were funded at $900,000. There were no other federal funds legislated for direct services to deaf people. Clearly, deaf individuals in the first broad category are receiving substantial financial attention to assist them in well-deserved educational pursuits. Deaf individuals in the second category will receive direct case service funds from the state vocational rehabilitation agency in their individualized rehabilitation programs, and some benefit from the federally funded postsecondary programs. Deaf individuals in the third category are not directly served in identified programs. Advocacy pursuits on behalf of this group need to be strengthened and focused.

The U.S. has a well-functioning system of special education for handicapped children from preschool through 12th grade. That system has been profoundly influenced by Public Law 94-142. Passed in 1975 and implemented through regulation in 1977, this legislation has dramatically changed the manner in which most handicapped children receive their education. It has created changes in the activities of parent groups, public school classrooms, residential schools for the deaf, local boards of education, state boards of education, professional organizations related to the handicapped, classroom teachers, and so on. The effects of this landmark legislation on those with hearing impairment are debated wherever people concerned with deafness gather. National organizations in the field of deafness have provided congressional testimony on the impact of PL 94-142. Persons interested in in-depth analysis of the multiple issues surrounding the implementation of this law should consult their national organizations or their members of Congress for further information. Of particular interest are the congressional oversight hearings that have been held by the Senate Subcommittee on the Handicapped.

Similarly, the U.S. has a functioning system of rehabilitation that has been profoundly influenced by Section 504 of the Rehabilitation Act of 1973. As PL 94-142 continues to be debated, so does the implementation of Section 504. The National Center for Law and the Deaf at Gallaudet College has played a leadership role in this area. Agencies such as LAPHIP (Legal Advocacy Program for Hearing-Impaired Persons) in Minneapolis work on a local level to seek enforcement of Section 504. The issues are complex, and several cases have reached the U.S. Supreme Court.

Historically, rehabilitation has encompassed more than the federal-state partnership in vocational rehabilitation. Rehabilitation has been an industry that encompasses numerous service delivery systems. These include social, welfare, employment, legal advocacy, and mental health services in addition to the more traditional rehabilitation services.

In 1983, Congress approved the Education of the Handicapped Act Amendments (PL 98-199) which could significantly affect the lives of all handicapped citizens of the U.S., including those who are deaf. Section 626, Secondary Education and Transitional Services for Handicapped Youth, provided for improved transitional services for handicapped school graduates as they move to postsecondary education, vocational rehabilitation, continuing education, employment, and independent living. [See Appendix A for a 1984 congressional report on H.R. 3435, including remarks on Section 626, and Appendix B for the text of Section 626 as approved in 1983.]

As the foregoing indicates, the federal role in education and rehabilitation of handicapped citizens has been significant. However, efforts to secure equivalent services for multihandicapped people have been less successful. Those few programs that were initiated with federal dollars folded when federal support was withdrawn. Hence, most hearing-impaired developmentally disabled people lack equal opportunity in the U.S.

In addition, legislation on developmental disabilities has had little impact on the field of deafness, although the legislative definition of developmental disabilities (see Chapter 2) clearly applies to hearing-impaired people as described in this chapter. One thrust of this chapter has been to examine why this legislative overlap has been so minimal and to issue a challenge to those who work with deaf people to examine thoroughly the implementation of developmental disabilities legislation to determine whether hearing-impaired people who meet the criteria of developmental disabilities can benefit more significantly from the legislation.

Summary

Estimates of the hearing-impaired developmentally disabled population in the U.S. hover around one million individuals of all ages. Preschool through 12th grade education is provided by a combination of federal, state, local, and some private funding. Attempts to provide services locally for those who are hearing-impaired and developmentally disabled meet with variable success. The Five New Basics, as proposed by the National Commission on Excellence in Education, and the recommendations of the Carnegie commission on literacy provide a stark contrast with the demonstrated achievement levels of individuals with impaired hearing and developmental disabilities. The U.S. needs to preserve and strengthen public policy that provides all of its citizens the opportunity to become productive citizens.

A critical phase of life for handicapped youth is the transition period between high school and adulthood. Career education programs in the schools and vocational rehabilitation services enhance the transition phase. When such services are absent, transition to adult life can be fraught with problems. If schools have not provided structured career education programs, students/clients are less able to make effective use of vocational rehabilitation services. Referral networks among educators, rehabilitation providers, postsecondary educators, and other human service providers need to be strengthened.

Families of hearing-impaired developmentally disabled people may face a lifetime of dependent adult children, with all the accompanying frustrations, economic loss, and family disruptions, if those children lack resources for gaining independent living and economic status. Federal legislation is pending that will facilitate transitional programming for handicapped youth. Entry into adult life may be through employment, postsecondary education, or such rehabilitation services as work evaluation, work adjustment training, sheltered workshop activities, group living in half-way homes, and other kinds of activities. Those entering directly into employment may face the dilemma of immediate "dead end-ing" with no promotional potential if they do not have competitive work skills or if their employers do not provide training.

There are three broad categories of deaf individuals—those with postsecondary academic potential, those who would benefit primarily from goal-oriented technical vocational education and other vocational rehabilitation services, and those who are less able and who have one or more additional handicaps. It is this third category that is of interest here. For individuals in this category, the necessary kinds of intensive continuing special education, rehabilitation services, and lifelong follow-along services are not available. During the late 1960s and the 1970s, attempts were made through grants of vocational rehabilitation monies to provide services. Federally funded programs were established in Hot Springs, Arkansas; St. Louis, Missouri; Indianapolis, Indiana; and Boston, Massachusetts. Those programs demonstrated that severely handicapped deaf individuals profit from specialized intensive programs of rehabilitation. Like other efforts initiated with federal funds, each was terminated, unable to continue upon the expiration of federal funding. In the early 1970s, legislation was introduced that had the potential for providing long-lasting programs of service to combat the debilitating effects of multiple disabilites. Unfortunately, that legislation did not gain the necessary momentum to become law. Also in the 1970s, the Administration on Developmental Disabilities funded a program of national significance at the University of Arizona. It was successful in providing information about and model programs for hearing-impaired developmentally disabled people and further heightening awareness of the special needs of this population. Statistical data, census information, and heightened awareness are all beneficial. They do not, however, replace direct and ongoing services to individuals in need. Communication barriers and language deprivation have grave consequences for those trying to meet their vocational needs. These problems can be ameliorated given staff expertise, facilities, and funding with open-ended, flexible policies that program for the individual.

Developmental disability legislation, rules, and regulations hold the hope for a beginning in solving the all-pervasive needs of hearing-impaired developmentally disabled people. The questions are simple: Do deaf individuals meet the definitions for eligibility for developmental disability services? And do existing legislation, rules, and regulations at long last contain the flexibility for mounting a significant effort on behalf of those who are hearing impaired and developmentally disabled? If hearing-impaired individuals can be served under existing legislation, an aggressive campaign must be waged to ensure equality of access for this group of disabled people. If they cannot be so served, then new legislation must be enacted to facilitate such services.

References

American Annals of the Deaf. (1983, April). Programs and services for the deaf in the United States. *128*(2), p. 210.

Bolles, R. N. (1983, December). Life/work planning: Change and constancy in the work force. *The Futurist, 7*(6).

Boyer, E. L. (1983). *High school: A report on secondary education in America* (The Carnegie Foundation for the Advancement of Teaching). New York: Harper and Row.

Hoyt, K. B. (1975). *An introduction to career education: A policy paper of the U.S. Office of Education.* Washington, DC: U.S. Government Printing Office.

National Commission on Excellence in Education. (1983). *A nation at risk: The imperative for educational reform.* Washington, DC: U.S. Government Printing Office.

Ouellette, S., & Lloyd, G. (Eds.). (1980). *Independent living skills for severely handicapped deaf people* (Monograph No. 5). Silver Spring, MD: American Deafness and Rehabilitation Association.

Peterson, E. W. (1981). The two sides of habilitation/rehabilitation services for the deaf. *Journal of Rehabilitation of the Deaf, 14,* 18–25.

Rawlings, B. W., Trybus, R. J., & Biser, J. (Eds.). (1983). *A guide to college/career programs for deaf students.* Washington, DC: Gallaudet College Office of Demographic Studies.

Schein, J. D., & Delk, M. D., Jr. (1974). *The deaf population of the United States.* Silver Spring, MD: National Association of the Deaf.

Stewart, L. (1978). *Hearing impaired developmentally disabled persons: A model demonstration program.* Tucson: University of Arizona College of Education.

Updegraff, D. R., & Egelston-Dodd, J. (1982). The national project on career education: Past, present, and future. *Directions, 2*(4).

Updegraff, D. R., Steffan, R. C., Jr., Bishop, M. E., & Egelston-Dodd, J. (1979). *Career development for the hearing-impaired: Proceedings of two working conferences.* Washington, DC: Gallaudet College Pre-College Programs.

Watson, D. (1976). *Deaf evaluation and adjustment feasibility: Guidelines for the vocational evaluation of deaf clients.* New York: New York University Deafness Research and Training Center. (Available from the National Association of the Deaf, Silver Spring, MD.)

Appendix A
Education of the Handicapped Act Amendments of 1984 (H.R. 3435)

[Excerpts from U.S. House of Representatives Report No. 98-410, Committee on Education and Labor (98th Congress, 1st Session), pp. 3–5, 29–30]

Legislative History

H.R. 3435, the Education of the Handicapped Act Amendments of 1984, was introduced in the House of Representatives by Rep. Austin J. Murphy on June 28, 1983, and referred to the Subcommittee on Select Education of the Committee on Education and Labor.

A hearing on H.R. 3435 was held by the Subcommittee on July 14, 1983.

Among the witnesses testifying at this hearing were Ms. Madeleine Will, Assistant Secretary for Special Education and Rehabilitative Services, U.S. Department of Education, accompanied by Dr. Edward Sontag, Acting Director, Special Education Programs; Dr. Eleanor Chelimsky, Director, Institute for Program Evaluation, U.S. General Accounting Office; Dr. Philip R. Jones, Professor and Coordinator, Administration and Supervision of Special Education, Virginia Polytechnic Institute; and Dr. Brian McNulty, Supervisor of Special Education and Early Childhood State Coordinator, Colorado Department of Education.

On July 21, 1983, following the introduction of amendments, the Subcommittee on Select Education met in open executive session and reported H.R. 3435 with amendments to the Committee on Education and Labor by unanimous voice vote.

On July 26, 1983 the committee on Education and Labor ordered reported H.R. 3435, with amendments, by a voice vote.

Background

The Education of the Handicapped Act is the principal mechanism for providing Federal aid to State and local school systems for educational and related services to handicapped children. Central to the Act is the State-formula grant program (Public Law 94-142), authorized under Part B, which requires each State receiving Federal funds to provide a free appropriate public education to all handicapped children in that State.

In addition to the State-formula grant program, this legislation authorizes ten discretionary grant programs aimed at supporting and improving the direct services provided under Public Law 94-142. These are designed to support a variety of research, technical assistance, demonstration, dissemination, training and model project activities.

In the Elementary and Secondary Education Amendments (ESEA) of 1966, Congress added a new Title VI creating both a program of grants to the States to assist in the education of handicapped children as well as a Bureau of Education for the Handicapped within the Office of Education, and establishing a National Advisory Committee on Handicapped Children (NACHC).

The Elementary and Secondary Education Amendments of 1970 (Public Law 91-230) consolidated into one act a number of previously separate Federal grant authorities relating to handicapped children, including Title VI of ESEA. This new authority was entitled the "Education of the Handicapped Act."

The Education Amendments of 1974 (Public Law 93-380) authorized a sharp increase in funds to assist States in educating handicapped children in the public schools. It required States to establish a goal for providing full educational opportunities for all handicapped children and to submit a plan and timetable for achieving this goal. It further provided procedural safeguards for use in identification, evaluation and placement for these children and elevated the administrator of the Bureau of Education for the Handicapped.

In 1975, the Education for All Handicapped Children Act (Public Law 94-142) expanded the Part B program. This part, which received a permanent authorization, was a significant milestone in the nation's efforts to provide full and appropriate educational and related services to handicapped children.

In 1977 the discretionary programs—parts C–F of the Education of the Handicapped Act were extended for five additional years. The National Advisory Committee on the Handicapped was not reauthorized in 1977 because the then Bureau of Education of the Handicapped was providing effective leadership in the area of handicapped education and, as a result, a separate advisory committee to also provide such leadership was no longer necessary.

The Bureau of Education for the Handicapped became part of the Office of the Assistant Secretary for Special Education and Rehabilitative Services in the Education Organization Act of 1979. The Bureau is now called Special Education Programs (SEP).

The Omnibus Reconciliation Act of 1981 (Public Law 97-35) extended the authorization of appropriation for the Education of the Handicapped Act through fiscal year 1983. Part B, the State Grant Program (Public Law 94-142), although permanently authorized, had its authorization ceiling capped from fiscal year 1981 through fiscal year 1984 in the Omnibus Reconciliation Act. Under Section 414 of General Education Provisions Act, the discretionary programs werc automatically extended for one additional year. The 1977 amendments did not include reauthorization of appropriations for Part G: Special Programs for Children with Specific Learning Disabilities on the grounds that the passage of Public Law 94-142 amends the definition of "handicapped children" to include "children with specific learning disabilities" therefore permitting potential grantees with projects addressing the service needs of specific learning disabled children an opportunity to apply for funds under any of the discretionary programs authorized by the Education of the Handicapped Act. Under the terms of a floor amendment, however, authority was provided for the continuation of model specific learning disability projects under Part E: Research.

*   *   *   *

Part C—Section 626: Secondary Education and Transitional Services

The Committee recognizes that while educational programs for elementary age handicapped children are fairly well developed in most areas of the country and are proving to be successful in meeting the unique educational needs of these children, this is hardly the case with secondary education programs. Research indicates that handicapped students at this level need more individualized instruction, counseling, practical daily living and socialization skills, as well as specially designed programs to assist them in improving their various career and academic skills. Appropriate vocational training is essential, the Committee believes, if handicapped students are going to be successful in making the transfer from the educational system to the "world of work."

In order to begin to address this need, H.R. 3435 authorizes the Secretary to make grants or enter into contracts to develop projects to improve secondary education programs, to coordinate with other federal activities serving this population and to provide training and related services to assist handicapped youth in the transitional process from the educational system to the wide range of postsecondary environments including but not limited to college [and] competitive and sheltered employment.

The Committee believes that the coordination among all educational and adult service agencies, including mental health, mental retardation, public employment, vocational rehabilitation and employers themselves is needed to facilitate the development of transitional services to handicapped youth. It is the Committee's intent that the Office of Special Education and Rehabilitative Services assist States with the administration of both special education and rehabilitation services in order to improve secondary, transitional and postsecondary opportunities for handicapped persons.

In order to promote the broadest possible participation of agencies which could contribute to successful transition of handicapped students from school to work and from home to independent living, Section 626 specifically references the State Job Training Coordinating Councils and Service Delivery Area Administrative Entities of the Job Training Partnership Act [JTPA], Public Law 97-300.

The inclusion of these entities as potential participants under Section 626 grant and contract activities is viewed as a positive step by the Committee to apply maximum resources to the needs of handicapped youth. However, if such entities do receive grants or contracts under Section 626, they can only be provided in a manner which is consistent with provisions of the JTPA.

It has come to the attention of the Committee that in many parts of the country, local school districts fail to provide adequate evaluations and individualized education programs for secondary handicapped students. The Committee anticipates that these new provisions will assist public agencies to be more responsive to the needs of handicapped youth in secondary programs.

Appendix B
Education of the Handicapped Act Amendments of 1983

[Excerpt from Public Law 98-199 (98th Congress, 1st Session), approved December 2, 1983]

Secondary Education and Transitional Services for Handicapped Youth

"Sec. 626. (a) The Secretary is authorized to make grants to, or enter into contracts with, institutions of higher education, State educational agencies, local educational agencies, or other appropriate public and private nonprofit institutions or agencies (including the State job training coordinating councils and service delivery area administrative entities established under the Job Training Partnership Act (Public Law 97-300) to—

"(1) strengthen and coordinate education, training, and related services for handicapped youth to assist in the transitional process to postsecondary education, vocational training, competitive employment, continuing education, or adult services; and

"(2) stimulate the improvement and development of programs for secondary special education.

"(b) Projects assisted under this section may include—

"(1) developing strategies and techniques for transition to independent living, vocational training, postsecondary education, and competitive employment for handicapped youth;

"(2) establishing demonstration models for services and programs which emphasize vocational training, transitional services, and placement for handicapped youth;

"(3) conducting demographic studies which provide information on the numbers, age levels, types of handicapping conditions, and services required for handicapped youth in need of transitional programs;

"(4) specially designed vocational programs to increase the potential for competitive employment for handicapped youth;

"(5) research and development projects for exemplary service delivery models and the replication and dissemination of successful models;

"(6) initiating cooperative models between educational agencies and adult service agencies, including vocational rehabilitation, mental health, mental retardation, public employment, and employers, which facilitate the planning and developing of transitional services for handicapped youth to postsecondary education, vocational training, employment, continuing education, and adult services; and

"(7) developing appropriate procedures for evaluating vocational training, placement, and transitional services for handicapped youth.

"(c) For purposes of subsections (b)(1) and (b)(2), if an applicant is not an educational agency, such applicant shall coordinate with the State educational agency.

"(d) Projects funded under this section shall to the extent appropriate provide for the direct participation of handicapped students and the parents of handicapped students in the planning, development, and implementation of such projects.

"(e) The Secretary, as appropriate, shall coordinate programs described under this section with projects developed under Section 311 of the Rehabilitation Act of 1973."

Chapter 17

Program Evaluation and Quality Assurance

Sandra Raymore Wright and Karoldene Barnes

This chapter will address the issue of quality assurance at the systems level, giving attention to program monitoring and evaluation procedures. Several formal systems will be described that offer formats for evaluating and achieving quality specifically in educational settings.

In the broadest sense, quality assurance involves paying systematic attention to all aspects of a service delivery system: (1) initial system design (selection of personnel, equipment, procedures); (2) standard-setting (agreeing on parameters of service); (3) periodic monitoring to determine whether actual service meets the standards; and (4) establishing a feedback loop to ensure corrective action when performance falls below standard. Documentation that the service provided has been appropriate and effective requires detailed attention to the recommendations that have evolved from the diagnostic, educative, and rehabilitative efforts of the interactive interdisciplinary team. In the past, individual professionals, clinics, and educational programs have lacked formal systems for documenting plans and progress for specific clients. Similarly, few service programs have had mechanisms in place for overall program evaluation. Due to recent regulatory changes and enhanced public awareness, program administrators have sought systematic methods for evaluating the quality of their programs and the progress of the clients they serve.

The quality assurance concept is one that historically relates to consumer issues in the industrial market place. However, this same concept has been generalized to the educational and health fields, largely in response to federal legislation such as Public Law 94-142 (the Education for All Handicapped Children Act) and Public Law 92-603, which resulted in Professional Services Review Organizations (PSROs). Educational service consumers (such as students, parents, administrators) and local, state, and federal agencies now may expect that service providers demonstrate and document accountability, i.e., assurance that the service being provided to disabled populations is of the highest quality possible (Diggs, 1983). This need for the documentation of quality prompts service providers to seek techniques or systems that assist in the planning, development, management, and evaluation of services.

To fulfill the PL 94-142 mandate requiring documentation of the appropriateness and effectiveness of provided services, special and regular educators, supervisors, and administrators must be knowledgeable and skilled in management systems that

- identify and provide appropriate services for all handicapped children;.
- ensure efficient program management strategies;
- accurately evaluate pupil progress; and
- demonstrate program and service accountability and cost effectiveness to boards of education, parents, state and federal agencies, and the public.

However, most preservice education programs for professionals dealing with handicapped populations focus on the clinical and educational skills necessary for service delivery rather than on program management skills. Nevertheless, the current focus on programming for the handicapped under PL 94-142 and the required documentation of services suggest that systems training at the preservice level is not only appropriate but also necessary in order to facilitate efficient accountability procedures. The lack of academic training in program management often extends beyond practitioners to those in supervisory and administrative positions. In a 1982 membership survey (Fein, 1983) conducted by the American Speech-Language-Hearing Association (ASHA), only 33 percent of the supervisor and administrator respondents reported receiving managerial training as part of their college or university coursework. Instead, inservice conferences, seminars, and workshops were by far the most common type of administrative, management, or supervisory training modes reported.

The ASHA collected supporting data in a professional self-study project in 1982 (Rees & Snope, 1983). Practitioners without ASHA Certificates of Clinical Competence at the bachelor's degree level, as well as those at the ASHA-certified master's degree level, responded to questionnaires designed to survey professional competencies. Of the 38 competencies surveyed, these practitioners rated themselves lowest in management skills. Less than 30 percent of the respondents with graduate degrees described themselves as competent in program management skills. Special educators also have identified inservice training needs in program evaluation (Bale, Hanley, & Grant, 1981). Randomly selected educators and educational administrators indicated their priorities among 10 training needs related to communication disorders. School principals earmarked four of their top five needs in the areas of development and evaluation of programs for communicatively handicapped students.

In 1981, ASHA members employed in school settings were randomly asked to participate in a national caseload survey (ASHA Staff, 1981). The specific data from this survey are addressed in a later section of this chapter. Two relevant points emerged from results generated by the 899 respondents.

- Almost one-third of the students served in their caseloads received less service than was needed.
- Eighty-eight percent indicated that a total of nearly 5,000 speech-impaired students were "identified but not served," and nearly 3,000 were "referred but not evaluated."

These data suggest that practitioners perceive weaknesses in their caseload management procedures, namely, that some communicatively impaired populations are either inappropriately served or not served at all under the present system of caseload management.

In both the 1981 and 1982 surveys, service providers, educators, and administrators indicated several training concerns relating to the assurance of quality services for speech-, language-, and hearing-handicapped students. These concerns pertained specifically to program management, quality assurance, caseload accountability, and data collection. Models for program management in these areas for use by both service providers and administrators do exist. The remainder of this chapter will address four such programs as well as applicable information derived from Quality Circles, a Japanese industrial management technique used by many American corporations.

Figure 1 describes the four management skill areas—program management, quality assurance, data collection, and caseload accountability—and examples of programs developed by ASHA through specially funded projects.

Management **Skills**	Management **Program**
Program Management	Essentials of Program Planning, Development, Management, Evaluation (PDME)
Quality Assurance	Child Service Review System (CSRS)
Data Collection	Comprehensive Assessment and Service Evaluation (CASE)
Caseload Accountability	Caseload Accountability Seminar: How to Make Better Decisions

Figure 1. Primary management skills with examples of programs. Copyright 1983 by the American Speech-Language-Hearing Association.

Although each of the four management programs in Figure 1 is designed to be used independently, given a work setting with few or no existing management systems, all programs are supportive and, indeed, complementary. A brief discussion of their interrelationship follows a summary of each.

Program Management and the PDME

In anticipation of a comprehensive plan for improved services for all handicapped children by the 1980s, various professional groups met in the early 1970s to discuss the concept of program accountability and the application of formal systems to achieve and demonstrate such accountability. Sponsored by ASHA's School Affairs Program, these workshops involved more than 3,000 school, university, and state department of education professionals. In the foreword to the program manual generated from this project, Healey (1973) stated:

> The consensus among school personnel favoring the development of a management-by-objectives system for speech, hearing and language programs and the momentum toward requiring a formal systems approach in educational programming suggested that a nationally developed manual for program planning, development, management,

and evaluation utilizing the best components of existing systems could provide appropriate technical assistance to speech, hearing and language specialists. (p. iii)

To this end, the PDME program was developed. The full name of the program and manual describes the nature of its focus: *Essentials of Program Planning, Development, Management, Evaluation: A Manual for School Speech, Hearing and Language Programs.* Figure 2 shows steps toward implementation of the PDME and the interrelationships of these steps.

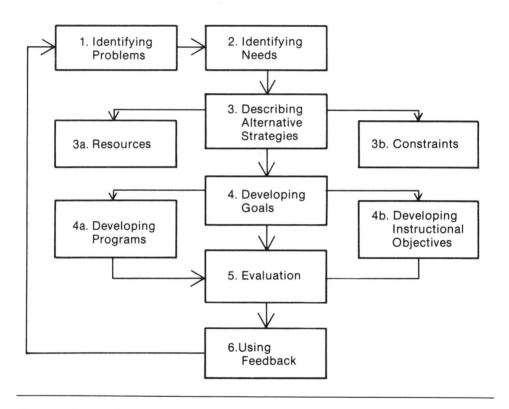

Figure 2. Schema for the PDME program. From *PDME Manual,* 1973 (DHEW, Office of Education, Bureau of Education for the Handicapped, Division of Research, Grant No. OEG-0-9-302169-4324(607), PL 91-230 Title VI), Rockville, MD: American Speech-Language-Hearing Association. Copyright 1973 by American Speech-Language-Hearing Association.

Five of the basic steps may be briefly described as follows:

1. Identifying Problems. Utilizing PDME procedures, program staff begin by analyzing the status of services to handicapped children. Major problems are identified as well as verified by reviewing available information. The unmet needs of pupils, the problems and concerns of staff, the extent to which facilities meet program needs, the financial resources available, the effects of program policies, and the existing case management practices may be identified. Once problems are indicated, a needs assessment is initiated. The magnitude of the identified problem(s) is determined through questionnaires, interviews, and data analysis.

2. Identifying Needs. Once problems are identified and validated by determining their magnitude, program strengths and limitations are outlined. Program needs are then determined and placed in a hierarchical arrangement. Next, the current program status in the identified need area is analyzed in relation to the determined need level. An example is offered to clarify the process.

Where we want to be: *All* speech/language pathologists and audiologists work together as a *team* with classroom teachers to provide language stimulation activities on a *regular* basis to hearing-impaired developmentally disabled students.

Where we are now: Some speech/language pathologists and audiologists have *independently* worked with classroom teachers to develop *limited* language stimulation activities for hearing-impaired developmentally disabled students.

Need: Increase the scheduling of uniform language stimulation activities in the classroom for hearing-impaired developmentally disabled children.

3. Describing Alternative Strategies. Once the need is identified, several possible solutions are outlined. The feasibility of each possible solution is evaluated. That is, the resources and constraints that affect the quality of the solution are identified. Do the constraints outweigh the resources? After reviewing the possible solutions, weighing the resources versus constraints, and considering the ultimate benefit to clients, a strategy is selected as a solution that reflects the highest potential for the best possible outcome in the least amount of time at the lowest cost possible.

4. Developing Program Goals. With the solution to the problem determined, the next step is to develop program goals. By deciding what is going to be done, and when, the criterion for success becomes specific, measurable, and directive. For example:

By March 15, 1984, implement the team-developed classroom language stimulation program in each elementary school classroom for hearing-impaired developmentally disabled students.

4a. Developing Program Objectives. The development of program goals leads to the next step in the PDME process, development of program objectives. As the objectives relate to the activities created to achieve the previously stated goals, they are measurable components of the program which address these details: *when* the objective will be complete, *who* will complete the objective, *what* will be done, *to whom* it will be done, the *criterion* for success, and the method of *evaluation* to be used to determine if the objective is completed. To carry the earlier mentioned example one step further, the following shows one objective of several involved in the process of developing a language stimulation program.

By October 1, 1984, each speech/language pathologist and audiologist will complete the Teacher Survey for all kindergarten teachers in schools he or she serves and submit the Teacher Survey to the supervisor.

4b. Developing Instructional Objectives. The same components exist for instructional objectives as for program objectives with the exception that the content relates specifically to activities in which the student is engaged. These objectives may be developed for long-range, monthly, weekly, or daily use. An example of a long-range instructional objective:

> By December 1, Michael will demonstrate an ability to get the attention of at least five classmates by saying or signing their first names in the teacher's presence. The classroom teacher will record the correctly identified names in Michael's work folder.

Through the use of instructional objectives, the practitioner is able to collect information that may be used to evaluate program component effectiveness.

5. Program Evaluation. The purpose of evaluation is to analyze and determine the effectiveness of the stated goals and objectives. The components of the objectives assist in the definition of the evaluation method. The PDME program describes several levels of evaluation based on the stated objectives. Upon completing the evaluation of objectives specific to a given goal, the evaluator is able to make appropriate program decisions for the future.

Quality Assurance and the CSRS

While the PDME process focuses on a general program management system, the following discussion describes a second system which focuses on improvement strategies for a single unit within a system, that of quality assurance. To be more specific, once a system for general program management is in place, what system can be used to identify and seek solutions to problems related to quality?

The Child Services Review System (CSRS) addresses the mandates of PL 94-142, which requires the provision of appropriate individualized services, documentation of services provided, team management for handicapped pupils, and personnel development for service providers. The CSRS meets these requirements by

- developing criteria for identifying and evaluating appropriate and effective services in the local setting;
- reviewing individual records or Individualized Education Programs (IEPs);
- including all service providers in various elements of the process; and
- involving providers in assessing and improving services.

The CSRS is designed to demonstrate that services meet identified standards of quality and do improve the abilities of pupils who receive the services. The system is designed to move sequentially through a series of activities which

- identify an area for review;
- establish desired standards within the chosen area;
- audit selected records germane to the chosen area;
- identify service delivery trends; and
- improve the quality of services.

Services provided to a specific pupil by a specific specialist are not appropriate for CSRS review. Instead, CSRS focuses on general outcomes of the intervention process and highlights those services that are effective and efficient as well as those that would benefit from modification.

Figure 3 illustrates the sequence of nine steps involved in the CSRS process. The following discussion briefly describes the primary components of each step.

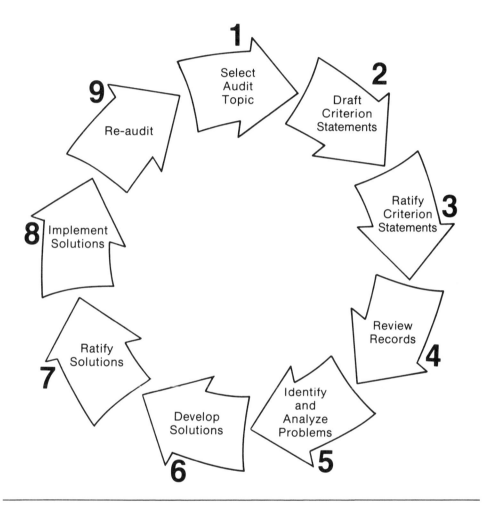

Figure 3. CSRS audit cycle. From *CSRS Manual*, 1981, Rockville, MD: American Speech-Language-Hearing Association.

The CSRS process begins with the selection of an audit committee, i.e., three to five direct service providers from the program staff who are trained in the CSRS system. The consensus process is a unique one in that it substitutes a participatory management procedure for the typical hierarchical decision-making process. Once the committee is established, the process, or cycle, begins with the selection of an audit topic, as shown in Figure 3.

1. Select Topic. The committee may select any topic specific to service delivery for review. Once the topic is identified, the focus or purpose of the audit is defined as well as the population for which records will be reviewed and the time period from which the records will be drawn.

2. Draft Criterion Statements. The committee drafts several statements that will serve as quality standards against which actual performance can be measured. Included in the statements are the expected levels of performance, which identify the specific components that outline the quality of the performance being reviewed. Each statement is given a threshold for action which specifies the number of reviewed records that must meet the expected level of performance. Records that fail to meet the established criteria are designated for action by the committee.

3. Ratify Criterion Statements. This step involves ratification by the staff member(s) whose records will be reviewed. Each criterion statement and threshold for action is reviewed by the staff member, who is encouraged to propose changes to those statements or thresholds that are unacceptable.

4. Review Records. From the population identified by the audit committee, the staff members review a sample of pupil records to determine if the conditions established in the ratified criterion statements have been met. Those records that do not pass the specified screening criteria are referred to the committee for further review. The committee then determines an actual level of performance for each criterion statement.

5. Identify and Analyze Problems. At this level, the audit committee compares the actual level of performance to the threshold for action for each criterion statement. After the committee verifies a performance deficiency, possible problems causing discrepancies between the threshold for action and actual level of performance are identified and rank ordered.

6. Develop Solutions. The committee next develops a remedial action plan based on the causes. This plan defines the parameters for action, personnel, and time involved, as well as the data for re-audit.

7. Ratify Solutions. Staff members whose records were reviewed are then asked to ratify the remedial action plan or to propose changes in the plan.

8. Implement Solutions. This step involves the program staff in taking the action specified in the plan. In this process, they complete new records, which are monitored by the audit committee.

9. Re-audit. Using the original criterion statements, the program staff re-audits at the time specified in the remedial action plan. The purpose of this step is to determine if services to the specified population have improved.

This description of the CSRS procedure is decidedly simplistic; however, the systematic nature of assessing and delivering quality services by a team of professionals is illustrated in this step-by-step problem-solving approach. Full and appropriate use of the procedure is possible only after completion of the CSRS training workshop, available from trainers who have participated in inservice training provided by ASHA.

To effectively plan, develop, and evaluate a program or the quality of any of its components, both the PDME and CSRS programs require that data be collected. As necessary as all data collection is, administrators and supervisors often face overburdened service providers when a request for data is made. An oft-heard response is "Not *another* form!" The following section addresses this critical area of data collection.

Data Collection and the CASE

As indicated, professionals working with handicapped children face increasing demands for data from educational consumers, administrators, and agencies at the local, state, and national levels. For example, data now must be collected on larger numbers of students due to child-find and child-count requirements. Also, the complexity of data gathering has increased due to several factors, e.g., discrepancies between federal and state needs, team evaluations, departmental concern for accountability, and student placement decisions. A PL 94-142 impact study (Dublinske & Karr, 1984) revealed that, due to increased data collection requirements, direct service providers spent 9 percent less time dealing with students. In addition, supervisors spent 62 percent more time in collecting, analyzing, and reporting data.

A 1972 project supported by ASHA at the local, state, and national levels to collect data on children with communication handicaps revealed further information related to the need for improved data gathering systems. The project, titled NEEDS (National Evaluation of Education Districts Services), identified several deficiencies in the existing data systems. Several pertinent findings emerged which gave direction to service providers (Snope, Duran, & Dublinske, 1981).

- No state department of education or federal agency had developed a student management data system that would permit the systematic collection of data to evaluate the progress made by handicapped students receiving special services.
- In local education programs, student management data were often absent.
- Few school districts routinely used any formal system to summarize and evaluate program and student management data.

In an effort to determine the feasibility of a student management system that would address the findings of the NEEDS survey, a field study was implemented. Data were generated by comparing items and procedures used in existing systems with those that would be required in a prototype. The feasibility study revealed that

- Record-keeping systems varied among school districts and among service providers.
- Student records were often difficult to locate.
- In at least 50 percent of the student cases surveyed, record forms being used did not provide for (1) a child's enrollment in other special education programs, (2) information related to services being provided by an outside agency, (3) identification of the referral source, (4) the date of the referral, or (5) screening of test results.

- Diagnostic test results were not present in 47 percent of the surveyed records.
- Student management data that would affect the evaluation of services as well as programmatic decisions varied greatly from school district to school district.

To provide speech/language/hearing service providers with a system to deal with the record-keeping problems and increases in demand and complexity of descriptive data, the *Comprehensive Assessment and Service Evaluation Information System* (CASE) was developed. Through a series of processes and model forms, the system is used to collect, store, and facilitate retrieval of student and program data. The CASE provides materials and guidelines for (1) evaluating and planning a program, (2) increasing program efficiency, (3) documenting program and staff practices, and (4) analyzing the appropriateness and effectiveness of services.

The CASE model was developed to help identify data needs, formalize data collection procedures, and help speech/language/hearing practitioners evaluate and upgrade existing systems. For those service providers implementing computer programs, CASE includes a computerization component that allows the development of an automated information system. This section of the system is designed to guide program designers to determine whether to use a manual or automated system, select an appropriate approach to computerization, and develop a computerized information system.

Figure 4 shows the flow of information provided by the CASE Information System. This data collection system consists of three program manuals which include systems specific to student management, program management, and system implementation.

Student Management. The processes at this level (see Figure 4) involve student identification, parent contact, referral, screening, assessment, placement, intervention, and case coordination. The activities are designed to collect, store, and retrieve information on the delivery of services to speech-, language-, and hearing-disabled individuals. Materials are provided for referral, screening, assessment, placement, and intervention. In addition to individual student information, student summary records are provided to document comprehensive information specific to individuals receiving services.

Program Management. The processes at this level involve student information, cost analysis, and special reports. Like the student management system, this system is designed to collect, store, and retrieve information. Its focus, however, is at the program level so that the data can be used for planning, designing, implementing, managing, and analyzing program functions, services, and outcomes. The system facilitates compilation of information by grade, school, and school district (Local Education Agency, LEA on the flow chart, Figure 4). Items pertinent to program cost and time allocations for personnel are also included.

Implementation Guide. A guide delineates seven implementation steps for use of CASE within a school or school district setting. Included are materials to be used as transparencies or handouts for inservice programs or data collection.

Forms. Data collection forms, available for each component, are flexible and additive in their application. More specifically, information components which might meet

STUDENT MANAGEMENT LEVEL

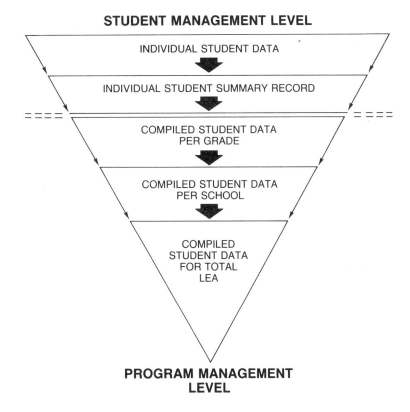

Figure 4. CASE information system flow chart. From *CASE Implementation Guide*, 1981, Allen, TX: Developmental Learning Materials. Copyright 1981 by Linc Services, Inc. Reprinted by permission.

the individual needs of a program can be added without altering the applicability of the component or the system.

Data collection is critical to the determination of caseload appropriateness. Administrators and service providers alike must document the number of students being seen, contact hours, etc. The following section outlines some of the problems and solutions for making caseload decisions.

Caseload Accountability

Caseload selection and size have always been of primary concern to specialists employed in school settings; PL 94-142 has brought this problem into sharper focus by requiring that practitioners account for the services they provide. In response to these concerns, the ASHA Governmental Affairs Department reviewed 1983 data received from a state educational consultant survey (Dublinske & Karr, 1984). The review revealed that only 28 states designated a maximum caseload, with a reported range from 15 to 80 students per practitioner. The ASHA Committee on Language, Speech, and Hearing Services in the Schools reviewed 1981 data and found that, in most instances, mandated caseload sizes were established with little or no rationale. In determining a specific caseload size, limited attention was given to (1) differences in disorder, type, or severity; and (2) the types of service delivery models that could be used (ASHA Staff, 1983).

In the national caseload survey conducted by ASHA in 1981 (ASHA Staff, 1981), 899 ASHA members reported the following:

- The average weekly caseload during the survey period was 43, while the average caseload for the entire school year was 53 students.
- Respondents indicated a total of 4,986 communicatively impaired students who were identified but not served and 2,897 who had been referred but not evaluated.
- Some respondents (31.4 percent) said they were not allowed to indicate in the Individualized Education Programs (IEPs) all the special education and related services needed by a child.
- Respondents indicated that 31 percent of the students served in their caseloads received less service than needed.

These data indicate that all communicatively handicapped children are not receiving an appropriate education as required under PL 94-142. This is due in part to the large caseloads that are mandated in some states. Although PL 94-142 does not recommend specific practitioner-student ratios, state and local policies in many instances do. As noted previously, maximum caseload size can exceed 80 students. Those concerned with quality of services must consider criteria for determining appropriate caseload size and composition; that is, a program with consistently large caseloads over a long period runs the risk of lowered service quality as well as service provider burnout. The ASHA has developed guidelines for four levels of service programs, number of times served per week, and caseload size (Committee on Language, Speech, and Hearing Services in the Schools, 1984, p. 56).

- Consultation (1 to 5 times/week): Up to 15–40 students
- Itinerant (2 to 5 times/week): Up to 25–40 students
- Resource Room (4 to 5 times/week): Up to 15–25 students
- Self-Contained (full-time placement): Up to 15 students with aide;
  up to 10 students without aide

In response to the needs of practitioners for training in caseload selection and dismissal, the ASHA national office staff developed a two-day seminar package. The seminar was designed to identify current caseload issues and problems, provide sample problem-solving/decision-making strategies to address the issues, and help participants identify methods to solve problems associated with case selection/dismissal and related areas. To supplement the seminar, a manual (ASHA, 1984) was developed, complete with fact sheets, suggested techniques, sample severity rating scales, synopses of seminar presentations, references, and methods for developing caseload selection material criteria. Included in the manual are

- facts about caseload on local, state, and national levels;
- issues and problems surrounding case selection and dismissal;
- solutions from experts who have dealt with caseload problems;
- methods to develop local or statewide entry and dismissal caseload criteria;
- strategies for gaining administrative support for caseload decisions and plans; and
- techniques to control caseload to maximize effectiveness.

Interrelationship of the Systems

As shown earlier in Figure 1, the described programs are designed to function as resources in four separate areas: program management (PDME), quality assurance (CSRS), data collection (CASE), and caseload accountability (Caseload Accountability Seminar).* To clarify the application of these programs, it is helpful to show their interrelationship in the process of providing quality services to hearing-impaired developmentally disabled students. The following example illustrates these interrelationships.

One Specific School District (OSSD) is a rural local education agency with a newly formed special education department. The director of the special education program, Ms. X, determined that, since no program management system was in place, she would implement the PDME program. She reasoned that its systematic nature would assist her in the planning, development, management, and evaluation of the special education department.

While completing the PDME evaluation process over the course of a year, Ms. X learned that members of her staff felt that the services being offered to the students, while adequate, could be improved. In an effort to identify the special education

---

*Readers interested in obtaining copies of the program manuals mentioned in this chapter may request purchase or other information from the following sources:

PDME, CSRS, Caseload Accountability
  Publications Office, American Speech-Language-Hearing Association,
  10801 Rockville Pike, Rockville, MD 20852

CASE
  DLM Teaching Resources, One DLM Park, Allen, TX 75002

Further information is also available through a program sponsored by the American Speech-Language-Hearing Association and partially funded by the U.S. Department of Education (Division of Personnel Preparation—Special Education Programs). The program, the PDQ Project, is fully titled "Planning and Development of Quality Services in the Schools." The focus of the PDQ Project is to provide management system information for professionals working in special education school settings. The project featured 50 one-day workshops during the 1984–85 school year throughout the U.S. School professionals likely to benefit from these experiential, problem-solving workshops include speech/language pathologists, audiologists, local level special educators (i.e., program supervisors, coordinators, and directors), and state level special educators. For further information, contact Sandra Raymore Wright, PDQ Project Director, ASHA, 10801 Rockville Pike, Rockville, MD 20852.

program's strengths and weaknesses, Ms. X used the CSRS system with the support of the CASE system to collect the necessary data. At the CSRS audit cycle level, which focuses on identification and analysis of problems, the audit committee determined that caseload issues were priority problems. Intervention on the basis of information received in the Caseload Accountability Seminar was proposed, and the solution was ratified and implemented. As a result of the CSRS re-audit, Ms. X and the special education program staff determined that the caseload problem was alleviated. Other departments in the school district, encouraged by the results of Ms. X's efforts, applied quality assurance systems to their programs.

The example illustrates the interrelated application of (1) PDME as a total program management technique, (2) CSRS as a system to evaluate the quality of a single component of the program, (3) CASE as a system of data collection strategies and forms, and (4) Caseload Accountability as a model for decision making related to entry/exit criteria and size.

Each of the four management systems implies or specifically addresses (as does PL 94-142) the need for interdisciplinary team interactions. The PDME suggests a total program strategy which implies team involvement in the various components of the system. The CSRS, pinpointing a specific program component for quality review, specifically addresses techniques for consensus-building for team members during the nine-step audit cycle. As a data collection system, CASE inherently involves teams of professionals in the gathering and analysis of data. Again, in the area of caseload accountability, teams of professionals working together to solve problems related to caseloads can effect change more readily than can individuals working separately. The next section focuses on this issue of team involvement in quality assurance.

Quality Assurance and Teaming

As Matkin pointed out earlier (Chapter 5), interactive interdisciplinary teams are particularly effective for evaluating and making placement decisions for hearing-impaired developmentally disabled children within the requirements and intent of PL 94-142. In addition to the use of teaming for student management, another benefit is the team's ability to gauge progress for program management purposes.

On the individual level, bridging the gap between identifying and evaluating a hearing-impaired developmentally disabled child or youth and initiating effective programming to maximize the social, emotional, and educational growth of that individual is a difficult task. Some common barriers to program implementation include

- limited availability of appropriate programs within a reasonable distance from home;
- limited availability of personnel to provide specific needed services in the program chosen by the family;
- inadequate space for delivery of service;
- large caseloads;
- failure to designate a team leader responsible for ensuring consistent service delivery;

- less than optimal parent/guardian participation in the educational and treatment plan; and

- inability or unwillingness of the school or other service system to assume the
  excess costs (beyond the average per capita cost) of programs for hearing-
  impaired developmentally disabled students.

The interactive interdisciplinary team consists of professionals whose common goals
are elimination of programmatic barriers and successful implementation of recommendations. An effective team needs to demonstrate supporting, participating, clarifying, and mediating behaviors and be skilled in group process techniques (e.g.,
brainstorming, consensus achievement). An effective team leader should be skilled in
managing the team and helping it achieve its goals within a given time frame. Defining
the goal, encouraging full expression of contrasting viewpoints, keeping the group on
task, guiding but remaining in the background, establishing group operational guidelines, summarizing discussions, promoting resolution of conflict, remaining neutral
during discussions, eliciting contributions to clarify areas of confusion, and allowing the
group to make final decisions are skills an effective facilitator or group leader must
possess.

Unfortunately, the responsibilities for team leadership and participation are often
informally assumed without training in the dynamics and skills for group participation
or leadership. However, with the addition of administrative sanction and priority
acknowledgment, a facilitator or group leader will be able to participate in training that
emphasizes creation of a group atmosphere which encourages input and discourages a
conflict mode of operation or the "playing out" of hidden agendas. Groups with this
type of open, production-oriented interaction achieve quality programming more
readily than do groups without administrative support or leadership training.

Teams require training in group participation as well as in leadership skills; team
leaders can then be chosen with the knowledge of what is needed for successful leadership. A team leader should have responsibility for calling all meetings, notifying all
participants, preparing a format and agenda, acting as facilitator, and summarizing the
meeting as to necessary follow-up and delegation of tasks to individual members. A team
leader may also have responsibility for supervising designated task completion for
specific cases; thus, the traditional "case manager" role may be one part of the team
leader's function. Realistically, the team leader is an advocate both for the individual
whose program is under consideration and for the personnel who have the responsibility
of carrying out the program plan agreed upon by both parents and professionals.

Quality Circles

A relatively new concept in management systems in the U.S., the Quality Circle,
emphasizes teamwork in participatory management. The Quality Circle (QC) process
stresses participatory decision making (O'Hanlon, 1983) and traditionally has been used
in business and industry to maximize productivity; educational institutions are beginning to adopt QCs as a means of quality assurance through group participation.

An overview of QCs developed by Bandy (personal communication, 1983) described
their development in Japan in 1961 under the guidance of Dr. Kaoru Ishikawa, an

engineering professor at Tokyo University. By combining components of Maslow's Hierarchy (Maslow, 1954) and the management theories of Herzberg (1966) and MacGregor (1960, 1966), as well as North American statistical quality control practices, Dr. Ishikawa conceived the Quality Circles system. Circles now operate throughout Japan and, since the 1960s, throughout parts of the Western world. The QCs are used in banks, hospitals, governmental and service organizations, and large U.S. corporations, e.g., Lockheed, General Motors, Westinghouse, Polaroid, and Honeywell, as well as in the U.S. Navy. Several educational institutions have also made use of QCs, e.g., the Muskegon, Michigan, school system; Lane Community College in Eugene, Oregon; and the Tulsa, Oklahoma, public schools. By spring 1983, more than 4,000 organizations had implemented QCs (Chase, 1983).

Based on the belief that people are the most important resource in a business or educational institution, the QC is a group of 5 to 12 people who voluntarily meet on a regular basis to discuss common problems and solutions in their work area. Through participatory management, the process aims to improve employee attitudes, motivation, and, ultimately, production. Those familiar with management theory will recognize that the people-oriented focus of Quality Circles bears a resemblance to Theory Z, a management style developed by William Ouchi (1981) that promotes not only greater employee productivity but also higher degrees of employee satisfaction, company loyalty, and performance (O'Hanlon, 1983).

Using a process similar to that of the Child Services Review System (CSRS) mention earlier, the successful operation of a QC involves the use of several steps and techniques. Figure 5 (facing page) graphically illustrates the Quality Circle operation. Briefly, these processes and techniques include the following steps (Bandy, 1984).

Problem Identification and Selection. Through the guidance of a specially trained group leader, the QC identifies several problems using brainstorming techniques. After group consideration of each problem, the group chooses a specific problem for the focus of its attention.

Problem Verification. To verify that the selected problem is indeed an existing area of concern, the circle members gather, display, and analyze data critical to the problem. External advisors may be asked to assist in the analytical component of this step.

Cause and Effect Analysis. Using cause and effect analysis techniques, circle members identify the major cause(s) of the selected problem. The techniques, specially designed for QC use, are basic cause and effect analysis (incorporating a fishbone diagram) and process cause and effect analysis (activities which include brainstorming and voting techniques).

Cause Verification. At this stage of problem solving, circle members collect and analyze data to verify the identity of the primary cause(s) of the problem. Data collection, analysis, and display techniques are similar to those used at the problem verification stage.

Solution Generation and Selection. Through the use of brainstorming and voting techniques, the circle members generate solutions to the problem. By setting priorities for their brainstormed solutions, members vote on the best solution(s) to the problem. That solution is then researched so that information supporting it may be presented to management.

Management Presentation. All circle members participate in the verbal presentation to their supervisor. The presentation includes a review of the QC process with data charts that were developed in the problem-solving process. The supervisor is then given a specified period of time in which to respond in

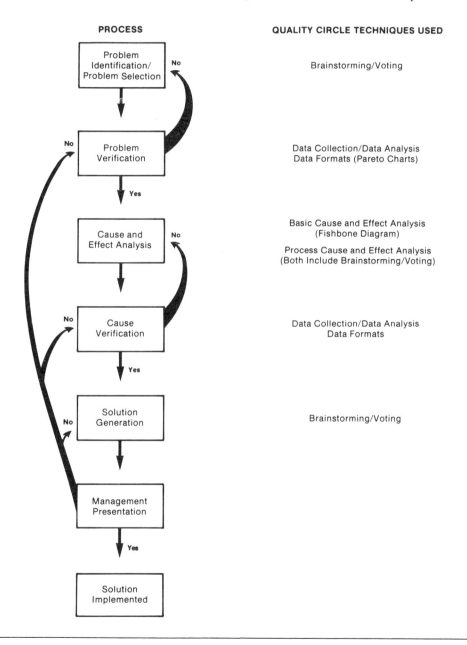

Figure 5. Flow chart of quality circle operation. From Beth R. Bandy, Director of Special Projects, Illinois State Board of Education. Reprinted by permission.

writing to the circle indicating his or her acceptance or rejection of the members' recommendation(s).

Solution Implementation/Rejection. If the supervisor accepts the circle recommendations, the next step, solution implementation, is enacted as quickly as possible. If, however, the supervisor rejects the recommendations of the circle, specific reasons must be provided. The circle then returns to the problem verification, cause verification, or solution generation stage to initiate the process again on the basis of the supervisor's written rationale. (p. 4)

Several techniques are used to facilitate the QC's specialized people-oriented problem-solving strategy. Before the actual problem-solving process is initiated, all Quality Circle members are trained in seven techniques.

1. Formal brainstorming
2. Data collecting
3. Data presenting formats and graphs
4. Decision analysis
5. Basic cause and effect problem analysis
6. Process cause and effect problem analysis
7. Management presentation

As in the earlier systems, obtaining administrative support is critical to the successful operation of Quality Circles. Management personnel must favor and accept the concept of participatory decision making. If there is a union, it is recommended that a representative be included as a member of the QC.

In the development of a QC program, a steering committee must be appointed by the administration to select and provide training for a facilitator, develop program goals and policies, and select an area for implementation. It is important that the program remain voluntary and have a regular meeting time and place (one hour per week is recommended). The facilitator is encouraged to maintain communication, to allow the program to grow slowly, to develop recognition methods (e.g., certificates), and to maintain publicity regarding the program.

The need for Quality Circle or Theory Z-like approaches (i.e., those approaches that involve long-term development of personnel, trust between workers, participative decision making, and a shared philosophy) in education is becoming apparent. Professionals are learning more about personnel burnout and stress and their negative impact on the education process. Moretz (1983) reported the results of a circle member reaction survey regarding the use of QCs in education. She found

- improved attitude factors (e.g., trust, communication, cooperation) in the group;
- generally improved problem-solving skills (e.g., goal setting, problem identification, consensus development); and
- mild to moderately improved interaction factors (e.g., confidence in administration's support and communication with the administration).

Ninety percent of the members recommended continuation and expansion of the QC process.

Implementation problems were found to include skepticism about the applicability of the QC in an educational setting; tendency of supervisors to arbitrarily merge different QC groups; tendency of highly trained members occasionally to spend time philosophizing and "hair-splitting;" slowdown at the end of the school term; lack of budget flexibility to allow the QC group to redirect its funds; inability to define *productivity* in education and to control the variables; and expression of "hopelessness," defined as the feelings of teachers and other educators that change will not occur.

However, Moretz contended that there is hope for application of Quality Circles in education. Larger educational institutions appeared more conducive to participation than did smaller educational settings, where greater adaptation was required. Citing funding of QCs as a major problem, Moretz described the cost of facilitator and group leader training and materials as possible deterrents. By suggesting "adoption" of smaller educational settings by larger institutions, Moretz focused on a possible solution: well-established QC programs could provide training and implementation guidance for new ones.

The Quality Circle process seems to hold promise for the educational field. Clearly, obtaining administrative support and training potential members are critical variables for ensuring success of this novel approach to quality assurance and stress management in the educational milieu.

References

ASHA. (1981). *Child services review system.* Rockville, MD: American Speech-Language-Hearing Association.

ASHA. (1984). *Caseload issues in schools: How to make better decisions.* Rockville, MD: American Speech-Language-Hearing Association.

ASHA Staff. (1981, July). The speech-language pathologist in the public school: A current profile. *Governmental Affairs Review, 2*(2), 77–81.

ASHA Staff. (1983). Recommended service delivery models and caseload sizes for speech-language pathology services in the schools. *Asha, 25*(2), 65–70.

Bale, R., Hanley, T. Z., & Grant, W. (1981). *An assessment of inservice training of regular classroom teachers: Final report* (Contract No. 300-79-0775). Washington, DC: U.S. Department of Education, Office of Program Evaluation.

Bandy, B. (1984). Operation: An overview of quality circles. Material for workshop conducted in Springfield, IL.

Chase, L. (1983, February). Quality circles. *Educational Leadership,* pp. 18–26.

Committee on Language, Speech, and Hearing Services in the Schools. (1984). Guidelines for caseload size for speech-language services in the schools. *Asha, 26*(4), 53–58.

Diggs, C. C. (1983). Professional accountability: Present and future directions. *Seminars in Speech and Language, 4,* 169–185.

Dublinske, S., & Karr, S. T. (1984). *State education agency consultant results.* Rockville, MD: American Speech-Language-Hearing Association.

Fein, D. J. (1983). Survey report: 1982 ASHA omnibus. *Asha, 25*(3), 53–57.

Healey, W. C. (1973). Foreword. In S. Jones & W. C. Healey, *Essentials of program planning, development, management, evaluation: A manual for school speech, hearing and language programs.* Rockville, MD: American Speech-Language-Hearing Association.

Herzberg, F. (1966). *Work and the nature of man.* New York: World Publishing.

Jones, S., & Healey, W. C. (1973). *Essentials of program planning, development, management, evaluation: A manual for school speech, hearing and language programs.* Rockville, MD: American Speech-Language-Hearing Association.

MacGregor, D. (1960). *The human side of enterprise.* New York: McGraw-Hill.

MacGregor, D. (1966). *Leadership and motivation.* Boston: Massachusetts Institute of Technology Press.

Maslow, A. H. (1954). *Motivation and personality.* New York: Harper and Row.

Moretz, H. L. (1983). QC teams in education: Experience and prospects. *1983 Transactions: Fifth Annual Conference of the International Association of Quality Circles,* 178–179.

O'Hanlon, J. (1983, February). Theory Z in school administration? *Educational Leadership,* pp. 16–18.

Ouchi, W. (1981). *Theory Z.* Reading, MA: Addison-Wesley.

Rees, N., & Snope, T. (1983). *Proceedings of the 1983 National Conference on Undergraduate, Graduate and Continuing Education* (ASHA Reports No. 13). Rockville, MD: American Speech-Language-Hearing Association.

Snope, T., Duran, J., & Dublinske, S. (1981). *CASE: Comprehensive assessment and service evaluation. Implementation guide.* Allen, TX: Developmental Learning Materials.

Chapter 18

Stress Management and Professional Burnout

Judith S. Johnson

As stated throughout this text, a team approach can improve services to handicapped individuals. Planning, implementing, and evaluating services in this manner allows for the best possible programming and monitoring for each individual in a caseload. However, the team approach to quality assurance is sometimes inhibited because of the inability of one or more individuals to function effectively in groups, inadequate experience and training in group dynamics, or a lack of familiarity with the needs of the hearing-impaired developmentally disabled population.

In any discussion of quality assurance, it is helpful to look at the needs of the individual who provides services. This person, who is a member of a team providing services, may be responsible for determining the most effective strategies for bridging the gap between diagnosing and programming for children with special needs. Quite often, due to the intense nature of their work, the members of the human services professions, and particularly special education teachers, experience occupational stress and burnout.

Madeline Hunter (1977) said that the three potentially most stressful occupations in the world were air traffic control, surgery, and teaching. Teachers bear the brunt of many ailments of the modern world—vandalism, physical assault, drug abuse, economic setbacks, scorn, and lack of public respect. It is frequently suggested that teachers suffer also from the belief that they must surely be in the most degrading and menial of all professions (Bardo, 1979; Mace, 1979; Zabel & Zabel, 1980).

Recent changes have increased teachers' burdens. The Education for All Handicapped Children Act of 1975 (Public Law 94-142) mandated increased involvement of regular classroom teachers with handicapped children and youth through the placement of such students in the public schools. This involvement, which includes the need to develop Individualized Education Programs with parental participation, has resulted in large numbers of teachers being overwhelmed with bureaucratic red tape each year before they have even begun to teach. These responsibilities, added to a workload expanded by larger classes, many hours spent in planning and preparation, mandatory school reports and forms, and a diminishing ability to maintain control over disrespectful and unruly students, have made the school environment an unpleasant place in which to work (Alley, 1980; DuBrin, 1979; Gray, 1979; Hendrickson, 1979; Kraft & Snell, 1980; Pattavina, 1980; Smith & Cline, 1980; Werner, 1980).

Public Law 94-142 has affected special education teachers in a similar manner—bringing them a changing student population, increased paperwork, and the imposition of greater accountability for their teaching (Bensky, Shaw, Gouse, Bates, Dixon, & Beane, 1980; Cook & Leffingwell, 1982; Foster, 1980; Shaw, Bensky, & Dixon, 1981; Weiskopf, 1980). Thus, the already considerable stress caused by the intense nature of their work with handicapped students is compounded further by these regulations. Such stress becomes even more pronounced when the students demonstrate slow, or little, improvement after a long period of remediation (Foster, 1980). Teachers of severely and profoundly handicapped children are believed to experience greater stress than those who teach nonhandicapped children (Moracco, Gray, & D'Arienzo, 1981). It is suggested that the degree of stress experienced is in direct proportion to the severity of the handicapping conditions. Students who are only mildly handicapped usually demonstrate the greatest academic advancement. Progress tends to decrease as handicapping conditions increase in severity and degree, resulting in a proportionately greater degree of teacher stress (Zabel & Zabel, 1980).

Hearing impairment, particularly in very young children, is one of the most debilitating of handicaps, one that requires an intensive, highly individualized educational program. Even so, such students often terminate their school years with poor academic achievement and, as adults, are often underemployed and function below normal levels within the structure of society. Teachers of the hearing impaired, fully aware of this fact, cannot help but experience stress both in their work and in the knowledge that the end results of their efforts may be subnormal performance (Meadow, 1981).

Hearing-impaired individuals who have additional handicaps require even more intensive schooling. Their teachers require different types of training, and they must approach their teaching fully cognizant of the problems that will confront them. Nevertheless, they are also affected by the crisis situations which dominate their work, and they suffer the inevitable consequences.

In short, educational and supportive personnel whose work entails extensive interaction with other people—particularly with those for whom the quality of life may be poor and whose problems are never fully remediated—experience a high degree of cumulative stress (Foster, 1980; Griffin, 1982; Weiskopf, 1980).

Stress and Burnout

Occupational stress can be described as resulting from conditions in the environment that are perceived as placing excessive demands on the individual employee. When constant occupational stress is experienced, physical or mental exhaustion may occur. "When the emotional stress continues without relief, the teacher, unable to cope with stress, begins the process of burning out" (Weiskopf, 1980, p. 19).

Stress can be perceived as a condition of life. It is an integral part of living, and, in spite of the bad publicity it receives, is not something to be eliminated from life. Stress is the driving force that enables people to meet the challenges of day-to-day living (Alley, 1980).

Hans Selye (1978) wrote that "stress is the spice of life," and that no individual can live without experiencing some degree of stress as a constant throughout life. The events of life—crossing a busy street, the cooling winds of a summer day, the return of the soldier from the battlefield—activate the body's stress mechanism to some extent. Stress is not necessarily bad for an individual, as any activity, any emotion, causes stress. Stress that causes illness in one individual can be an exhilarating experience for another. It is only when there is excessive stress that it becomes a threat to the very quality of life. Thus, stress is viewed as a problem only when it interferes with one's ability to effectively carry out day-to-day tasks.

The effects of excessive stress vary in severity from a gain or loss in appetite (Collins & Masley, 1980; Harlin & Jerrick, 1976; Hendrickson, 1979; Meadow, 1981) to total physical or emotional breakdown (Harlin & Jerrick; Hendrickson). Some of the more common physiological effects experienced by teachers are frequent headaches (Collins & Masley; Harlin & Jerrick; Hendrickson; Walsh, 1979), colds and flu (Harlin & Jerrick; Hendrickson), stomach problems (Gray, 1979; Walsh), heart problems (Walsh), sleep-lessness (Gray; Meadow), fatigue (Collins & Masley; Gray; Hendrickson; Weiskopf, 1980), dizziness (Hendrickson), shortness of breath (Gray), and increased blood pressure (Collins & Masley; Gray; Walsh).

In addition to the physiological effects of stress, teachers also experience a variety of psychological effects. Hendrickson (1979) stated that "teachers who feel physically unwell soon find themselves depressed by their symptoms" (p. 37). Common psycho-logical effects of stress are depression (Collins & Masley, 1980; Foster, 1980; Harlin & Jerrick, 1976; Weiskopf, 1980), low self-esteem (Alley, 1980; Kyriacou & Sutcliffe, 1978), and irritability (Collins & Masley; Gray, 1979; Harlin & Jerrick; Weiskopf). Stress has also been linked to addiction to alcohol and other drugs, including excessive smoking (Harlin & Jerrick; Hendrickson; Walsh, 1979; Weiskopf; Zabel & Zabel, 1980).

Stress and the Special Education Teacher

Cook and Leffingwell (1982) reviewed common work stressors experienced by special educators. They postulate that while each stressful situation should be evaluated individually, and no two individuals respond identically to similar situations, a common pattern of stressors, which can be remediated by school systems, does exist.

Both role conflict, or role ambiguity, in which the teacher is faced with conflicting demands from others, and role overload, where the workload becomes too great in volume or too difficult, contribute to the degree of stress experienced by the teacher. The teacher's role perceptions of his or her work are greatly influenced by previous education and training and by personal values and expectations. Those perceptions often come into conflict with role perceptions held by school administrators and fellow teachers. Difficulty in achieving consensus produces teacher stress. Lack of time to complete work during the normal school day is perceived as stress-producing, because teachers perceive that school-related work infringes heavily on their personal time.

Special populations require materials and equipment specifically designed to facili-tate individualized instruction. The inadequate provision of such materials by school administrators means that teachers must purchase or create their own individualized materials. This further contributes to the overall level of stress among teachers.

Physical plant accommodations influence the facility with which a program can be implemented. All too often, special education teachers are relegated to space not designed for classroom use. They are placed in hallways, equipment rooms, temporary empty classrooms, conference rooms, and locations far removed from the mainstream of school life.

Cook and Leffingwell also addressed the issue of teacher relationships with others in the school environment. Professional constraints, such as the lack of opportunity to participate in school decision making and overall policy development, create stress, as do incompetent administrators and inadequate relationships with other teachers. Lack of recognition, lack of appreciation, and low teacher pay are cited as major sources of job dissatisfaction.

Bensky et al. (1980) investigated whether the requirements of PL 94-142 are stressful for teachers. Their findings, based on responses from 114 regular classroom teachers, special education personnel, and administrators, indicated that major stress factors for educators were (1) writing Individualized Education Programs and completing due-process paperwork, (2) dealing with parents, (3) after-school work requirements and related activities, (4) excessive pupil load, (5) diagnosis and assessment, and (6) dealing with other teachers.

Stress and Teachers of Hearing-Impaired Children and Youth

Meadow (1981) reported on a study involving 240 teachers, administrators, support personnel, and dormitory workers working with hearing-impaired children and youth. Subjects were asked to complete the Maslach Burnout Inventory (Maslach, 1981) as well as a sheet containing demographic information and four supplemental questions related to career motivation and job satisfaction. Findings indicated that teachers of hearing-impaired children scored significantly higher on the emotional exhaustion scale than teachers of nonhandicapped children. Among school personnel taking the inventory, classroom teachers experienced the greatest emotional exhaustion in connection with their job.

Respondents in the oldest age group—older than 35 at the time of the study—experienced the lowest degree of emotional exhaustion. Respondents aged 21 through 26 ranked second; those aged 31 through 35 ranked third; and respondents aged 27 through 30 indicated the highest degree of emotional exhaustion. Respondents who had been in the field for only a year or two registered the least emotional exhaustion. Those who reported between 7 and 10 years of experience with hearing-impaired students indicated the most emotional exhaustion, while those individuals with 11 or more years of experience ranked second.

Meadow postulated that the oldest group represents "those staunch souls who remain in the field after their more exhausted colleagues have retired or have changed careers" (p. 17). While the survey was limited in scope and coverage, Meadow suggested:

> It would seem that there is a "critical period" in the career of teachers of deaf children when they are likely to experience particular feelings of stress. Teachers and others with the most intensive day-to-day contact with students are most likely to succumb to burnout, as do those personnel located in demonstration schools and residential schools. (p. 20)

Meadow concluded her report by suggesting that the problem of stress and burnout among professionals working with hearing-impaired students is one that needs serious attention. She reminded us that the general education establishment is already acutely aware of these needs.

Johnson (1983) investigated the occupational factors perceived to be predominant sources of stress by teachers of hearing-impaired students; she also determined what relationships existed among those perceptions when they were compared to a variety of demographic and school environment characteristics. Results of the study indicated that the majority of the teachers of hearing-impaired children and youth perceived teaching to be stressful. Twenty-seven percent considered teaching to be either very stressful or extremely stressful, while 45 percent of the respondents perceived teaching to be moderately stressful. The remaining 27 percent considered teaching to be either mildly stressful or not at all stressful.

The predominant sources of occupational stress as perceived by more than half of the teachers of hearing-impaired children and youth were poor working conditions in the school environment and poor support systems in the teaching environment. In contrast, other studies report that sources of stress for teachers stem mainly from dealing with pupil-related problems.

The majority of the responding teachers reported no change in health or in the use of tobacco, caffeine, or alcohol. However, those who reported higher levels of stress tended to report increased use of caffeine or alcohol. The most frequent symptom of stress experienced by teachers of hearing-impaired children and youth was fatigue. Other symptoms reported included upset stomach, headaches, colds and flu, irritability, depression, and loss of appetite.

Based on the findings of Johnson's study (1983), several conclusions were drawn about teachers with high levels of stress.

1. Personal characteristics
   a. Male teachers reported more stress than did female teachers.
   b. Teachers between 31 and 40 years old experienced more stress than did those in other age categories, while those over 40 experienced the least stress.
   c. Teachers with more than five years of teaching experience reported more stress than did teachers with less experience.
   d. Hearing-impaired teachers reported more stress than did hearing teachers.

2. School environment characteristics
   a. Teachers who taught in schools where the total school population was 401–500 reported more stress than did teachers who reported fewer children in the total student body.
   b. Middle or junior high school teachers reported the most stress, while preschool teachers reported the least.
   c. Teachers employed in rural area schools reported higher levels of stress than did teachers working in urban or suburban area schools.

3. Demanding working conditions
   a. Teachers who taught more than 40 different students a day reported more stress than did those who taught fewer students.
   b. Teachers with more than 40 hours per week of direct contact with students experienced more stress than did those with less contact.
   c. Teachers who took continuing education courses for certification or a

salary increase experienced more stress than did those who took no courses, or who took leisure-type courses.

 d. Teachers who spent more than 60 hours per week in school-related activities reported more stress than did teachers who spent fewer hours in such activities.

 e. Teachers required to supervise extracurricular activities reported more stress than did teachers without such assignments.

 f. Teachers without classroom aides reported more stress than did those with aides.

4. Experience with multihandicapped hearing-impaired students

 a. Teachers who spent more than 25 percent of their instructional time with multihandicapped hearing-impaired students reported more stress than did those who spent less time with such students.

 b. Teachers who had not been trained to work with multihandicapped hearing-impaired students reported more stress than did teachers who had been trained to work with these students.

Teachers were asked whether they would stay in the same job or leave, if they were free to choose. The majority of teachers (58 percent) indicated they would change fields completely if they were free to choose another occupation. This group was composed predominately of individuals who experienced high stress levels. Teachers who indicated that they would like to change to another job, but remain in the field of education, experienced less stress, while those who indicated that they would prefer to stay in the same job reported very little stress.

To the extent that the subjects who participated in the Johnson study (1983) were representative of teachers of hearing-impaired children and youth, one can conclude that a large percentage consider teaching to be a stressful occupation, indicating a definite need to explore effective stress-reduction strategies for use with this population. Miller and Potter (1982) similarly found that, of 123 randomly sampled speech/language pathologists, 43 percent said they were experiencing "moderate to severe" burnout.

The role of preservice training is crucial to the whole issue of stress alleviation. The majority of the stress sources identified by teachers in the Johnson study dealt with poor working conditions, time pressures, and poor support systems in the schools. This indicates that teacher-training institutions need to focus attention on instructional material that realistically portrays the school environment and those interactive societal influences that have great impact on the teacher.

Teachers need to develop skills in identifying potentially stressful situations and in generating appropriate responses to those situations. Familiarity with the problems normally encountered in the special education setting enables the teacher to be more effective. Teacher preparation, therefore, should include the realities of uncertainties and potential failures that will be encountered on the job.

Addressing Burnout Personally

Once teachers and administrators in programs for hearing-impaired developmentally disabled populations recognize and acknowledge the symptoms and effects of stress and burnout, several strategies for dealing with the problem on a personal and programmatic basis are available.

Stress first needs to be recognized and reduced from a personal perspective. Individual teachers need to develop awareness of possible stress-producing conditions in their work environment and to become familiar with their own personal stress indicators. They must recognize when they begin to move into the sustained stress area that precedes burnout. This implies "acknowledging personal vulnerabilities and setting realistic standards of performance" (Zabel & Zabel, 1980, p. 25). It also means that teachers who spend a great deal of time intensely involved in the lives of others must learn to focus on their own needs. They must set aside time for a life outside the school. They must also be prepared to demand changes in those situations in the school environment that consistently produce excessive stress (Zabel & Zabel, 1980).

Setting realistic standards of performance means that planning for success in teaching is necessary for the well-being of both teachers and children. The delegation of paperwork and nonteaching duties to classroom aides and parent volunteers is one method that both lightens the noninstructional workload and relates directly to the goals and priorities a teacher sets as part of the overall workload.

Long hours of direct contact with students are a definite invitation to teacher fatigue. Teachers need to break up continuous contact by encouraging administrators to consider team teaching, rotation of classes, and the greater use of parent volunteers and classroom aides during the school day. Similarly, variation in the routine of the school day is crucial to avoid burnout. Teachers need to avoid repetitious activities and should introduce variety into their lessons as often as possible. Isolation from other staff members should also be avoided. Support from other service providers in the work environment helps to prevent burnout.

Outside the immediate school environment, developing a full, active life is also crucial to the prevention of burnout. Teachers need to engage in mentally stimulating activities as well as physical exercise because both can contribute to the relief of the stress and tensions that build up during the school day. Many schools have swimming pools, exercise rooms, and gym facilities that can provide excellent outlets for physical tension.

The likelihood of encountering a relatively stress-free teaching environment is quite remote. For this reason, it is imperative that teachers maintain a continuous personal effort to avoid burnout. Some teachers will require a variety of stress-reduction strategies; for others, a single strategy may be sufficient. Each teacher must select the strategies that suit him or her best.

Addressing Burnout Administratively

Public educators acknowledge, and school administrators concede, that they must assume responsibility for stressful conditions in the educational environment and provide assistance in alleviating those conditions (Dixon, Shaw, & Bensky, 1980; Werner, 1980). Dixon, Shaw, and Bensky also suggested that as administrators attempt to improve the mental health status of their staffs and organizations, they do so with both local and external environmental conditions in mind. They further noted that the administrator's role in such a program closely follows the Individualized Education Program process and involves four basic tasks.

1. Diagnosis of the environmental conditions influencing the organization or individual.

2. Planning and designing possible intervention strategies that focus on stress situations.

3. Implementing appropriate change strategies aimed at eliminating or minimizing stress conditions.

4. Evaluating the effectiveness of the implemented strategies and the mental health status of the organization or individual. (p. 32)

There is a proliferation of literature that identifies stressful conditions in the school environment. Administrators, aware of such factors, need to be cognizant of those that they have authority to change. They should be aware that stress control and stress reduction are components of the normal, daily administrative process.

Stress control should not be considered as just one of many activities in the school program, but rather as part of a school administration's primary concern for the well-being and productivity of the staff, upon which all other program activities depend. Too frequently stress management tends to be handled in a peripheral manner, rather than as an integral part of the core administrative philosophy. To be effective, the school's commitment must be well planned, forward thinking, and total. Support systems that focus on supervisory personnel responsiveness to teacher concerns, improvement of general working conditions, better management of student-related problems, and the avoidance of management by crisis must become key factors in policy development.

The provision of opportunities for teachers to engage in team communication with other service providers is a major factor in the alleviation of stress. Professional interaction can have a significant positive impact on morale and provides increased opportunities for sharing problems on a routine basis.

Additional change strategies designed to eliminate or minimize stress conditions in the school environment should include the reduction of excessive workload and time pressures. Workload and time pressures weigh heavily on teachers; current administrative practices, therefore, should be examined with an eye to minimizing the scheduling of activities that create undue stress. Administrators need to ensure that consideration is given to heavy student caseloads, the number of subjects taught per day, the amount of extracurricular responsibility, the amount of paraprofessional help that is available, the amount of noninstructional paperwork, and the severity of each student's handicapping condition (Cook & Leffingwell, 1982).

The extra paperwork involved in federal- and state-mandated Individualized Education Programs (IEPs) can also generate stressful situations. Administrators need to consider the feasibility of release time for IEP development, committee meetings, and the administrative paperwork associated with IEPs. Time management techniques should also be examined as potential mechanisms for relieving job overload.

"Teachers require the tools of their profession in order to be effective" (Cook & Leffingwell, p. 56). School administrators should provide teachers with appropriate materials and equipment to help them do their jobs properly. Teachers should be assigned classroom space that is appropriate for the number and types of children in the class.

In addition, teacher support should include the provision of adequate "other" staff to assist teachers in the performance of their teaching responsibilities. Parent volunteers and classroom aides, for example, should be available to substitute for the teacher in a variety of situations.

The provision of financial assistance to teachers to further their education at local colleges and universities is another way to benefit not only the teacher but also the school. Opportunities for upgrading teacher skills in teaching and managing children will in the long run contribute toward the alleviation of stress.

The provision of professional support to teachers who are experiencing excessive stress could prevent burnout. Existing support service personnel in the system can frequently provide teachers with stress-reduction strategies and also assist in the implementation of such strategies on a schoolwide basis (see Chapter 13 for further discussion).

Still another factor in the alleviation of stress is the provision of the opportunity for teachers to engage in team communication with other service providers. Administrators must understand that this type of professional interaction can have a significant positive impact on morale and provide their staffs with increased opportunities for sharing problems on a routine basis.

Future Research

Investigations into teacher stress as perceived by teachers of hearing-impaired children and youth should go beyond the self-report questionnaire. In-depth interviews with teachers who have permanently left teaching should be conducted to isolate avoidable departures from the profession. The effect of stress on teacher performance in the classroom is also an area for further research. Fruitful areas for investigation include: How is teacher performance affected by stress? At what point do teachers begin to lose effectiveness in the classroom as a result of stress? What relationships are there between teacher stress and student performance?

Administrators' perceptions of teacher stress are yet another area of potential research. How do administrators perceive teacher stress, and are their perceptions different from those of teachers?

It may be presumed that other personnel involved with educating hearing-impaired children and youth also experience stress on the job. There is a need to determine stress levels among dormitory counselors and teachers' aides, for example. Occupational stress factors involving other personnel who work with hearing-impaired students have not been identified. Once those factors have been reported, how might they compare with those identified by teachers?

The majority of the responding teachers in the Johnson study (1983) indicated that, if they were free to change their occupation, they would prefer to be doing something other than teaching. A study of individuals in other helping professions, to compare their level of job satisfaction with that of teachers of hearing-impaired children and youth, is another area worthy of investigation.

References

Alley, R. (1980). Stress and the professional educator. *Action in Teacher Education, 2*(4), 1–8.

Bardo, P. (1979). The pain of teacher burnout: A case history. *Phi Delta Kappan, 61*(4), 252–254.

Bensky, J. M., Shaw, S. F., Gouse, A. S., Bates, H., Dixon, B., & Beane, W. E. (1980). Public Law 94-142 and stress: A problem for educators. *Exceptional Children, 47*(1), 24–29.

Collins, J. J., & Masley, B. A. (Eds.). (1980, June). Stress/burnout report. *Share and Exchange, A Newsletter for Teachers, 8*(4), 1–28. Worcester, MA: Worcester Public Schools.

Cook, J. M., & Leffingwell, R. J. (1982). Stressors and remediation techniques for special educators. *Exceptional Children, 49*(1), 54–59.

Dixon, B., Shaw, S. F., & Bensky, J. M. (1980). Administrator's role in fostering the mental health of special services personnel. *Exceptional Children, 47*(1), 30–36.

DuBrin, A. J. (1979). Teacher burnout: How to cope when your world goes black. *Instructor, 88*(6), 56–62.

Foster, R. E. (1980, Winter). Burnout among teachers of severely handicapped, autistic children. *The Pointer,* pp. 24–28.

Gray, L. J. (1979). Slow down: You move too fast. *Teacher, 96*(8), 52–53.

Griffin, B. (1982). Beating burnout. *Rehab Brief, 5*(3), 1–4.

Harlin, V. K., & Jerrick, S. J. (1976). Is teaching hazardous to your health? *Instructor, 86*(1), 55–58, 212, 214.

Hendrickson, B. (1979). Teacher burnout: How to recognize it; what to do about it. *Learning, 7*(5), 37–39.

Hunter, M. (1977). Counterirritants to teaching. *Instructor, 87,* 122–125.

Johnson, J. S. (1983). *Stress as perceived by teachers of hearing impaired children and youth.* Unpublished doctoral dissertation, Gallaudet College, Washington, DC.

Kraft, S. P., & Snell, M. A. (1980, Winter). Parent-teacher conflict: Coping with parental stress. *The Pointer,* pp. 29–37.

Kyriacou, C., & Sutcliffe, J. (1978). Teacher stress: Prevalence, sources, and symptoms. *British Journal of Educational Psychology, 48,* 159–167.

Mace, J. (1979). Teaching may be hazardous to your health. *Phi Delta Kappan, 60*(7), 512–513.

Maslach, C. (1981). *The Maslach burnout inventory.* Palo Alto: Consulting Psychologists Press.

Meadow, K. P. (1981). Burnout in professionals working with deaf children. *American Annals of the Deaf, 126*(1), 13–22.

Miller, M., & Potter, E. (1982). Professional burnout among speech-language pathologists. *Asha, 24*(3), 177–181.

Moracco, J. C., Gray, P., & D'Arienzo, R. V. (1981, March). *Stress in teaching: A comparison of perceived stress between special education and regular teachers.* Paper presented at the Eastern Educational Research Association Annual Meeting, Philadelphia.

Pattavina, P. (1980, Winter). Bridging the gap between stress and support for public school teachers. *The Pointer*, pp. 89–94.

Selye, H. (1978). *The stress of life.* New York: McGraw-Hill.

Shaw, S. F., Bensky, J. M., & Dixon, B. (1981). *Stress and burnout. A primer for special education and special services personnel.* Reston, VA: Council for Exceptional Children.

Smith, J., & Cline, D. (1980, Winter). Quality programs. *The Pointer*, pp. 80–87.

Walsh, D. (1979). Classroom stress and teacher burnout. *Phi Delta Kappan, 61*(4), 253.

Weiskopf, P. E. (1980). Burnout among teachers of exceptional children. *Exceptional Children, 47*(1), 18–23.

Werner, A. (1980, Winter). Support for teachers in stress. *The Pointer*, pp. 54–59.

Zabel, R. H., & Zabel, M. K. (1980). Burnout: A critical issue for educators. *Education Unlimited*, 23–25.

Chapter 19

Advocacy: Attitudes, Ethics, and Strategies for the Professional

Jerome D. Schein

An advocate pleads another's cause. It may seem somewhat strange, then, that disabled people need advocates. After all, is anyone opposed to giving aid to those who have physical and mental impairments that limit their functioning in our society? Sadly, the answer must be yes. Hence, the importance, if not the necessity, of advocates to assist disabled people in obtaining the services they require to achieve their maximum potential within our society. Advocates are needed not because disabled people are inherently weak and incapable, but because they are members of an unfavored minority group.

This chapter will address the history of services for disabled people, taking the broad worldwide perspective first, then narrowing the focus to a historical survey of rehabilitation legislation in the United States. That introductory material will lay the foundation for the balance of the chapter, which will discuss specific issues and propose strategies to meet present and near-future assaults on the welfare of disabled people.*

Hierarchy of Attitudes toward Severe Disabilities

Public attitudes toward severe disabilities advance through five stages to form an instructive hierarchy (see Figure 1). The five stages do not necessarily exhaust the range

---

*Throughout this chapter, the term *disabled* is used in preference to *handicapped*. The latter term implies more than impairments that limit or impede functions; handicapped individuals also have social adjustment problems. Because these problems arise from the way that societies treat disabled people, the term *handicapped* would be inappropriate in the context of this paper. However, it is used, inescapably, when it is part of a title such as the Education for All Handicapped Children Act. *Disabled,* on the other hand, means only that functions have been lost. Whether these functions lead to serious problems of life adjustment depends upon how the individual and the society react to the disabilities.

This chapter is based on a speech commissioned by the American Speech-Language-Hearing Association and delivered in Haverhill, Massachusetts, August 14, 1982.

of attitudinal variations, nor do they have some essential veridicality. They are abstractions that ignore much detail for the purposes of exposition. The five stages provide a framework on which to array observations about the administrative, legislative, and judicial events of concern to advocates. If it is useful in facilitating discussion and thought, the framework serves its purpose.

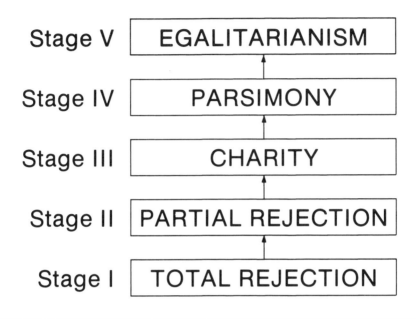

Figure 1. Hierarchy of attitudes toward disabled people.

Stage I: Total Rejection

The most primitive attitude is outright hostility toward disabled people. Many ancient peoples considered physical disabilities as evidence of sin, of evil spirits, of the Devil's work. Others saw disabled people as threats to survival of their society. The Spartans exemplified that attitude; they preached that severely disabled infants should be left on the hillsides to die. Nomadic tribes justified abandoning their disabled tribe members to near-certain death by noting the burden they imposed on the movements of the tribe. Armies in retreat often adopted the same attitude toward wounded soldiers, sometimes killing them rather than leaving them to the mercies of the enemy. But whether seen as the moral right of the majority or as protection for the safety of the group, an acceptable reaction to disability in some societies at some times has been to kill the disabled individual.

Deadly reactions to severe disabilities are not solely a matter of the distant past. Hitler ordered the destruction of physically and mentally handicapped individuals. Some were gassed; others were sexually sterilized. The enormity of the Holocaust has obscured the Nazis' antipathy toward disabled people. It is real enough for the survivors, among whom are deaf people who testified recently to the permanence of the scars from the brutality they suffered.*

Now that we have almost reached the twenty-first century, have we set Stage I attitudes firmly behind us? Unfortunately, no. A British jury recently acquitted a physician charged with murder because he had allowed a neonate with Down's syndrome to die 69 hours after birth by prescribing large doses of a morphine-like drug and not feeding the child (Lasagna, 1982). In March of 1983, in Indiana, the story was repeated with minor variations. Again, the newborn baby was diagnosed as having Down's syndrome. In addition, the child had an operable defect of the trachea, one that prevented food from reaching its stomach. The parents refused consent for the operation, giving as the reason for their refusal their unwillingness to raise a defective child. The case was taken to court, where the Indiana judge ruled that the parents had the right to make a decision that would lead to the child's death. Before the state's attorney general could bring the case to the U.S. Supreme Court, the baby died of starvation. The federal Department of Health and Human Services responded with the so-called Baby Doe rule that requires hospitals to post notices warning that failure to properly care for a disabled infant violates federal law and that further forbids hospitals from permitting such practices on penalty of losing federal dollars. The regulation has already been challenged in court and temporarily withdrawn. Its pertinence here, however, rests on the fact that, in 1983, total rejection persists as a reaction to disability.

Over the centuries of recorded history to our very day, then, societies have had aversions to disabilities so strong that they have justified killing. Primitive urges to destroy the weak members of the tribe still exist in our country.

Stage II: Partial Rejection

From open hostility, society's attitudes toward disabled individuals move to partial rejection. The severely disabled individuals are either ignored or placed out of sight. This attitude improves upon killing, though slightly, by relegating the disabled person to lifelong incarceration in human warehouses that would often fail an examination for storage of domestic animals.

Many countries still maintain leper colonies. In the U.S., victims of Hansen's disease (as leprosy is now named) live in an isolated area in Louisiana. Despite what is known about how leprosy is transmitted and how uncontagious it is, we consign its victims to lonely lives away from the view of the general community. Of course, lepers in this country are not forced to live in Carville. They are free to leave once they are found to be uncontagious, and some do. But many stay because they lack the financial resources to move elsewhere. They are poor, a condition related to leprosy. The visitor to Carville aware of these facts must still be nagged with a queston: Why are these sick people sent to so remote a location? Why are they not treated close to their homes?

Severely disabled persons have found themselves literally discarded by society, often being put out of sight where they do not offend public sensibilities. Many of our

---

*The New York Society for the Deaf sponsored a conference on this topic titled "Crying Hands." A report of the meeting can be obtained from the society, 344 East Fourteenth Street, New York, NY 10003.

institutions for mentally ill people have not provided treatment, only imprisonment. The courts have confirmed this assessment and ordered that inmates be released unless some form of appropriate therapy is undertaken. Mentally retarded children have been placed in facilities that barely sustain their lives and that are devoid of any educational efforts to develop their self-care skills. The U.S. Congress reacted in 1975 with the passage of Public Law 94-142, making the education of all children, regardless of physical or mental condition, mandatory. For what remains of Stage II attitudes, one can say that they are better than Stage I, but not by much.

Stage III: Charity

In the next stage, disabled people arouse society's sympathy but not action. Society deplores the impairments, but it does nothing to relieve their burdensome effects. An excellent example of this attitude is displayed by Scrooge, in Dickens's *A Christmas Carol*. When Scrooge observes Tiny Tim, the old man's response is typical of his time: Heartbroken, he rushes out to purchase a turkey for the family's Christmas dinner. Scrooge becomes solicitous to Tiny Tim's father, but Scrooge does not try to help Tiny Tim to grow.

In Stage III, the response to disability is charity. The crowd drops coins in the blind man's cup. Eleemosynary institutions send food baskets to feed the man who lost his legs in an industrial accident. To display a "tsk-tsk" attitude toward a severely disabled person—with some temporary succor and nothing more—exemplifies Stage III thinking.

Stage IV: Parsimony

Next, compassion for severely disabled persons is joined by the realization that educating and rehabilitating disabled people makes good economic sense, that helping them to become partially or wholly self-sustaining adds to the welfare of all, in the way that ignoring them or palliating their difficulties does not. Under the leadership of the late Mary Switzer, rehabilitation blossomed in the U.S. Her arguments before Congress on behalf of the rehabilitation administrations she headed were generally of this form: It costs less in the long run to rehabilitate disabled persons than to provide them with charity. She subscribed to the ancient wisdom, "Give a man a fish and he will eat for a day; teach him to fish and he will eat for all of his days." Members of Congress on both sides of the aisle applauded Mary Switzer and annually voted greater sums for her programs.

Special education has learned from rehabilitation's successes. From 1966, with the establishment of the Bureau of Education for the Handicapped, to the present, leaders in special education have often sounded like carbon-copy Mary Switzers. They, too, have attempted to increase congressional appropriations by arguing the economic soundness of their programs. They have maintained that it costs less to educate a disabled child than to pay for a lifetime of custodial care. Until very recently, that economic theme has dominated special education's philosophy. It is particularly evident in the Vocational Education Act that mandated 10 percent of all funds be devoted to education of disabled people. The intent was clear enough: Teach these children through education to become self-sufficient adults. It is not an argument that appears initially obnoxious. Yet it has its philosophical critics.

Stage V: Egalitarianism

Society reaches the hierarchy's pinnacle when it concludes that its disabled members should receive educational and rehabilitation services because they have a right to them. The services need not be justified on moral, religious, or economic grounds. The services are provided because disabled people are citizens. Stage V thinkers consider all citizens equally deserving. If physical or mental disabilities interfere with citizens' rights, then society must make the changes that will enable them to enjoy those rights—regardless of costs. Special education and rehabilitation services are not charity; these services should not be supported only because they are economically sound. They usually are economically sound, but for Stage V thinkers that is not their raison d'etre. These programs help disabled people to overcome their disabilities and to become fully participating members of society. Disabled people must be afforded equal opportunities *because they are citizens,* no more and no less.

Progress Clearly in Jeopardy

These five attitudes—total rejection, partial rejection, charity, parsimony, and egalitarianism—coexist in our society today. Some people hold views representing one stage, while others have views at other stages. The same person may vacillate from stage to stage. Since our government responds to the wishes of the electorate, advocates must contend with the relative preponderances of these various views. Until recently, the majority seemed to be moving up to Stage V, believing that disabled individuals should have the accommodations and services that allow them to function at a high level in our society as a matter of citizenship. Maybe most people do embrace that viewpoint, whether as a matter of enlightened self-interest or from even higher motivation, but loud voices are shouting slogans that awaken echoes from as far back as Stage I. Progress is clearly in jeopardy.

Consider an essay that appeared on the op-ed page of the July 30, 1982, *New York Times,* written by Harry Schwartz, former member of its editorial board and now writer-in-residence at a medical school.

> The Supreme Court recently handed down what will probably become a landmark decision when it denied deaf 11-year-old Amy Rowley a full-time sign-language interpreter to help her at school. What it did, in effect, was to lay down a principle for rationing scarce social services for those who cannot afford them. . . . We Americans don't like the concept of rationing. That fact probably explains why we have tried to avoid the basic problem opened up by the vast expansion of Government-financed social services begun in the Johnson Administration and continually expanded until these still-young parsimonious 1980's.
>
> The problem is that our resources are finite and therefore limited. But the needs and desires for "free" social services—that is, Government-financed education, health care, welfare, aid to the handicapped and all the rest—are potentially infinite. They cannot all be met and therefore we must work out principles on how to spread our inadequate resources as best we can, to ration them among the many and diverse claimants. (p. A21)

Chilling words for egalitarians. Of course, Mr. Schwartz's logic can be attacked and probably defeated. Whether resources are scarce or abundant is not an absolute, as his argument would demand. By scrapping plans for the MX missile, a doubtful weapon at best, all of the state and federal rehabilitation programs could be financed for the next decade, with ample monies left over to support special education for the same period. But the emotions expressed by Schwartz reflect a dismaying prospect for those who advocate on behalf of severely disabled individuals. The position he presents falls between Stages III and IV. The writer ignores the economic benefits of education and rehabilitation. He almost falls in Stage II, saying that our purse may not have enough coins to dispense charity to all. Some will need to be ignored. Should they be destroyed? The essayist does not go beyond cautioning against too firm a commitment to the civil rights of disabled people. At the least, he challenges disabled people's entitlement to full citizenship, even though his rationale is couched in pseudoeconomic terms. Were the essay found in a less prestigious journal than the *New York Times,* it might be ignored. It cannot be ignored, because it comes from a member of a group toward which advocates for disabled people usually look for support, intellectuals. To have them make such attacks must alert everyone to the dangerous state of our present attitudes. The essay represents a retreat from hard-won victories for disabled people, victories in which papers like the *New York Times* played a significant, supporting role. These arguments pose an increasing danger to advocates; in responding to such arguments they may grant them undeserved cogency. To persuade with the egalitarian philosophy requires a full commitment to it.

Federal Legislation

Let us look briefly at the history of federal legislation for vocational rehabilitation. The National Defense Act of 1916 was the first recognition of this nation's obligation to disabled veterans. That law provided vocational training—but only for wounded soldiers. In 1920, Congress expanded the vocational rehabilitation programs to include nonmilitary persons. The inclusion of all disabled adults slowly expanded through successive legislative acts. However, the services were limited to job training and placement.

The quarter century from 1943–68 was particularly fruitful. In 1954, for example, the Vocational Rehabilitation Act Amendments provided for training grants to develop rehabilitation personnel. The 1967 amendments established the National Center for Deaf-Blind Youth and Adults, the first federal recognition of this severe disability, previously considered unfeasible for vocational rehabilitation. Successively, the Congress advanced from Stage III thinking into Stage IV for all disabilities, regardless of their severity.

In 1973, and more so in 1978, the U.S. moved legislatively into Stage V— rehabilitation services as the right of disabled people, regardless of economic return to society. Congress changed the name of the legislation in 1973 by dropping "vocational" from its title. Changing the title to the Rehabilitation Act signaled Congress's shift from economic to social motivation for rehabilitation. The law added provisions for independent living services, removed age restrictions for services by federally funded rehabilitation agencies, and broadened the range of services to cover telecommunications and recreation.

The greatest innovation in the law was Title V, with its now-famous Section 504. Title V is sometimes called "The Bill of Rights for Disabled People." Its power derives, in part, from its brevity. The full text of Section 504 consists of one sentence: "No otherwise qualified handicapped individual . . . shall . . . be excluded from participation in, be denied the benefits of, or be subjected to discrimination under any program or activity receiving federal financial assistance." The lack of equivocation in that sentence made clear Congress's egalitarian stance. You can see why the Rehabilitation Act of 1973 and the 1978 amendments to it indisputably placed congressional thinking in Stage V.*

Shortly after passing the Rehabilitation Act, Congress enacted further landmark legislation in Public Law 94-142, the Education for All Handicapped Children Act. Like the rehabilitation legislation, the special education act aimed to provide services to disabled children not as a privilege, not as charity, not as a sympathetic gesture, not for the economic good of the community, but as a civil right. Emerging from a series of lawsuits by parents in various states, the act codified what the courts had been saying up to that point, that if society provides free education for some of its citizens, it must provide it for all.

The legislative period from 1973 to 1978 will certainly be looked upon as one of great social advances. Today, however, the rationale for equal opportunities for all citizens—able-bodied and disabled—is being challenged. Serious critics of rehabilitation and special education are asking if it does not cost too much to accommodate people who are different. The question assumes a Stage IV attitude and betrays the regressive thinking of those who raise the question. It can be dealt with on those terms, seeking economic justification, or it can be answered by exposing its reasoning and confronting its dollars-and-cents logic with the higher objectives of universal human rights. Before taking up the challenge that these critics, and even more regressive ones, pose, let us try to find the bases for the downward shifts in attitudes. Why has there been a retreat from Stage V to earlier stages?

Causes of Discontent with the Egalitarian Position

What has gone wrong? What events have driven, and may still be driving, public attitudes away from Stage V? Why are regulations for the administration of special education and rehabilitation being weakened? Do some recent court decisions signal a long-term shift away from the civil rights position? Make no mistake, the current administration in Washington acts with the support of many voters. The courts, too, are not unmindful of public sentiments. What has happened between the high-minded behavior of Congress in the 1970s and its less noble action in recent days? Some conjectures about the underlying causes of public disaffection for the rights of disabled people, while not complete explanations, may serve as stepping stones to counter strategy by advocates of the egalitarian position. These hypotheses may provide some direction to the efforts of those who support continued progress for disabled people.

---

*Unfortunately, Congress did not appropriate funds for all of the services it authorized, particularly independent living. Nonetheless, these laws show that congressional attitudes had advanced beyond Stage IV, even if its fiscal policies had not caught up with its social ambitions.

Distrust and Overreaction

As any school child should know, our government is designed as a system of checks and balances. Underlying that system is a deep distrust of governments—all governments. The founders of our nation divided power among the branches of government because they did not wish any one branch to have supreme power. The highest authority is the most dispersed: It resides in the people.

The suspiciousness of authority and its broad dispersion lead to many problems with which students of our history are familiar. Less apparent is that the lack of trust often extends from one branch to another, and correctly so, if we respect the wisdom of the Constitution.

Over the years of expansion of social services, Congress has demanded more and more proof that the various programs it has authorized and funded are producing the benefits they are designed to produce. The federal administrators have, in turn, pressured the states to provide evidence of good works. Congress has cried for *accountability*, and it has written the concept into the social service laws. The term comes from cost accounting; it emphasizes that which can be enumerated. So accountability has come to mean counting things: How many people rehabilitated? How many disabled children enrolled in educational programs? Accountability tends to ignore how well services are delivered. The qualitative aspects of service delivery slip behind the quantitative.

That circumstance, favoring quantity over quality, has led critics to complain, often justifiably, that disabled people have been caught in a "numbers game." In trying to reach numerical goals, officials have sacrificed program quality. The costly cases have been put aside; many more people could be served and the resulting report to Washington improved by concentrating on the easier cases. In vocational rehabilitation, the term "Band-Aid rehab" came increasingly into prominence. In education, seriously disabled children were denied places in classrooms by administrators who argued that they did not have the resources to serve them properly. These administrators used Stage IV arguments to frustrate the attempts of parents to obtain an education for their disabled children by discussing the children's right to education in terms of the costs of providing it.

As a result of these decisions in the field, Congress ordered in 1973 that priorities in rehabilitation be changed to give preference to the most severely disabled individuals. In education, Congress mandated free, appropriate education for all disabled children. As noted above, Congress went even farther to redress the grievances of disabled people in terms of participation in their government, employment, access to public facilities and telecommunications, and so on.

The Congress unfortunately overreacted to the instances of neglect that had occurred. Aroused by occasional examples of abuse, Congress wrote extensive procedural safeguards into the education and rehabilitation acts. Federal administrators, as required by Congress's intent, added more paperwork designed to ensure that the agencies receiving federal funds used them in accordance with the law. The result was an explosion of regulations generating tons of paper fallout. Agencies had to employ monitors within their agencies to meet with the monitors from the state and federal governments. The National Association of Rehabilitation Facilities, for example, points out that its members' workshops are regulated by at least 46 different local, state, and federal agencies. Community-based residential programs must conform to regulations and prepare for audits from 33 government agencies, which impose an incredible 255 inspections, audits, and approvals annually!

Such instances of massive duplication of authority waste money and damage morale. The administration in Washington knows about these ridiculous distortions of the principle of accountability. Indeed, it has used them to frustrate efforts to promote Stage V approaches to social services. In response to the ridiculous tangle of regulations, the administration has proposed an equally ridiculous solution: To reduce unnecessary paperwork, abolish the programs! It is like a physician who proposes to cure a patient's headache by cutting off his or her head.

The public has been told repeatedly that present social service programs do not work, that they lead to outrageous abuses and yield little benefit to those for whom they have been enacted. These attacks have taken their toll. They may be simplistic, only partially accurate, and obfuscate larger issues. Nonetheless, the persistent assaults threaten the principle of civil rights that the programs have promoted and the federal laws have protected.

Waste and Fraud

The case of the Rudd (Iowa) Public Library's confrontation with Section 504 gained widespread publicity in 1976. It became a symbol of wasteful practices imposed upon local agencies by Washington. The library had been denied funds because people in wheelchairs lacked access to its facilities. Television news reporters gleefully interviewed the Rudd officials, who pointed out that not a single person in Rudd (population 700) used a wheelchair. The reporters made considerable fun of the cost of a ramp that would be used by no one. Unreported was the offer by a nearby lumber company to build the ramp without charge. Nor did any of the commentators point out that Rudd ought not deny access to people who may wish to come there. Furthermore, and most tellingly, none of the pundits who made sport of the situation bothered to remind their audiences that Congress does not legislate for Rudd alone. The regulator agency may have been overzealous in its application of the law to that community, but Rudd had remedies—remedies it forsook in favor of the publicity campaign against a principle.

When a case of fraud by welfare recipients is brought to public attention, it is likely to receive more violent reactions than the embezzlement of a bank's funds. Corporate crimes do not seem to arouse the same degree of hostility among the public as abuse of food stamps by elderly people who try to avoid proscriptions against using them for purchasing certain forbidden luxuries. Yet the bank fraud may result in much greater public cost. Equally puzzling for some is the contrast in attitudes toward mistakes made by officers in the social and military services. Poor planning that leads to misallocation of social services generates a cry to abolish the system. Poor planning that results in military planes unable to fly because they lack parts stirs the appeal for larger appropriations. When a military expedition fails because it has been badly managed, the officers responsible, like as not, will be promoted. Such is hardly the case in social service delivery. Notice that the huge cost overruns of military suppliers find defenders in Congress and the administration. When a Lockheed or Chrysler face bankruptcy, the federal government lends them money in open defiance of "free enterprise." Similarly bad management by a state welfare agency arouses no sympathy for the poor people whose lives are being threatened; rather, some critics scream to punish them further by doing away with all social services.

Why is military spending considered essential and social services not? President Reagan's 1982 budget message stated that defense expenditures were "untouchable" and then proposed slashing education and rehabilitation appropriations by 25 to 50 percent. Should the reasoning behind those decisions go unchallenged?

Commitment

One more element of the public's shifting attitude toward social services has been the failure of many of the leaders of voluntary agencies to react strongly to these attacks. Instead of proudly showing the value to our society of Stage V thinking, instead of at least arguing the merits of Stage IV approaches, instead of mounting a forceful counter-attack against undisguised attempts to destroy a half-century of significant social progress, many leaders seemingly have deserted to the other side.

Last year the superintendent of a school for disabled children published a statement opposing Social Security Disability Income payments to his students. He argued that it was wrong for the students to have money that the school could not control. He further stated that most of the students did not need the money, that their needs were provided for very well. A few months later, a national magazine published by an organization of disabled people carried an editorial supporting the superintendent's position and expanding upon it. Shortly thereafter the medical director for the Social Security Administration announced that he was reconsidering the decision to classify the disability as severe, thereby cutting off funds to all individuals similarly disabled. After seeing the editorial in the national magazine, the medical director (who will remain anonymous) wrote to me, "If [disabled] leaders do not believe that [disability] creates serious problems, why should this agency?" So far that ruling has not been made, but the threat is there; if carried out, its effects could seriously disrupt all services for children and adults with that disability.

Most leaders of disabled people are not traitors. Most are strong, self-sacrificing people who accept stewardships of their organizations reluctantly. What they can be faulted for is lack of commitment to Stage V. They either do not understand what the disabled community has been fighting to attain or they lack confidence in the principle. They need the armor of great faith to wear in the face of the heavy, sometimes insidious attacks on that principle.

Points of Counterattack

The present difficulties in holding the line against regression from the egalitarian position can be partially laid on three points: (1) suspicions inherent in the structure of our government, (2) flaws in the delivery of social services, and (3) lack of commitment on the part of some leaders in the disabled community. Doubtless there are other factors, such as the declining economy, that can account for altered public attitudes toward disabled people, but these three factors seem to be amenable to counterattack by those who desire to advance disabled people's rights. Bolstering our sagging economy, on the other hand, is a task that strains the entire government.

What can be done to restore lost momentum and to further improve the position of disabled people in our society? Wise politicians say, "You can't beat something with nothing." Disabled people need to adopt a strong, positive platform. They and their advocates must decide what position they take with respect to their status in our society. History argues for Stage V. The civil rights position has the best opportunity to defend disabled people against any circumstances, short of total destruction. Economic conditions change; sympathies shift; but the individual's rights, under the U.S. Constitution, are inviolate.

Having agreed upon that position, disabled people must be prepared to challenge illogic and to fight against demagoguery. They and their advocates can tease out the threads of unreasoning passion from the fabric of arguments that cloaks attacks upon them. If a service is a right, then its abuse cannot lead to abolishing it. A person who drives recklessly loses his or her license, but the rest of the community continues to drive autos without feeling the need to defend their right to drive. If a disabled person abuses social services, that person—not all disabled people—should be disciplined. The responses to these attacks upon disabled people come more easily once the civil rights principle is adopted. If the abuse challenges the right to services, then advocates have a terrible problem; but if the abuse is dealt with aside from the services being abused, then advocates have reasonable grounds.

What Is an Advocate?

The preceding discussion has taken up an analysis of attitudes toward disabled people, has searched for relevant evidence in U.S. history, and has concluded that an optimistic view of what can be done by advocates is justified. How does one apply these ideas to advocacy on the local level? And there is a prior question: What is an advocate?

An advocate is generally defined as one who pleads the cause of another. Its first dictionary meaning is "lawyer" or "counselor." An advocate is one who gives support to a particular cause. In that sense, the etymology of the word is revealing and most apt in this application: The word derives from the Latin *avocare,* "to summon." So the advocate is one who is called upon to provide aid.

There are two types of advocacy, *case* and *class.* Case advocacy usually refers to the representation of a single individual, while class advocacy describes support for a group of individuals sharing some characteristic(s). Case and class advocacy may be subdivided by the types of workers and by the services they perform (Goldenson, 1978).

Case advocacy may be carried out by

- unpaid volunteers, "citizen advocates," who may often be part of a voluntary agency or members of a consumer group;
- government officials selected to represent the interests of disadvantaged and disabled citizens, often called ombudsmen;
- lawyers, who may or may not be connected with agencies;
- case managers, who typically are employees of service agencies, whether voluntary or government, and who oversee all aspects of particular clients' cases; and/or
- guardians or trustees appointed by a legal body to protect disabled individuals.

Class advocates may be subdivided into the functional categories of

- legislative advocate, or lobbyist, who represents the clients' interests in lawmaking;
- community advocate, who develops action within a community or state;
- program broker, who works between government and private agencies to obtain services for a client group;
- protector, who provides guardianship for a group; and
- consumer advocate, who is both an advocate, in any of the above four senses, and a member of the group. (p. 137)

Those types are not mutually exclusive; a particular individual may fill more than one role. The purpose of the classification is to reveal the extent of advocacy and to give it some functional coherence. Any of these advocates may seek for their clients professional treatment and care, education and training, transportation, trusteeships, removal of environmental barriers, and housing. They work in a variety of arenas with a broad spectrum of the public and government. They must obviously have considerable skills to be successful—skills that are not presently taught but come with experience. Yet advocates may be professionals (like lawyers) or lay people, paid or volunteers. Clearly, the range of functions and personnel covered by the term *advocate* is broad.

Suggestions for Effective Advocacy

What follows are ideas gleaned from a large number of successful advocates. The order of presentation does not indicate their importance in the process. Though they may not be equally important, each idea makes a substantial contribution to successful advocacy.

Being Informed

An advocate loses critical ground when unable to answer pertinent questions. Equally devastating can be a failure to be aware of significant events relating to the issue being pursued. Those the advocate must convince often look upon the advocate as an expert on the disability. That does not mean that if certain information is unavailable the advocate should invent data or lie. To the contrary, an honest response that a certain topic has not been studied and that the answer is not known to anyone can be disarming—and helpful.

Take the question of the size of the deaf population. In the late 1950s, a federal official invented an answer to that nagging gap in the then-available data. Asked by the head of his agency to provide testimony for Congress, he used the rate of deafness from the 1930 decennial, a rate not supported by the Bureau of the Census which had determined it. The head of the agency rejected the rate as "too small to justify the budget line." The harried official then went back to his office, thought it over, and returned with the rate of deafness that remained in the literature for the next two decades: 1 per 1,000. The head of the agency was satisfied. What, then, was wrong with that bit of inventiveness?

It was an educated guess; it was picked up by authors on deafness, who incorporated it in their books and articles. But it was not identified as a guess in testimony before Congress and in subsequent material produced by that agency. The federal agency had an answer, so it would not support a study to get up-to-date empirical data (Schein, 1982).

In 1971, a national study was financed, and a very different answer emerged. The rate of deafness was twice as large as the guess—2 per 1,000 (Schein & Delk, 1974). The guess that stood in lieu of empirical data underestimated the deaf population by half. Because federal funding had been based on the lower figure, that guess probably cost deaf people dearly over the years. The advocate, by claiming expertise he did not have, actually hurt the very people he had been engaged to assist.

Similar instances occur when advocates appear before legislative committees. A few years ago I had a call from a federal agency that wanted to know the prevalence of Meniere's disease in the U.S. I explained that the figure could not be known, since no one had attempted to count the victims of this cruel disorder at that time. The impatient caller explained to me that the head of her agency was due to testify the following morning and that he had written something about "the _____ sufferers of Meniere's disease in the United States." Her job was to fill in the blank. It was 5:00 p.m., she pointed out, and she wanted to go home. I remained adamant and refused to invent a number. However, the next day a figure appeared in the testimony. Where did it come from? You are correct if you conclude that it was made up.

Do advocates have to become experts? Not at all. They need to know where to find experts, and they need to use them. Such agencies as the American Speech-Language-Hearing Association (ASHA) and the Gallaudet College National Information Center on Deafness stand ready to provide answers to pertinent questions if the answers are available. These national agencies and numerous others on the state and local level can provide authoritative information on almost any aspect of hearing impairment.* They can point out conflicts in opinions and gaps in information. Thus armed, the advocate can make an impressive presentation before any group.

Getting the Act Together

Nothing sabotages advocacy quicker than opposition from those whom the advocate is supposed to represent. Authorities seem to delight in confronting advocates with opposing views from within their own ranks and saying, "How can you expect me to support that action when your own people do not agree that it should be taken?" It is a difficult ploy to manage. Of course, an advocate can respond that there is no more reason to expect unanimity among a special population than among the general population. Still, the point is somewhat blunted by the dispute in the ranks of advocates. This may be avoided by gaining consensus before approaching the legislators or administrators from whom some action is desired. But how?

---

*Presently, 16 states have legislatively mandated commissions for their deaf and hearing-impaired residents. Some states have established official advocates for disabled people. In addition, many cities have commissions devoted to the problems of the disabled. These agencies all have a role to play in advocacy as well as being prime sources of information about hearing impairment.

One method that has proved unusually effective is the needs assessment. The name misleads somewhat, because "needs" are usually not essential to life, but rather are desirable things that are lacking. A needs survey, then, establishes what a group wants and, in that sense, is a device for gaining consensus. The needs assessment also aids in establishing priorities and, thereby, directing the group's energies. Deciding what to work for in any given period is a difficult task, because someone's prized goals must be placed second. Assuring those whose favorites are set aside that they will have their turn in the near future can be a powerful move to maintain cohesion among members of a group with opposing wishes.

How does one conduct a needs assessment? There are a number of techniques, but, for the purposes of advocacy, they should all involve as much grassroots input as feasible. Because the process of interviewing each individual in a large group is not economical, representatives of segments of the population are selected. Those representatives must be given ample opportunity to express their views in an atmosphere that is conducive to gaining agreements, not encouraging disruption. In the deaf community, for example, there tends to be a division between the communication moderates and the communication liberals (sometimes described as aural/oralists and aural/manualists). A conference held in 1977 to establish priorities for advocacy brought representatives of the two groups together for a two-day meeting. Considerable staff work preceded the conference; representatives were provided ample information about the matters to be discussed. Care was taken throughout the meetings to avoid acrimony. Then the results were published simultaneously in the (somewhat conservative) *Volta Review* and the (more liberal) *Deaf American* (Schein, 1977a, 1977b). How well did this strategy work? The reader is invited to review the priorities and consider how many have actually been attained, most within three years of the publication dates.

Consensus is valuable, but sometimes all that can be obtained on a particular issue is an agreement from those who do not support it not to actively oppose it. Advocates cannot always expect, nor should they strive for, unanimity on every issue. For example, not everyone in a given state may be in favor of the educational policies of the state school for hearing-impaired students. If, however, those who do not wish to send their children to that school agree merely to forgo testifying against it, the school's supporters, in turn, should be willing to remain silent on some issues favoring alternative educational programs in the state. Such compromises in other fields are common—and effective.

There are other methods for achieving a harmonious public face on behalf of hearing-impaired people. One that was tried, and unfortunately partially failed, was the Council of Organizations Serving the Deaf (COSD). The COSD tried to provide a forum that would bring together all of the diverse groups that had any interest in hearing-impaired people. In the COSD meetings, opposing views could be heard and then agreements reached on major issues of general interest. The idea was and is meritorious. It failed nationally for a reason extraneous to the basic purpose of COSD. Faced with cuts in its federal support, COSD began to solicit individual memberships and to seek other grants. Those actions placed it in direct competition with the organizations it was to bring together, and they naturally rebelled, eventually destroying the national organization. The idea—bringing into contact all of the diverse views of hearing impairment—is still a good one; this may be attested to by the fact that a few states still have COSD chapters operating a decade after the national organization collapsed. Whatever the mechanism, some way should be found in every state to keep all interested parties—professionals, consumers, and parents—in continuous, meaningful contact with each other.

Hearing-impaired people have a right to expect empathy, if not support, from other physically disabled people. On some issues, the interests of hearing-impaired citizens do not differ from those of citizens with other disabilities. Of course, the same holds true for those with other disabilities: They should have the support of hearing-impaired people. Occasionally, administrators respond to requests for aid from one disabled group with the argument, "If we do that for you, we must do it for all disabled people" (with the implied conclusion that the "it" would then be too expensive for the state). At such times, it is critical for the success of advocacy that the other disabled groups be in a position to argue either that, indeed, they also wish the same or that, no, they do not. To go it alone in such a case would be foolhardy.

To counter the reluctant administrator, agreement in advance among the interested disability groups is clearly advised. An organization of advocates for disabled people can be invaluable to the separate groups represented, as well as to disabled people in general. Connecticut, for example, has a COSD chapter and the Connecticut Coordinating Committee of the Handicapped. The former group provides a communication base for all people interested in hearing impairment and the latter for all interested in disability. From those two bases highly successful advocacy can be launched.

Presenting the Case

What stance do you take when you meet with administrators or legislators? Some advocates feel that a highly aggressive, openly hostile approach works. Others believe in tugging at heart strings. With respect to the former, first, how well does a militant stance work? Listen to a candid state administrator of vocational rehabilitation (paraphrased here to protect anonymity).

When I first took office, I was contacted by the state's association of the deaf. They asked for a meeting, and I was able to arrange one in a reasonable period of time. They arrived with a delegation of 15 or 16 people. I was a bit taken aback, but I quickly arranged to have the meeting moved out of my office and into an empty conference room on another floor. That took a few minutes, and I was terribly pressed for time. The president began with a recitation of things that had gone wrong or not been done since the beginning of the century. I do not exaggerate. For almost the entire hour, during which the speakers kept interrupting each other to get in another jab at VR, I heard about what a lousy outfit we were.

Finally, I had to leave. No one had presented me with a plan of action. They had not given me a chance to say a word. All I could say was that I was sorry about any past difficulties, but I could neither do anything about them nor could I assume responsibility for them, since I had only taken office in the last few months. The entire session was most unsatisfactory to me; it wasted my time. Maybe the catharsis was worth it to the people who came, but they certainly did not help their cause. To the contrary, I refused to meet with them again for almost a year. I could see no reason to waste my time again.

The quotation is not invented. It happened. And it happens to legislators, too. Sometimes advocates, long frustrated, build up a huge head of steam and, when finally given the opportunity to meet with a significant person, explode. It is understandable but inexcusable. The result, as noted by the quoted administrator, is usually counterproductive. Instead of a forward-looking, effective relationship, the recitation of past ills only sets up an adversary relationship between the potential helper and the advocates. In such an encounter, the advocate seldom has the advantage. The losers, of course, are the disabled people who are often known to the administrators and legislators only by way of their advocates.

The civil rights marches and other dramatic acts led by Martin Luther King, Jr., dramatized the plight of minority groups. These bold acts also stirred disabled groups; they pointed a way to go. In early 1977 the American Coalition for Citizens with Disabilities (ACCD) greeted the newly appointed Secretary of Health, Education, and Welfare, Joseph Califano, with a sit-in designed to force his signature on regulations implementing Section 504. On April 28, 1977, he signed, acknowledging the impetus given his action by ACCD. The publicity had brought the distress of disabled people to the top of his agenda from the far lower place it had occupied when he took office. The tactic worked then. But it can be overdone.

Of course, advocates must show concern for their clients' problems and enthusiasm for the solutions. They may be forced to take extreme actions on occasion. However, high energy need not generate hostility. Passion can be kindly.

A far better way to address potential helpers is with the belief that they are basically honest and fair, that they will certainly help, if they know what is wrong and how to fix it. In short, you should meet administrators and legislators in the spirit of a shared responsibility: You understand your group, you know its needs, and you have reasonable proposals for meeting these needs. You believe the potential helpers, for their part, want to assist those in need and will do so, so long as they have a sensible plan and the resources to implement it. That approach gives the administrators and legislators room in which to offer other options. It enlists their sympathies and, most likely, will lead to strong positive actions. Even when it does not, the approach keeps the door open, a door that hostile approaches slam.

Some advocates have found that in seeking cooperation from employers it is often fruitful to say, "Let us help you obey the law." The gambit has worked with organizations confronted by Section 504. The advocate offers to show the employer how to comply with that federal statute and similar legislation, while at the same time maintaining productivity and generating public approval. These positive ideas have been effective in working with large and small companies, though they are by no means foolproof.

There are administrators who prefer to assert their presumed rights over those of others, and even to interpret the law idiosyncratically. In such instances, gentle persuasion stands little chance of success. What then?

Using the Courts

When administrators prove recalcitrant or when they cannot provide desired changes or services within existing mandates, advocates have sought relief in the courts.

In the 1950s and '60s there were some notable victories for civil rights activists, beginning with the Supreme Court's decision in *Brown v. Board of Education.*

Court actions, however, are often slow and not always satisfactory. Attempts to obtain educational rights for disabled children led to dozens of cases pursued in a bewildering array of courts. Though most cases ended in victories for the parents who brought the actions, practical results were not realized until Congress passed PL 94-142, which had as one of its aims relief for parents from more court battles. By making it a matter of explicit federal law and by providing incentives to obeying the law, Congress obviated the necessity for parents to establish their rights in each state.

But there have been a number of disappointments. The first came from the assumption that winning a court decision assures obtaining the outcomes one seeks. Parents have found that a court decision does not always translate into immediate and favorable actions by government administrators. Courts lack the machinery to oversee the execution of their orders on a day-to-day basis.

A second disappointment came from poor selection of cases. In the attempts to determine the precise meaning of Section 504, deaf people have had some unfortunate results. Cases have been lost on technical points that do not illuminate the statutory intent. Lawyers have an epigram that every advocate should keep uppermost in mind when litigation is being considered: "Bad cases make bad law." If the case chosen to test a statute has complications that might obscure the verdict, whether favorable or unfavorable, the clients should be discouraged from pursuing the case in court, at least early in the history of the law.

These cautionary statements should not dissuade the vigorous pursuit of justified claims in the courts. However, like the reaction to seeming injustice, "There oughta be a law," the cry of "Sue the offenders" should not become a reflex to every denial of a desire. The good advocate will choose the time and the occasion for legal action carefully.

Monitoring

Advocates must be prepared for backsliding. Some victories must be won again and again. Where feelings in opposition are strong, renewed efforts to reverse previous decisions may occur, whether in court, the legislature, or executive offices. Persistence is an essential part of advocates' repertoires. Monitoring is an essential activity. Conditions change, personnel change, even the needs of disabled clients change. The advocate must be prepared to make the fight for basic principles repeatedly.

Minimizing Burnout among Professional Advocates

In the struggle to assert the rights of their clients, advocates themselves can be victimized. The person who directs a large group of advocates, professional and volunteer, must not take their morale for granted. The staunchest advocates become tired, discouraged, and, occasionally, disillusioned. They need to know that their organization not only supports a disabled group but also supports them. They need to know that they do not lose their rights while struggling for the rights of others. Advocates, if they are to succeed, need to be comfortable advocating.

How does the leader of advocates manage this? Like any good leader, he or she must be alert to the tell-tale signs of disaffection among those on the firing line. Signs of stress should not be ignored. Usually, frank discussions between advocate and advocate's leader will suffice. Having the opportunity to express feelings and to resolve doubts helps to maintain morale. Advocates also respond well to recognition for their achievements and to encouragement that comes from even minor gains that result, directly or indirectly, from their efforts. Maintaining morale is important because dedicated advocates do the best job. An unhappy, uncertain advocate is usually an ineffective advocate. (For a full discussion of the burnout problem, see Chapter 18.)

The Consumer Advocate

Ultimately, hearing-impaired people should be their own advocates. The aim of the advocate should be to step aside and let the clients manage their own affairs. This thought has been very well expressed by Dr. Frank Bowe, himself deaf and, at the time he wrote these words (1978), the director of American Coalition of Citizens with Disabilities: "In the past women have spoken for women, Blacks for Blacks, and Indians for Indians. By contrast, children and disabled people have always relied on others to be their representatives" (p. 140).

Does this view mean that there is no role for nondisabled advocates? It might seem so, but that assumption would only be a first approximation. True, deaf people have been remarkably independent, historically preferring to manage their own affairs. The National Association of the Deaf, founded in 1880, is the oldest organization of disabled people in the U.S. It came into being as a reaction to the Milan Conference's proclamation against the use of sign language in the education of deaf children. Nonetheless, the strongest leader that the organization has had in its 100-plus year history, the late Dr. Frederick C. Schreiber, argued for cooperation with nondeaf people.

> One of the main ways the NAD operates is through the support and assistance of many people [he names several nondeaf persons]—all of whom can and do come to the assistance of NAD when requested, cheerfully and quickly. Conversely, when these same people request the assistance of the Executive Secretary—the same quick and cheerful response is given—must be given—if we are to expect continued support. (Schein, 1981, p. 40)

What Schreiber espoused—reciprocity between disabled and able-bodied people— seems as valid today as when he said it nearly a decade ago. Disabled people have much to offer the general community. They should seek and be afforded opportunities to contribute to, as well as gain from, the commonweal. Developing and maintaining the independence of disabled people does not conflict with providing advocacy. On the other hand, advocacy that does not strive to free the disabled individuals of the need for support becomes oppressive in itself. Advocates should recall that the Latin derivation of their name means "to summon." The client calls for the advocate when one is wanted; advocates should not impose themselves on the clients.

364 Bridging Assessment and Programming

Discussing the advances made by disabled people in the U.S., Bowe (1978) concluded, "Their progress, recent as it is, reflects the basic appropriateness of their conviction that they must speak for themselves" (p. 140). And to those wise and forceful words could be added . . . with the vigorous support of their most sincere advocates.

Conclusion

Will these strategies work? If disabled people assert their claims to services as a matter of civil rights, are they likely to succeed? Can the egalitarian view prevail against harsh assaults?

An account of a little publicized, highly dramatic incident in U.S. history may inspire some confidence. It took place during the Civil War. The city of Washington had recently been under siege. The Confederate Army was only a few miles from the Capitol. A less auspicious time to petition Congress on behalf of disabled people could hardly be imagined. What is more, the petitioner had the effrontery to be seeking a social service that flew in the face of established wisdom. What he wanted from the Congress was higher education for deaf people. Imagine, at a time when many people thought that those who were deaf were also dumb (stupid), this man wanted Congress to charter a college for deaf students!

Well, the Congress did just that. In 1864, the Columbia Institute for the Deaf, Dumb, and Blind (later renamed Gallaudet College) was established in Washington, D.C., and funded by the Congress. Edward Miner Gallaudet had presented Congress with sound arguments in favor of higher education for deaf people, and the Congress agreed (Atwood, 1964). Gallaudet's arguments rested largely on the basis of the deaf students' rights. He presented essentially the egalitarian position. Today, Gallaudet College stands as a monument to the civil rights of disabled people, a monument before which every U.S. citizen should stand in awe, not because this is the only country in the world that has founded a liberal arts college for deaf students, which it is, but because the country took that forward step on behalf of some of its disabled citizenry when its own existence was in jeopardy.

The arguments in favor of disabled citizens' rights need not be pressed shyly, need not be held back because the times are inauspicious or the wrong group is in power. For civil rights, the appropriate time is, and will long continue to be, now.*

---

*I wish to acknowledge the substantial contribution to this chapter by Dr. Craig Mills. Over the years he has instructed me patiently, by word and deed, about rehabilitation in its broadest sense. He read this chapter in draft and suggested corrections of a number of errors and infelicities. While expressing my gratitude for his emendations, I accept sole responsibility for any mistakes that remain.

References

Atwood, A. W. (1964). *Gallaudet College. Its first one hundred years.* Washington, DC: Gallaudet College.

Bowe, F. (1978). Consumer rights for the disabled. In R. M. Goldenson (Ed.), *Disability and rehabilitation handbook.* New York: McGraw-Hill.

Goldenson, R. M. (Ed.). (1978). *Disability and rehabilitation handbook.* New York: McGraw-Hill.

Lasagna, L. (1982). Murder most foul. *The Sciences, 22*(6), 7–8.

Schein, J. D. (Ed.). (1977a). Current priorities in deafness. *Volta Review, 79,* 162–174.

Schein, J. D. (Ed.). (1977b). The demographics of disability. *The Deaf American, 29*(6), 21–25.

Schein, J. D. (1981). *A rose for tomorrow.* Silver Spring, MD: National Association of the Deaf.

Schein, J. D. (1982). The demographics of deafness. In *Special seminar on deafness.* Austin: Texas Commission for the Deaf.

Schein, J. D., & Delk, M. T. (1974). *The deaf population of the United States.* Silver Spring, MD: National Association of the Deaf.

Schwartz, H. (1982, July 30). Rationing medicine. *New York Times,* p. A21.

Part V
Resources and Opportunities

Chapter 20

Networking:
A Critical Strategy

No man is an island, entire of itself;
every man is a piece of the continent,
a part of the main. . . .

  —John Donne,
  Devotions upon Emergent Occasions, 1624

The editors and authors of this book have intentionally gathered and presented current philosophies and methods related to service delivery that stress professional-professional and professional-client interaction. We believe that interactive practice yields greater fruits for our labor. Our perspective is that clients and professionals pay a price when an isolated service delivery tack is chosen, whether this strategy is perpetuated within a system by a single staff member, by a group of specialists from a particular discipline, or by separate professional groups in the human service delivery system. The price paid involves multiple losses. Not only does the opportunity for growth of a professional and personal nature become elusive, but also, and equally critical, the tools and knowledge for enhancing professional expertise and service delivery may be bypassed. Prevention or amelioration of career burnout is certainly difficult, if not impossible, to achieve in such a framework.

We are witnessing two trends in the United States in the 1980s that are altering the course of human service delivery. The first is economic. Funding for many programs that serve the disabled population has been cut despite heralded legislative and regulatory mandates to improve services and the quality of life for these same individuals. The second trend is the steadily increasing application of computer technology in the fields of education and rehabilitation.

The educator, rehabilitation specialist, or program administrator is caught in the convergence of these powerful trends. In addition, and often as a result, the same professional may be vulnerable to and experiencing symptoms of burnout. Significant changes related to trends of this magnitude, whether imposed or voluntary, tend to foster adoption of an isolationist posture. Professionals in service delivery systems, for reasons of practicality, desire to minimize information overload and, seemingly, to maximize time usage. A rather reasonable approach, some might concur; with limited funds, how can a program provide its staff and clients with costly technology? And, are the changes worth the time and money necessary to re-educate staff?

Another impetus for maintenance of isolationism among professionals who work with hearing-impaired individuals has been the dogmatic and opposing points of view about the appropriate choice of communication and education methodology. Historically, two major camps evolved, and most professionals were inclined to pledge allegiance to one or the other. Those individuals tending toward a more eclectic approach often were viewed skeptically and usually were assumed to lean toward one or the other of the ideologies. What price have we and our clients paid over the years to maintain such a divisive system in which the needs of the professional rather than those of the client take precedence?

As David Yoder stated in the Foreword, we still have much to discover about maximizing the human potential of individuals who have both hearing impairment and developmental disabilities. Areas targeted for concerted and coordinated exploration include a broad range of diverse topics.

- Increased forums in which families of individuals with disabilities can receive support, information, and respite;
- Strategies for improving staff morale and longevity;
- Innovative interdisciplinary training at the preservice level of education;
- Incorporation of mental health principles into training for clinicians and special educators;
- Disability-oriented training models for mental health professionals;
- Development of population-appropriate assessment instruments; and
- Leadership and materials development in career education for elementary and secondary school-age individuals with hearing impairment and developmental disabilities.

Networking is one proven strategy for tackling these and related issues. Fortunately, our country's human resources are rich and varied, and systems for tapping the network are often within reach.

The remainder of this chapter is devoted to providing the reader with a resource network—a potpourri of agencies, organizations, curricula, and materials that can facilitate excellence in the delivery of services to individuals with both hearing impairment and developmental disabilities. The listing is by no means all-inclusive or exclusive. Our hope is to provide a jumping-off place for gathering information or initiating dialogue. Such networking can only result in more creative and substantive programming for our target population as well as greater fulfillment in meeting our collective professional challenge.

John Naisbitt noted in his popular text, *Megatrends* (1982), that most social invention in the U.S. could be traced to five states—California, Florida, Washington, Colorado, and Connecticut. "It's difficult to say why," said Naisbitt, "other than to observe that all five are characterized by a rich mix of people. And the richness of the mix always results in creativity, experimentation, and change" (p. xxviii).

If Naisbitt's hypothesis is accurate, then our challenge, as a subgroup working toward a common purpose, is to activate and stimulate the mix. The only risk is gain.

EVELYN CHEROW

The Network

Advocacy

- National Center for Law and the Deaf. (1984). *Legal rights of hearing-impaired people* (2nd ed.). Washington, DC: Gallaudet College Press.

  Legal rights and strategies for hearing-impaired people seeking equal access to employment, education, medical care, government benefits, public facilities, and the legal system are explained in lay terms. The National Center for Law and the Deaf is a public service of Gallaudet College.

- Burgdorf, J. D., Jr., & Spicer, P. P. (1983). *The legal rights of handicapped persons: Cases, materials and text.* Baltimore: Brookes Publishing.

  This supplement provides full extracts of the latest judicial decisions and legislative enactments plus an analysis of current legal trends affecting handicapped people.

Assistive Devices

- The Physically Impaired Association of Michigan Information Clearinghouse and Referral Service on Assistive Devices

  PAM Assistance Center
  8011 West Maple
  Lansing, MI 48908
  (517) 371-5897

  The Center provides hands-on displays and information on more than 6,000 products from 1,000 companies and publishes a newsletter. Although primarily serving the Michigan area, it accepts requests from other areas of the country.

- ABLEDATA

  National Rehabilitation Information Center (NARIC)
  4407 8th Street NE
  Washington, DC 20017
  (202) 635-5826 (voice); (202) 635-5822 (TTY)

  ABLEDATA is an information service that collects, organizes, searches, and delivers information on rehabilitation products. The computerized data base lists some 6,000 product data entries. Product listings include information concerning personal care, home management, vocational educational management, communication, sensory disabilities, mobility, seating, transportation, recreation, and rehabilitative and therapeutic aids. The system is accessed through the use of information brokers who, in addition to providing access to the national data bank, develop local information resources.

- Fellendorf, G. W. (1982). *Current developments in assistive devices for hearing-impaired persons in the United States.* Washington, DC: Fellendorf Associates.

  This report is a current summary and information source for the field of assistive devices for the deaf and hearing impaired. In addition to existing devices, prototype new devices and trends in research and development are discussed.

- *Now Hear This* (videotape)
  Sertoma Foundation
  P.O. Box 17003
  Kansas City, MO 64132

  This videotape on assistive listening devices and systems was developed by Gwenyth Vaughn, Ph.D., Chief of Audiology and Speech Pathology at the VA Medical Center in Birmingham, Alabama, and Robert Lightfoot, M.S., a rehabilitative audiologist. Hardwire, infrared, FM, and loop systems are discussed and demonstrated.

- Rehabilitation Engineering Centers

  The rehabilitation engineering program of the National Institute of Handicapped Research is an outgrowth of the major research and training program in prosthetics and orthotics of the Rehabilitation Services Administration. The concept of rehabilitation engineering was formed at a workshop conducted by the National Academy of Sciences in 1970. The term *rehabilitation engineering* was used to represent the merging disciplines of science, technology, and medicine to benefit disabled individuals. In addition to pointing out the need for research and education with technological emphasis, the National Academy of Science recommended the formation of a series of rehabilitation engineering centers of excellence, so that specific areas of research could be addressed by clinical scientists and specialists in technology. Presently, there are 16 rehabilitation engineering centers in the U.S. with 3 collaborating centers overseas. The centers are generally located in clinical settings and have formal arrangements with university-level programs in medicine and engineering for scientific and educational collaboration.

Rehabilitation Engineering Centers	Core Areas of Research
Cerebral Palsy Research Foundation of Kansas, Inc. P.O. Box 8217 2021 North Old Manor Wichita, KS 67208	Vocational aspects of rehabilitation
Children's Hospital at Stanford 520 Willow Road Palo Alto, CA 94304	Controls and interfaces
Children's Hospital Medical Center 300 Longwood Avenue Boston, MA 02115	Neuromuscular control using sensory feedback systems
Gallaudet College 800 Florida Avenue NE Washington, DC 20002	Deafness and hearing impairment
Kruzen Research Center Moss Rehabilitation Hospital 12th Street and Tabor Road Philadelphia, PA 19141	Locomotion and mobility
Medical Rehabilitation R & T Center New York University 400 East 34th Street New York, NY 10016	Evaluation of functional performance of devices for severely disabled individuals

Medical Rehabilitation R & T Center Tufts University Box 1014, 171 Harrison Avenue Boston, MA 02111	Communication systems for individuals with nonvocal disabilities
Northwestern University 345 East Superior Street, Room 1441 Chicago, IL 60611	Internal total joint replacement
Rancho Los Amigos Hospital 7601 East Imperial Highway Downey, CA 90242	Functional electrical stimulation of paralyzed nerves and muscles
Smith-Kettlewell Institute of Visual Sciences 2232 Webster Street San Francisco, CA 94115	Sensory aids—blind and deaf
Texas Institute for Rehabilitation and Research 1333 Moursund Avenue Houston, TX 77030	Effects of pressure on tissue
Trace Center 314 Waisman Center 1500 Highland Avenue Madison, WI 53706	Communication systems for individuals with nonvocal disabilities
University of Iowa Carver Pavillion Iowa City, IA 52242	Low back pain
University of Michigan 208 W. E. Lay Automotive Lab 2320 Herbert Street Ann Arbor, MI 48109	Automotive transportation for the handicapped
University of Tennessee 532 South Stadium Hall Knoxville, TN 37916	Deafness and hearing impairment
University of Virginia School of Medicine P.O. Box 3368, University Station Charlottesville, VA 22903	Spinal cord injury

Burnout

- Building-Based Staff Support Team Model
  Fred Baars
  Division of Exceptional Children
  North Carolina Department of Public Instruction
  Education Building
  Raleigh, NC 27611
  (919) 733-6081

A building-based staff support team is a peer multidisciplinary problem-solving group whose purpose is to provide a vehicle for discussion of issues related to specific needs of teachers and students and to offer consultation and follow-up assistance. Activities focus on expediting the referral process, assessing and meeting inservice training needs of teachers, helping teachers with specific children, and networking individual schools to share promising practices.

- American Association of University Affiliated Programs. (undated). *Developing a community team.* Available from:

  Catherine Kessler
  Georgetown University Hospital
  Bles Building, Room CC-52
  3800 Reservoir Road NW
  Washington, DC 20007

  Developing a Community Team is the companion to *Community Workbook for Collaborative Services to Preschool Handicapped Children.* Like the workbook, it is especially useful for communities embarking on or involved in collaborative planning for handicapped children. Although it is aimed at preschool-age children, the document provides a useful generic framework for collaborative efforts on behalf of other special groups.

- Greenberg, S. F., & Valetutti, P. J. (1980). *Stress and the helping professions.* Baltimore: Brookes Publishing.

  This is a nonmedical, nontechnical text that confronts the negative effects of high-level job stress and provides practical guidelines for recognizing, coping with, and reducing that stress.

Career Education

- Office of Career Development for Special Populations
  345 Education Building
  1310 South 6th Street
  University of Illinois
  Champaign, IL 61820
  (217) 333-2325

  The office's mission is to expand and improve the career development and employment opportunities provided to special populations. This is achieved through research and development, training evaluation, dissemination, and technical assistance activities conducted jointly with various agencies and organizations operating in Illinois as well as nationally and internationally.

- New York State Office of Vocational Rehabilitation. (1983). *Model plan for services to deaf persons.* Albany, NY: State Education Department. Available from:

  Office of Vocational Rehabilitation
  State Education Department
  Albany, NY 12234

  The document is intended especially for OVR personnel, including personnel who determine and/or implement policies. The document covers issues and concerns relating to all deaf and hard-of-hearing populations. While greater emphasis has been placed on people who are severely disabled according to federal and state statutes, the plan can benefit all hearing-impaired people seeking OVR services.

- Cho, D. W. (undated). *Characteristics of the handicapped population in the United States: Demographics and economic status. A report based on the 1978 survey of disability and work.* Eugene, OR: University of Oregon Center on Human Development, Specialized Training Program.

  This report summarizes selected information on the adult handicapped population in the U.S. compiled from the 1978 Survey of Disability and Work. Included are demographic characteristics, work experiences, and program participations. The purpose of this report is to disseminate these data and relevant findings to policy makers, handicapped constituencies, and researchers.

Curricula and Special Projects

- Bulletins on Science and Technology for the Handicapped
  AAAS Project on the Handicapped in Science
  1776 Massachusetts Avenue NW
  Washington, DC 20036
  (202) 467-4497 (voice and TTY)

  This quarterly newsletter (from the American Association for the Advancement of Science) offers a unique combination of information on the latest science and technology projects, organizations, and programs for disabled people as well as those emanating from the work of disabled scientists. The bulletin is available on tape for visually impaired readers.

- Educational Programs for the Handicapped
  Joseph Nervi
  National Aeronautics and Space Administration
  Lewis Research Center
  Cleveland, OH 44135
  (216) 433-4000, Ext. 708

  This new project is designed to adapt selected educational programs related to air and space themes for use by the disabled. At present, four videotapes have been captioned at three different reading levels. Their topics are the solar system, the universe, pollution, and satellite sensing. The target audience for these materials is elementary through senior high school students. Materials are also in development for people with visual impairments.

- LINC Associates. (1984). *The SpecialWare directory*. Phoenix: Oryx Press. Available from:
  LINC
  1875 Morse Road, Suite 215
  Columbus, OH 43229
  (614) 263-2123

  This directory of courseware and software products for special education is updated annually. Listed are instructional, administrative, professional, and evaluation/testing materials for special education as well as product information concerning curriculum skill areas, educational levels, hardware compatibility, and warranty and preview policies of each product.

- Instructional Materials and Resource Center for Handicapped Children and Youth. (1983). *Special educators' guide to exemplary curricula results of a national field-based survey* and *Educators' guide to effective special education materials* (1983–84 ed.). Indianapolis: Division of Special

Education, Indiana Department of Public Instruction. Available from:
Instructional Materials and Resource Center for Handicapped Children and Youth
Box 100, Butler University
Indianapolis, IN 46208
(317) 927-0219

These guides are a result of a national, field-based survey designed to identify exemplary special education curricula. The Special Educators' Guide lists 179 curriculum guides reported as exemplary by more than 500 universities, state departments of education, and special centers. The Educators' Guide lists special education materials by exceptionality area, level, and curricular area as recommended by 500 special educators. User information is available as is a directory of selected publishers including current addresses.

- Stepp, R. E., Jr., & Reiners, E. (Eds.). (1983, September). *Proceedings of the 16th Symposium on Research and Utilization of Educational Media for Teaching the Deaf. American Annals of the Deaf, 128,* 507–782.

The symposium focused on the use of mainframe computers and microcomputers in teaching the hearing impaired. An update on the place of computer programs in educational programs for hearing-impaired children is also included. Also featured is an index by author and subject of all papers presented at these educational media and technology symposia since 1965.

Electronic Mail

- SpecialNet
National Association of State Directors of Special Education
1201 16th Street NW, Suite 404E
Washington, DC 20036
(202) 822-7933

The NASDSE manages this electronic mailbox which is available to anyone in the U.S. who has access to a computer terminal or microcomputer. The system allows message exchange between individuals, selected groups, or anyone on the network. SpecialNet Bulletin Boards provide current information on special education topics—federal legislative activities and budget, OSERS and SEP activities, litigation data, computer applications, employment opportunities, consultant resource bank, conference schedules, and assistive devices, to name a few.

- Middleton, T. (1983, September). DEAFNET—The word's getting around: Local implementation of telecommunications networks for deaf users. In R. E. Stepp, Jr. & E. Reiners (Eds.), *Proceedings of the 16th Symposium on Research and Utilization of Educational Media for Teaching the Deaf. American Annals of the Deaf, 128,* 613–618.

The computer-based telecommunication network for the deaf, DEAFNET, is described, and methods for establishing a self-supporting system at both local and national levels are discussed.

Family Information

- Moore, C., Morton, K. M., & Southard, A. (1983). *A reader's guide for parents of children with mental, physical or emotional disabilities.* Baltimore: State Planning Council on Developmental Disabilities. Available from:

Maryland State Planning Council on Developmental Disabilities
201 West Preston Street
Baltimore, MD 21201

This guide, prepared with support from the Montgomery County (Maryland) Association for Retarded Citizens, is a resource manual in four parts. The first covers general readings in all disability areas. Part two is geared to specific disabilities under such topics as the early years, personal accounts, and the adult years. Part three includes more concrete concerns including attitudes, genetic counseling, rights of children, and sexuality. The last section lists pertinent journals and directories.

- Family Resources Database

  Family Resource and Referral Center
  National Council on Family Relations
  1219 University Avenue SE
  Minneapolis, MN 55414
  (612) 331-2774

  This data base provides access to the core collection of information covering the literature, programs, and services of the family and allied fields. There are two parts: entries from such sources as books, audiocassettes, family study centers, government publications, conference proceedings, human resource bank, etc.; and the Inventory of Marriage and Family Literature Project, University of Minnesota.

- Perske, R., & Perske, M. (1980). *New life in the neighborhood: How persons with retardation or other disabilities can help make a good community better.* Nashville: Abingdon.

  This book is a touching account of changing times, describing different individual experiences and those of people with developmental disabilities interacting informally and formally in communities across the country.

- Parent Training Materials

  The Pacer Center, Inc.
  4701 Chicago Avenue
  Minneapolis, MN 55407
  (612) 827-2966

  The Pacer Center is a parent advocacy coalition for educational rights that has produced a series of materials, including a parent newsletter and a parent training model.

- Parent Respite Co-ops

  Care Co-Op Consultant
  2324 West Main Street
  Kalamazoo, MI 49007

  The program provides information on forming and operating a parent co-op.

- American Society for Deaf Children
  814 Thayer Avenue
  Silver Spring, MD 20910
  (301) 585-5400 (voice and TTY)

  The ASDC offers a network of personal support for families of deaf children and actively participates in matters of national and international importance to parents by working on national advisory boards and meeting with leaders to represent parents of children who are deaf.

- Deafpride, Inc.
  2010 Rhode Island Avenue NE
  Washington, DC 20018
  (202) 635-2050 (voice), (202) 635-2049 (TTY)

  Deafpride is a nonprofit organization which works for the human rights of deaf people and their families by bringing together deaf and hearing people and providing opportunities for them to develop their potential as advocates.

- Murphy, A. T. (Ed.). (1979, September). The families of hearing-impaired children [Monograph]. *The Volta Review, 81,* 265–384.

  This compendium offers parent and professional perspectives on the issues of rearing a child who has a hearing impairment.

- *Bridging the Gap*
  Videotapes with Kenneth Moses
  Association for Retarded Citizens/Illinois
  6 North Michigan Avenue
  Chicago, IL 60602

  These videotapes serve as a training resource for gaining insights into the dynamics of parenting an impaired person, as a stimulating medium to initiate group discussion regarding parent-professional interaction, and as part of an ongoing parent-professional development program.

  Tape 1: Mourning Theory—An optimistic and supportive guide highlighting the feelings of parents of impaired children. The tape was recorded with a live audience of parents and professionals and creates an intimate atmosphere and stimulus for discussion.

  Tape 2: Burnout/Re-ignition—A sociophilosophic presentation before a live audience aimed at producing an understanding that all human beings are united in a singular struggle to live in a world that is not necessarily just, sensible, or consistent.

  Tape 3: Questions & Answers/Discussion—A unique potpourri of reactions, sharings, questions, explorations, and genuine strugglings with the issues parents face. This moving and thought-provoking experience invites viewers to examine and share their own concerns.

  Training Manual: This is a compilation of theory, practical suggestions, and resources meant to guide individuals who are going to conduct meetings and discussion following the presentation of any or all of the videotapes.

- Resource Networks, Inc.
  930 Maple Avenue
  Evanston, IL 60202
  (312) 864-4522

  Inservice workshops and audiotapes are available for professionals who work with families of disabled individuals. The audiotapes cover the subjects of fundamental counseling and grieving states.

- Mulick, J. A., & Pueschel, S. M. (Eds.). (1983). *Parent-professional partnerships in developmental disability services.* Cambridge, MA: Ware Press. (Also available through Resource Networks, Inc., 930 Maple Avenue, Evanston, IL 60202.)

  This compilation of writings from a variety of professionals focuses on how families raising a disabled child can cope with their emotions and thereby mobilize their resources and enhance the chances for comprehensive follow-up care.

Inservice Training

- AAMD Staff Training Information (ASTI) in Developmental Disabilities
  American Association on Mental Deficiency
  1719 Kalorama Road NW
  Washington, DC 20009
  (202) 387-1968 or (800) 424-3688 for a search request

  The ASTI is a computerized collection of staff development materials consisting of more than 1,300 training and training-related items. Materials listed are for use in training programs for professionals, paraprofessionals, and parents serving people with developmental disabilities. Training items are cross-referenced by training setting, staff discipline, materials format, and by client age, kind of disability, and severity of disability. Examples of training subjects are feeding, prenatal counseling, sexuality, and behavior management.

- Blackman, J. A. (Ed.). (1983). *Medical aspects of developmental disabilities in children birth to three: A resource for special service providers in the educational setting.* Iowa City: University of Iowa.

  The purpose of this manual is to provide field-based medical information for early-intervention professionals in the educational setting. The focus is on those medical issues that may directly affect the developmental progress of young children. The information is presented in a way that helps to identify both the problems interfering with a child's growth and development and the provision of appropriate services and high quality care.

Mental Health Programs

- Trybus, R. J., & Edelstein, T. A. (1981). *Directory of mental health programs and resources for hearing impaired persons.* Washington, DC: Gallaudet Research Institute.

  This directory encompasses a broad spectrum of institutions and individuals who have indicated that they provide mental health services to hearing-impaired individuals. The listing is organized alphabetically by state and is subdivided into programs and resources.

Preservice Education

- Bogatz, B. E. (Ed.). (1983). Preservice education and leadership training. *Directions, 3*(3) [Published by Gallaudet College, Washington, DC].

  This issue of the journal includes a description of several preservice training programs offered by the School of Education and Human Services at Gallaudet College. An interview with Dr. Herman Goldberg, the Executive Administrator of the Office of Special Education and Rehabilitative Services, covers topics related to special education under the Reagan administration.

Professional Societies, Associations, Special Interest Organizations, and Agencies*

Administration on Developmental
  Disabilities
State Protection and Advocacy
  Agencies
Switzer Building
330 C Street SW
Washington, DC 20202

Alexander Graham Bell Association for
  the Deaf
3417 Volta Place NW
Washington, DC 20007

Alliance for Engineering in Medicine
  and Biology
4405 East-West Highway, Suite 402
Bethesda, MD 20814

American Academy for Cerebral Palsy
  and Developmental Medicine
2315 Westwood Avenue
P.O. Box 11083
Richmond, VA 23230

American Academy of Ophthalmology
1833 Fillmore Street
Box 7424
San Francisco, CA 94115

American Academy of Pediatrics
1801 Hinman Avenue
Evanston, IL 60204

American Association for Counseling
  and Development
5999 Stevenson Avenue
Alexandria, VA 22304

American Association for Health,
  Physical Education and Recreation
1201 16th Street NW
Washington, DC 20036

American Association for Maternal and
  Child Health
233 Prospect
La Jolla, CA 92037

American Association on Mental
  Deficiency
1719 Kalorama Road NW
Washington, DC 20009

American Association of University
  Affiliated Programs for the
  Developmentally Disabled
1234 Massachusetts Avenue NW,
  Suite 813
Washington, DC 20005

American Brittle Bone Society
1256 Merrill Drive
West Chester, PA 19390

American Civil Liberties Union
  (ACLU)
132 West 43rd Street
New York, NY 10036

American Cleft Palate Association
331 Salk Hall
University of Pittsburgh
Pittsburgh, PA 15261

American Coalition for Citizens with
  Disabilities
1200 15th Street NW, Suite 201
Washington, DC 20005

American College of Obstetricians and
  Gynecologists
600 Maryland Avenue SW, Suite 300
Washington, DC 20024

American Council of the Blind
1211 Connecticut Avenue NW,
  Suite 506
Washington, DC 20036

American Deafness and Rehabilitation
  Association
814 Thayer Avenue
Silver Spring, MD 20910

American Diabetes Association
2 Park Avenue
New York, NY 10016

American Epilepsy Association
710 West 168th Street
New York, NY 10032

---

*From *Children Who Are Different: Meeting the Challenges of Birth Defects in Society* (pp. 261–265) by R. B. Darling and J. Darling, 1982, St. Louis: C. V. Mosby. Copyright 1982 by the C. V. Mosby Company. Updated and expanded by permission.

American Epilepsy Society
179 Allyn Street, #304
Hartford, CT 06103

American Foundation for the Blind
15 West 16th Street
New York, NY 10011

American Foundation for Maternal and
   Child Health, Inc.
30 Beekman Place
New York, NY 10022

American Heart Association
7320 Greenville Avenue
Dallas, TX 75231

American Legion
National Child Welfare Division
P.O. Box 1055
Indianapolis, IN 46206

American Lung Association
1740 Broadway
New York, NY 10019

American Medical Association
535 North Dearborn Street
Chicago, IL 60610

American Occupational Therapy
   Association
1383 Piccard Drive, Suite 300
Rockville, MD 20850

American Pain Society
340 Kingsland Street
Nutley, NJ 07110

American Physical Therapy Association
1111 North Fairfax Street
Alexandria, VA 22314

American Psychological Association
1200 17th Street NW
Washington, DC 20036

American Public Health Association
1015 15th Street NW
Washington, DC 20005

American Society for Deaf Children
814 Thayer Avenue
Silver Spring, MD 20910
   (Formerly International Association
   of Parents of the Deaf)

American Speech-Language-Hearing
   Association
10801 Rockville Pike
Rockville, MD 20852

American Spinal Injuries Association
Northwest Memorial Hospital
250 East Superior, Room 580
Chicago, IL 60611

American Vocational Association
2020 North 14th Street
Arlington, VA 22201

Architectural and Transportation
   Barriers Compliance Board
330 C Street SW
Washington, DC 20202

Arthritis Foundation
3400 Peachtree Road NE, Suite 1101
Atlanta, GA 30326

Association for Children and Adults
   with Learning Disabilities
4156 Library Road
Pittsburgh, PA 15234
   (State chapters)

Association for Children with Down's
   Syndrome
2616 Martin Avenue
Bellmore, NY 11710

Association for Children with Retarded
   Mental Development
817 Broadway
New York, NY 10003

Association for Education of the
   Visually Handicapped
206 North Washington Street,
   Suite 320
Alexandria, VA 22314

Association for Persons with Severe
   Handicaps
7010 Roosevelt Way NE
Seattle, WA 98115

Association for Retarded Citizens
National Headquarters
2501 Avenue J
Arlington, TX 76011

Association for the Aid of Crippled
   Children
345 East 46th Street
New York, NY 10017

Association for the Visually
   Handicapped
1839 Frankfort Avenue
Louisville, KY 40206

Asthma and Allergy Foundation of
America
1707 N Street NW
Washington, DC 20036

Candlelighters Foundation
2025 Eye Street NW, Suite 1011
Washington, DC 20003
(For parents of children with
potentially fatal diseases)

Center for Sickle Cell Disease
Howard University
2121 Georgia Avenue NW
Washington, DC 20057

Center on Human Policy
Syracuse University
216 Ostrom Avenue
Syracuse, NY 13210

Council for Exceptional Children
1920 Association Drive
Reston, VA 22091

Cystic Fibrosis Foundation
6000 Executive Boulevard, Suite 309
Rockville, MD 20852

Deafness Research Foundation
55 East 34th Street
New York, NY 10016

Disability Rights Center
1346 Connecticut Avenue NW,
Suite 1124
Washington, DC 20036

Down's Syndrome Congress
Central Office
1640 West Roosevelt Road
Chicago, IL 60608

Education Commission of the States
444 North Capitol Street NW
Washington, DC 20001

Epilepsy Foundation of America
4351 Garden City Drive, Suite 406
Landover, MD 20785

Federation for the Handicapped, Inc.
211 West 14th Street
New York, NY 10011

Foundation for Child Development
345 East 46th Street
New York, NY 10017
(Orthopedic disorders)

Foundation for Children with Learning
Disabilities
P.O. Box 2929
Grand Central Station
New York, NY 10163

Goodwill Industries of America, Inc.
9200 Wisconsin Avenue
Bethesda, MD 20814

Independent Living for the
Handicapped
800 3rd Street NE
Washington, DC 20002

Information and Referral Service for
Autistic and Autistic-like Persons
306 31st Street
Huntington, WV 25702

International Reading Association
P.O. Box 8139
800 Barksdale Road
Newark, DE 19714

Joseph P. Kennedy, Jr., Foundation
1701 K Street NW, Suite 205
Washington, DC 20006
(Mental retardation)

League for Emotionally Disturbed
Children
171 Madison Avenue
New York, NY 10017

Library of Congress
Division of the Blind and Physically
Handicapped
Washington, DC 20543

Little People of America
P.O. Box 126
Owatonna, MN 55060

March of Dimes Birth Defects
Foundation
1275 Mamaroneck Avenue
White Plains, NY 10605

Maternal and Child Health
Parklawn Building
5600 Fishers Lane
Rockville, MD 20857

National Association for Hearing and
Speech Action
10801 Rockville Pike
Rockville, MD 20852

National Association for Visually
  Handicapped
305 East 24th Street, 17-C
New York, NY 10010

National Association of Developmental
  Disabilities Councils (NADDC)
1234 Massachusetts Avenue NW,
  Suite 203
Washington, DC 20005
  (Formerly National Conference on
  Developmental Disabilities)

National Association of Social Workers
7981 Eastern Avenue
Silver Spring, MD 20910

National Association of State Directors
  of Special Education
1201 16th Street NW, Suite 610E
Washington, DC 20036

National Association of State Mental
  Retardation Program Directors
113 Oronoco Street
Alexandria, VA 22314

National Association of the Deaf
814 Thayer Avenue
Silver Spring, MD 20910

National Ataxia Foundation
6681 Country Club Drive
Minneapolis, MN 55427

National Center for a Barrier Free
  Environment
1140 Connecticut Avenue NW,
  Suite 1006
Washington, DC 20036

National Center for Law and the Deaf
Gallaudet College
800 Florida Avenue NE
Washington, DC 20002

National Center on Educational Media
  and Materials for the Handicapped
154 West 12th Street
Columbus, OH 43210

National Clearinghouse for Mental
  Health Information
National Institute on Mental Health
15C-17 Parklawn Building
5600 Fishers Lane
Rockville, MD 20857

National Committee for Children
  and Youth
1145 19th Street NW
Washington, DC 20006

National Committee on Arts for the
  Handicapped
1825 Connecticut Avenue NW,
  Suite 418
Washington, DC 20009

National Council of Community
  Mental Health Centers
6101 Montrose Road
Rockville, MD 20852

National Council to Combat Blindness
139 East 57th Street
New York, NY 10022

National Cystic Fibrosis Foundation
3379 Peachtree Road NE
Atlanta, GA 30326

National Easter Seal Society
2023 West Ogden Avenue
Chicago, IL 60612

National Federation of the Blind
1800 Johnson Street
Baltimore, MD 21230

National Genetics Foundation, Inc.
555 West 57th Street
New York, NY 10019

National Hemophilia Foundation
19 West 34th Street, Suite 1204
New York, NY 10001

National Homecaring Council
67 Irving Place
New York, NY 10003

National Information Center on
  Deafness
Gallaudet College
800 Florida Avenue NE
Washington, DC 20002

National Institute on Mental Health
Parklawn Building
5600 Fishers Lane
Rockville, MD 20857

Office of Human Development
Administration on Developmental
  Disabilities
200 Independence Avenue SW
Washington, DC 20201

Parents' Campaign for Handicapped
   Children and Youth
1201 16th Street NW
Washington, DC 20036

Physical Education and Recreation for
   the Handicapped
Information and Research Utilization
   Center
1201 16th Street NW
Washington, DC 20036

Planned Parenthood
World Population Center for Family
   Planning
810 Seventh Avenue
New York, NY 10019

President's Committee on Employment
   of the Handicapped
Washington, DC 20210

Rehabilitation Engineering Society of
   North America
4405 East-West Highway, Suite 402
Bethesda, MD 20814

Rehabilitation International
432 Park Avenue South
New York, NY 10016
   (Formerly International Society for
   Rehabilitation of the Disabled)

Rehabilitation Services Administration
Switzer Building, Room 3090
330 C Street SW
Washington, DC 20202

Sickle Cell Disease Foundation of
   Greater New York
209 West 125th Street, Room 108
New York, NY 10027
   (Formerly Foundation for Research
   & Education in Sickle Cell Disease)

SIECUS (Sex Information & Education
   Council of the United States)
84 Fifth Avenue, Suite 407
New York, NY 10011

Social and Rehabilitation Services
Division of Developmental Disabilities
330 C Street SW
Washington, DC 20202

Society for the Protection of the
   Unborn through Nutrition
17 Wabash Avenue, Suite 603
Chicago, IL 60602

Spastic Children's Foundation
1307 West 105th Street
Los Angeles, CA 90044

Special Interest Group for Computers
   and the Physically Handicapped
c/o Association for Computing
   Machinery
11 West 42nd Street
New York, NY 10036

Spina Bifida Association of America
343 South Dearborn Street
Chicago, IL 60604

Technology and Media for Exceptional
   Individuals (TAM)
Institute for the Study of Exceptional
   Children
Department of Special Education
University of Maryland
College Park, MD 20742

United Cerebral Palsy Associations
66 East 34th Street
New York, NY 10016

U.S. Civil Service Commission
Washington, DC 20415

U.S. Department of Health and
   Human Services
Children's Bureau
Washington, DC 20201

U.S. Department of Health and
   Human Services
National Center for Child Advocacy
P.O. Box 1182
Washington, DC 20013

U.S. Department of Health and
   Human Services
Office of Child Development
P.O. Box 1182
Washington, DC 20013

U.S. Department of Health and
   Human Services
Rehabilitation Services
Washington, DC 20201

U.S. Social Security Administration
Division of Disability Operations
6401 Security Boulevard
Baltimore, MD 21235

Index

AAMD Adaptive Behavior Scales, 218–19

Academic vs. social skills: and the schools, 241–42

Accountability: and social services, 353, 354

Acoustic immittance measurement: acoustic reflex, 138, 139; for the developmentally disabled, 138–39; static compliance, 138; tympanometry, 138

Acoustic reflex measurement, 138–39; limitations of, 139

Adaptive behavior: assessment of, 214, 218–19

Adolescence: and daily living skills, 244; educational policy for, 243; identity development, 243; psychological development, 242–44; psychosocial problems of, 242–44

Advocacy: and burnout, 362–63; case, defined, 356; child psychiatrist's role in, 236–37; class, defined, 356–57; for clients, 14; code of ethics, 14; consumer as advocate, 363–64; in the courts, 362; for the disabled, 346–65; effects of approach, 360–62; and independence of disabled, 363–64; monitoring results of, 362; need for coordination, 360–61; need for information, 357–59; and needs assessment, 359; sources of information, 358–59, 371; and vision care, 163, 167

Advocate: defined, 356–57

Aided communication: defined, 271; examples of, 271

Allen Preschool Vision Test, 157, 158, 160

Alport's syndrome, 105, 116

Amblyopia, 155

American Coalition for Citizens with Disabilities, 361, 380

American Speech-Language-Hearing Association (ASHA), 381; NEEDS survey, 323–24; PDME program, 317–20; Position Statement on Infant Hearing, 119–21; Position Statement on Nonspeech Communication, 285–92; and professional self-study, 316; School Affairs Program, 317; school caseload study, 316, 325–26

Amniocentesis, 104, 107

Anger: parental, 84–85, 94

Annual Survey of Hearing-Impaired Children and Youth, 36–56; data sources, 36–37; education orientation of, 37; unevenness of coverage, 37

Antibiotics: aminoglycosides, 107, 110; and infant hearing loss, 107

Anxiety: appropriateness of, 91; uses of, 90–91

Apraxia of speech: and communication system, 275; defined, 274–75

ASHA Committee on Language, Speech, and Hearing Services in Schools: caseload study and guidelines, 316, 325–26

Assessment: adapting tests, 221–23; of adaptive behavior, 214, 218–19; of cognitive behavior, 211, 214; criteria for test selection, 212–14; developmental scales, 214–16; in the educational domain, 210–28; group administered tests, 214n; of intelligence/mental abilities, 216–18; interview techniques, 214; of motor development, 202–4; observational techniques, 214; organizing and presenting tests, 221; planning strategies, 221–23; process evaluation, 223–25; of psycho-educational skills, 214, 219–21; in the psychological domain, 210–28; of social-emotional behavior, 214, 218–19; standardization of tests, 212–13; testing-of-limits procedures, 222. *See also* Audiological evaluation; Communication evaluation; Evaluation; Psychiatric assessment; Speech discrimination assessment; Vision assessment

Assigning Structural Stage procedure, 179

Assistive devices: resources on, 371–73

Asymmetrical tonic neck reflex, 200; and communication, 206–7; effect on audiological evaluation, 132–33; relation to neuromotor dysfunction, 132–33

Audiological evaluation: alternate response modes, 135; behavioral assessment, 125–27; behavioral techniques, 124; child position in, 134; and cognitive ability, 132; data interpretation problems, 126; early assessment, 122; electrophysiological

This book was typeset in 11/13 Garamond by Barton Graphics, Hyattsville, Maryland. It was printed on 60 lb. Glatfelter Hi-Brite by The John D. Lucas Printing Company, Baltimore, Maryland. The cover and text were designed by Judith Bair.